Recent Advances in
HAEMATOLOGY

A. V. HOFFBRAND MA(Oxon) DM FRCP(Lond) FRCPath
Professor of Haematology and Honorary Consultant, Royal Free Hospital and School of Medicine, London since 1974. Previously, Senior Lecturer in Haematology at the Royal Postgraduate Medical School, London.

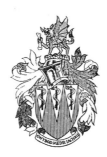
716

Recent Advances in
HAEMATOLOGY

EDITED BY

A. V. HOFFBRAND

NUMBER THREE

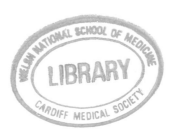

CHURCHILL LIVINGSTONE
EDINBURGH LONDON MELBOURNE AND NEW YORK 1982

CHURCHILL LIVINGSTONE

Medical Division of Longman Group Limited

Distributed in the United States of America by
Churchill Livingstone Inc., 19 West 44th Street, New York,
N.Y. 10036, and by associated companies,
branches and representatives throughout
the world.

First edition 1982

ISBN 0 443 02385 9
ISSN 0143-697X

British Library Cataloguing in Publication Data
Recent advances in haematology – No. 3
    1. Blood – Diseases
    616.1'5   RC636

Library of Congress Catalog Card Number 81–67471

Printed in Great Britain at The Pitman Press, Bath

Preface

In the four years since the second volume of Recent Advances in Haematology, there have been major developments in understanding of the physiological, biochemical and immunological processes that underly the normal functions of the blood and bone marrow. Many of the properties of the bone marrow stem cells have been elucidated as new techniques of bone marrow culture have been developed. Moreover, the range of treatment for patients with blood diseases continues to widen and improve. Many of these recent developments overlap with advances in medical oncology on the one hand, and with those in the understanding and treatment of cardiovascular disease on the other. This expansion in knowledge has been accompanied by publication of new journals and monographs and the appearance of many excellent review articles. Nevertheless, we feel there is still need for a single volume that brings the general haematologist up to date with developments over the whole area of the subject and which acts as a source of reference to the recent literature.

In the present volume, haematologists from the United Kingdom, United States and Australia, have combined to produce a general review of advances in Haematology since 1977. The Editor is grateful to all the authors who despite heavy clinical and laboratory commitments have spent much time in gathering together recent published information and have summarised this in such a lucid and authoritative form. The Editor also wishes to thank Miss J. Allaway and Mrs M. Evans for typing (and retyping) many of the manuscripts and to Andrew Stevenson and Claire McLeod and Churchill Livingstone for their constant encouragement, assistance and understanding during the assembly of this book.

Since this book is based on close trans-Atlantic co-operation, the chapters have largely been kept in the original spelling (American or English style) of the original manuscript.

London, 1982   A.V.H.

Contributors

JOHN W. ADAMSON MD
Professor of Medicine, Head, Division of Haematology, Department of Medicine,
University of Washington School of Medicine, Seattle

C. DEAN BUCKNER MD
Professor of Medicine, The Fred Hutchinson Cancer Research Center, University of
Washington, Seattle

C. N. CHESTERMAN DPhil (Oxon) FRACP
Reader, University of Melbourne Department of Medicine, St Vincent's Hospital
Fitzroy, 3065, Australia

REGINALD A. CLIFT FIMLS
Research Associate, University of Washington School of Medicine, Seattle

J. R. DUNLEAVY
Senior Systems Analyst, Regional Computer Unit, Oxford Regional Health Authority

M. P. ESNOUF MA BSc DPhil
Senior Research Officer, Department of Biochemistry, The Radcliffe Infirmary
Oxford

ALEXANDER FEFER MD
Professor of Medicine, University of Washington School of Medicine, Seattle

A. S. GALLUS FRACP FRCP(C)
Senior Staff Specialist in Haematology, Flinders Medical Centre, Bedford Park, 5042,
Australia

D. A. G. GALTON MA MD FRCP
Honorary Director, Medical Research Council's Leukaemia Unit; Professor of
Haematological Oncology, University of London, Royal Postgraduate Medical
School; Consultant Physician, Hammersmith Hospital, London

K. GANESHAGURU BSc PhD
Lecturer in the Department of Haematology, The Royal Free Hospital and School of
Medicine, London

H. H. GUNSON DSc MD FRCPath
Director of the National Blood Transfusion Service, North Western Regional Health
Authority, Manchester

A. V. HOFFBRAND MA DM FRCP FRCPath
Professor of Haematology The Royal Free Hospital and School of Medicine, London

ALLAN JACOBS MD FRCPath FRCP
Professor of Haematology at the Welsh National School of Medicine, University of
Wales, Cardiff

GEORGE JANOSSY MD PhD MRCPath
Reader in Immunology, The Royal Free Hospital and School of Medicine, London

H. E. M. KAY MD FRCP FRCPath
Consultant Haematologist, Royal Marsden Hospital, London

P. B. A. KERNOFF MD MRCP
Consultant Haematologist, Haemophila Centre and Haemostasis Unit, Royal Free
Hospital, London

JOEL D. MEYERS MD
Assistant Professor of Medicine, University of Washington School of Medicine Seattle

JEANETTE MLADENOVIC MD
Senior Research Fellow, Division of Haematology, Department of Medicine,
University of Washington School of Medicine, Seattle

MALCOLM A. S. MOORE DPhil
Member of the Sloane Kettering Institute for Cancer Research: Professor of Biology,
Sloane Kettering Division, Cornell Graduate School of Medical Sciences, New York

DAVID G. PENINGTON MA DM FRCP FRACP FRCPA
Professor of Medicine, University of Melbourne Department of Medicine, St
Vincents Hospital, Fitzroy, Australia

JANET D. ROWLEY MD
Professor, Department of Medicine, University of Chicago, Chicago

STANLEY L. SCHRIER MD
Professor of Medicine (Haematology), Chief, Division of Haematology, Stanford
University Medical Center, University School of Medicine, Stanford, California

RAINER STORB MD
Professor of Medicine, University of Washington School of Medicine, Seattle

KEITH M. SULLIVAN MD
Assistant Professor of Medicine, University of Washington School of Medicine,
Seattle

E. DONNALL THOMAS MD
Professor of Medicine, University of Washington School of Medicine, Seattle

E. G. D. TUDDENHAM MRCP MRCPath
Senior Lecturer in Haematology, Haemophilia Centre and Haemostasis Unit, Royal
Free Hospital and School of Medicine, London

D. J. WEATHERALL MA MD FRCP FRCPath FRS
Nuffield Professor of Clinical Medicine; Honorary Director MRC Molecular
Haematology Unit, University of Oxford, Oxford

PAUL WEIDEN MD
Clinical Associate, Professor of Medicine, University of Washington Medical School,
Seattle

R. G. WICKREMASINGHE BSc PhD
Research Fellow, Department of Haematology, Royal Free Hospital and School of
Medicine, London

ROBERT P. WITHERSPOON MD
Assistant Professor of Medicine, University of Washington School of Medicine,
Seattle

Contents

1. Disorders of iron metabolism

Allan Jacobs

During the four years since the subject was last reviewed in this series (Jacobs, 1977) a considerable amount of new information has led to modification of the conventional view of iron transport, its intracellular functions and the results of iron overload. The present account will be confined to these aspects and no account will be given of those areas where there has been little new development. A more detailed and comprehensive series of reviews may be referred to (Jacobs & Worwood, 1974 and 1980). Specific reviews will be mentioned under each heading.

Transferrin

Iron is transported through the plasma and the extravascular spaces bound to the β-globulin transferrin, a glycoprotein whose biochemistry and physiology has been recently reviewed (Aisen, 1980). There is still no complete agreement regarding the exact molecular weight of transferrin though the most reliable determination is probably that of MacGillivray et al (1977) which is based on a nearly complete amino acid sequence. The 676 residues together with the two carbohydrate chains give a molecular weight of about 81 000. The protein appears to consist of a single polypeptide chain with two binding sites, each of which can bind one atom of ferric iron. The plasma concentration of transferrin is normally about 1.8 to 2.6 g/litre. The similarity of the iron-binding sites and major areas of duplication in the two halves of the molecule suggest doubling of a structural gene during the evolutionary process (MacGillivray & Brew, 1975). Brock et al (1978) has shown that bovine transferrin can be cleaved into two monoferric fragments. While each fragment can bind iron they cannot act as donors to reticulocytes.

X-ray diffraction studies of diferric rabbit transferrin show the bilobed nature of the molecule (Gorinsky et al, 1979) and these two distinct halves may well correspond to the fragments produced on tryptic cleavage. The exact location of the iron binding sites is not known. About 6 per cent of transferrin is composed of carbohydrate in the form of two identical branched chains terminating in sialic acid. Loss of the sialic acid residues affects neither its iron-binding properties not its half life in the circulation. Each iron-binding site involves two imidazol and three tyrosyl groups and the attachment of an iron atom depends on the simultaneous binding of an anion which is normally bicarbonate. Neither can be bound in the absence of the other though other anions can substitute for bicarbonate under experimental conditions. At the pH and bicarbonate concentration in blood the apparent stability constant for Fe^{3+} binding to both sites is about $10^{23} M^{-1}$ (Aisen, 1974). Iron appears to be released from the transferrin molecule only at specific sites on receptor cells. It cannot be removed effectively by any of the pharmacological chelating agents alone. In vitro the transfer of iron atoms between transferrin molecules can be mediated by citrate (Aisen &

Leibman, 1968) and some anions may facilitate the detachment of the iron by desferrioxamine (Pollack et al, 1976).

The precise mechanism of in vivo detachment of iron from transferrin by cells is not known but may involve reduction of the iron or of the binding groups, chelation by an external ligand or displacement of bicarbonate. Egyed et al (1980) suggest that intracellular haem proteins may play a role. There has been considerable discussion of possible differences between the two binding sites, particularly since the demonstration by Fletcher & Huehns (1967) that the two behaved differently in donating their iron to reticulocytes in vitro. There is evidence of physio-chemical differences between the two sites (Aisen, 1980) though none that points clearly to a physiological difference. There has been little evidence of interaction between the two sites and Wenn & Williams (1968) using isoelectric focussing showed that apotransferrin, monoferric-transferrin and diferric-transferrin all coexisted with binding being an apparently random process, the balance shifting to the right with increasing iron saturation. Princiotto & Zapolski (1975) showed a difference in the pH dependence of iron dissociation from the two sites in vitro and suggested that a conformational change might make one site relatively unavailable at low pH and similarly more easily dissociated. However, these phenomena taking place between pH5 and 7.4 are an uncertain indication of biological differences.

In vivo evidence supporting the hypothesis that one site of diferric (Fe_2) transferrin molecules donates iron preferentially to the developing red cell and to the placenta has been produced by Awai et al (1975a, b) and Brown et al (1975). After the i.v. injection of a mixture of $^{59}Fe_2$-transferrin and $^{55}Fe_1$-transferrin in rats ^{59}Fe disappeared more rapidly from the plasma and was preferentially removed by red blood cells, bone marrow, liver and spleen in the first 3 hours. In a further experiment the A site (reticulocyte orientated) was labelled with ^{55}Fe and the B site with ^{59}Fe. Thirty minutes following the injection of this transferrin the ratio of $^{55}Fe/^{59}Fe$ in red cells and bone marrow haem was greater than 5 while in the liver the ratio was 0.1. The maximum difference in distribution between A and B site was obliterated by redistribution at later times. Similar results were obtained with iron-deficient or iron-loaded rats and in the presence of haemolysis or erythroid hypoplasia. Other experiments also showed that A site iron was selectively transported to the fetus across the placenta. Fletcher & Huehns (1968) predicted that iron absorbed by the small intestine was transported from there on the A site of transferrin thus diverting it specifically to erythroid cells. Portal plasma labelled by the instillation of radioactive iron into the duodenal lumen was found to donate its iron more readily to erythroid tissue than plasma labelled randomly (Brown, 1975). These studies lent support to the original hypothesis but Pootrakul et al (1977) suggest that the results can be explained largely on the basis of experimental artefact and they conclude that iron atoms from the two sites of transferrin have similar tissue distributions in vivo.

Harris & Aisen (1975a) found that rabbit Fe_2-transferrin is no more efficient than Fe_1-transferrin as an iron donor for rabbit reticulocytes. When doubly labelled transferrin was prepared there was no preferential iron uptake from the A site by reticulocytes. Similar studies in man have also failed to show functional differences between the two sites (Harris & Aisen, 1975b). It appears that in a homologous system of transferrin and reticulocytes from the same species there is no functional difference between the two binding sites. The accumulated experience of ferrokinetic experiments show that over 95 per cent of the plasma iron in man is cleared by a process accounted for by a single exponential function (Cavill & Ricketts, 1974), indicating that iron on both sites behaves similarly.

Attempts have recently been made to define the distribution of iron between the binding sites in vivo. In fresh human serum iron shows a preference for the N-terminal site (the B site) and on incubation at 37°C an even greater shift to this site occurs (Williams & Moreton, 1980). This preference appears to be related to a dialysable fraction of serum which may bind to the protein and alter the affinity of the binding site. In haemolytic disorders where plasma iron turnover is increased iron is found bound preferentially to the C-terminal site. This suggests that the two sites may not be physiologically equivalent and it has been deduced that iron is loaded preferentially on the C-terminal site but unloaded preferentially from the N-terminal site. It is suggested that chloride is the dialysable factor facilitating redistribution on the molecule (Williams, 1980).

Transferrin binding to specific cell surface receptor sites has been studied in reticulocytes by many workers (Morgan, 1974) and recent work with bone marrow cells gives similar results (Kailis & Morgan, 1974). However, evidence from EM autoradiography (Morgan & Appleton, 1969; Sullivan et al, 1976) and other tracer techniques (Sly et al, 1975) implies that the transferrin molecule may actually enter the cell together with its iron and there is even a suggestion that iron is transported directly to the mitochondria in this way where its release from transferrin is regulated by haem (Ponka et al, 1977). This does not, however, accord with the evidence of Barnes et al (1972) and some authors doubt whether transferrin ever penetrates the outer cell membrane (Loh et al, 1977). The precise nature of the iron release mechanism is still not clear and attempts have been made to characterise the erythroid binding site. Maximum transferrin and iron uptake occurs in early and intermediate normoblasts. Maturation of the erythroid cell is associated with a decrease in the number of transferrin binding sites (Nunez et al, 1977; van Bockxmeer & Morgan, 1979). When Friend erythroleukaemia cells are induced to differentiate with DMSO the number of transferrin binding sites increases (Hu et al, 1977). Solubilisation of the reticulocyte membrane with Triton X-100 has led to the identification of fragments which could be the primary transferrin receptor (Leibman & Aisen, 1977; Sullivan & Weintraub, 1978). These appear to be a glycoprotein with a molecular weight in the range of 350 000 and consisting of two unequal subunits. Transferrin binding appears to depend on the carbohydrate portion of the large subunit and binding can be blocked by an antibody raised against the purified receptor (Van der Heul et al, 1978). The interdependence of anion and iron binding by transferrin may be an important factor in its iron-donating function. The bicarbonate which normally forms part of the iron-transferrin complex can be experimentally replaced by oxalate (Aisen & Leibman, 1973) and the resulting iron protein is less than 35 per cent as effective as an iron donor to reticulocytes. The presence of oxalate does not prevent transferrin binding to the cell but prevents it from releasing its iron. Aisen (1974) has suggested that the iron-releasing mechanism of the reticulocyte involves an attack on the anion-binding site of transferrin. While bicarbonate can be removed easily by the reticulocyte with the subsequent release of iron, oxalate cannot be removed in this way and the iron remains bound to the protein.

The delivery of iron to non-erythroid cells has not been studied extensively. Jandl et al (1959) showed that iron uptake by liver slices increased only slightly with increasing transferrin saturation up to 60 per cent but above this level there was a marked and progressive increase in uptake. Bailey-Wood et al (1975) showed that iron uptake from transferrin by Chang liver cells in culture increased with increasing saturation of the protein in the medium throughout the range 30 to 100 per cent. Similar results have been obtained with thyroid tissue slices (Buchanan, 1971). The release of iron from perfused rat liver (Baker et al, 1975) and from Chang cells (White et al, 1976) is dependent on transferrin saturation and it seems likely that the process involves the presence of specific receptor sites on the cell surface. Iron uptake by human peripheral blood monocytes, lymphocytes and granulocytes is also directly related to the iron saturation of transferrin (Summers & Jacobs, 1976). Larrick and Cresswell (1979) found transferrin receptors to be twice as numerous on human T lymphocytes as on B lymphocytes. MacDonald et al (1969) showed that isolated macrophages from rabbits with turpentine-induced inflammation ingested more iron than normal macrophages. Later studies by O'Shea et al (1973) suggested that this might be due to uptake of the intact iron-transferrin complex with subsequent degradation of the protein.

The liver parenchymal cells are the major site of transferrin synthesis (Morgan, 1974) though human peripheral blood lymphocytes may be a minor source in man (Soltys & Brody, 1970). It is likely that transferrin is synthesised on the ribosomes of the rough endoplasmic reticulum but that its transit time through the liver cytoplasm is longer than that of albumin. Nutritional status, liver function, oestrogen level and hypoxia may all influence transferrin synthesis (Morgan, 1974) but the most important single factor is the level of iron stores. The increased plasma concentration found in iron deficient subjects is due to increased synthesis and this returns to normal soon after the start of iron therapy and before there is any significant increase in haemoglobin concentration (Lane, 1966). Tavill & Kershenobich (1972) have made direct measurements on the effect of iron in regulating transferrin synthesis in rats and Morton & Tavill (1977) have shown that synthesis is most closely related to hepatic concentrations of ferritin. A reduction of hepatic ferritin levels by the induction of haem enzyme synthesis with phenobarbitone resulted in increased transferrin synthesis though the mechanism is far from clear. Changes in plasma ferritin level did not produce any feedback effect on transferrin synthesis.

Lactoferrin

The iron-binding protein of milk has been known for many years and its properties have been reviewed (Masson, 1970; Malmquist et al, 1978). It is widely distributed in the body and is found in gastric mucosa, intestinal epithelial cells, mammary gland, bronchial epithelium and in granulocytes (Mason & Taylor, 1978). It is antigenically distinct from transferrin though there is some similarity in amino acid sequences (Spik & Mazurier, 1977). Its moecular weight is about 75 000 to 80 000. Estimates of normal plasma concentration in man vary from 0.2 to 3.0 mg/l (Malmquist et al, 1978). Plasma turnover studies show that following injection of the labelled protein it is eliminated with a mean fractional catabolic rate of 5.7/day, iron free lactoferrin disappears at a slower rate (Bennett & Kokocinski, 1979).

Bullen et al (1972) feel that lactoferrin (LF) derived from milk may play an important role in protecting infants against E. Coli gastroenteritis by depriving the micro-organism of iron. Similarly the LF of polymorphonuclear neutrophils may play an important role in the cell's antibacterial function (Bullen & Armstrong, 1979). Disintegration of leucocytes after migration to a focus of infection is followed by release of the protein into the interstitial fluid, where at a slightly acid pH, it may compete successfully with transferrin for iron. Animal studies have suggested that this may be followed by ingestion of the lactoferrin-bound iron by macrophages and its incorporation into ferritin, thus resulting in the low plasma iron concentration and increased ferritin stores characteristic of infection (Van Snick et al, 1974, 1977).

Broxmeyer et al (1978, 1980a) have shown that LF can function as a negative feedback regulator of granulocyte and macrophage production. It appears to decrease colony formation by decreasing the production of colony stimulating activity (CSA) by monocytes. It inhibits at very low concentrations (10^{-17} M) in vitro and its action depends on its degree of iron saturation, the apoprotein being without effect. More recent studies indicate a functional heterogeneity of peripheral blood neutrophils with respect to lactoferrin. When neutrophils are fractionated by a rosetting procedure using rabbit IgE antibody-coated sheep erythrocytes only lactoferrin obtained from the rosetting cells can supress CSA activity. LF from rosetting-negative neutrophils is inactive at concentrations as high as 10^{-5} M. (Broxmeyer et al, 1980b). There is a similar heterogeneity in human monocytes and it has been suggested that LF inhibits the production of CSA from an Ia antigen-positive subpopulation (Broxmeyer, 1979).

The functions of iron in non-erythroid tissues
There are a large number of iron compounds in the body which are not related to erythropoiesis (Wrigglesworth & Baum, 1980). Many are haem compounds and some are concerned with tissue respiration but a wide variety of metabolic processes in all cells involve enzymes which contain iron or require iron as a cofactor. While these are not, perhaps, the direct concern of the haematologist they play a key role in iron metabolism. Their maintenance depends on an adequate supply of iron and their depletion in iron deficiency has secondary metabolic effects. Detailed reviews have recently appeared of the cytochromes (Lemberg & Barratt, 1973; Nicholls & Elliott, 1974) and of the non-haem iron proteins (Hall, Cammack & Rao, 1974). Myoglobin accounts for about 15 per cent of the non-storage iron in the body (Akeson et al, 1968). Mitochondria in all animal cells contain an electron transport pathway which allows the eventual oxidation of intracellular substrates by molecular oxygen with the generation of ATP. This pathway contains a variety of iron compounds which transmit electrons by means of reversible valency changes in their iron atoms. Failure of this system due to lack of oxygen supply, enzyme depletion or block with metabolic inhibitors leads to failure of energy production, accumulation of metabolites and eventual cell ceath. There is evidence that iron is also necessary for mitochondrial protein synthesis through a mechanism independent of haem synthesis (Marcus et al, 1980) and this may be important in maintaining integrity of the organelle. Cytochrome P450 is found in endoplasmic reticulum and plays a major part in hydroxylation reactions associated with drug detoxication by the liver (De Matteis, 1980). Induction of a specific apoenzyme by administration of a drug such as barbiturate or benzpyrene is accompanied by stimulation of haem synthesis with consequent iron mobilisation. In rat intestinal mucosa cytochrome P450 concentra-

tion is highest in the upper intestine and in the most mature villous cells. Its synthesis is dependent on a direct iron supply from the gut lumen (Hoensch et al, 1976). The enzyme is also found in adrenal mitochondria where it takes part in steroid hydroxylation.

Iron is essential to a number of other processes only a few of which can be mentioned here. A role in cell division has been suggested by Robbins & Pederson (1970) and its specific requirement for DNA synthesis (Hershko et al, 1970; Hoffbrand et al, 1976) is probably based on the iron dependence of the rate–limiting enzyme ribonucleotide reductase. The iron dependence of globin chain synthesis in red cells was first noted by Rabinowitz & Waxman (1965) but it is known that the presence of haem is necessary for all chain initiation in reticulocytes. The general nature of this phenomenon is emphasised by its demonstration in the translation of exogenous messenger RNA added to reticulocyte extracts (Mathews et al, 1973) and in non-erythroid cells (Beuzard et al, 1973). More specific examples of iron dependence include the enzymes tyrosine hydroxylase (Moore & Dominic, 1971), monoamine oxidase (Youdim et al, 1975) and proline hydroxylase (Prockop, 1971). The sensitivity of enzymes such as the disaccharidases (Hoffbrand & Broitman, 1969) glucose-6-phosphate dehydrogenase and 6-phosphogluconate dehydrogenase (Bailey-Wood et al, 1975), are more difficult to explain.

The various influences of iron metabolism on lymphocyte function are still a matter of conjecture. The dependence of lymphocyte transformation on iron delivery by transferrin has been elegantly demonstrated by Phillips & Azari (1975) who showed that neither iron nor transferrin alone were effective. Lymphokine production may also be iron dependent (Joynson et al, 1972). Nishiya et al (1980a) have shown that E-rosetting by human peripheral blood lymphocytes is inhibited by iron, either as the citrate or bound to transferrin. This inhibition can be reversed by treating the cells with desferrioxamine. There is a suggestion that the increase in serum IgA and IgG in thalassaemic patients after splenectomy may be related to the serum iron concentration (Kapadia et al, 1980). T-lymphocyte function is also inhibited by ferritin in vitro with suppression of transformation induced by phytohaemagglutinin, concanavalin A, pokeweed mitogen and the mixed lymphocyte reaction (Matzner et al, 1979). Immunofluorescent studies suggest that T-cells have a greater capacity to produce ferritin than B-cells (Nishiya et al, 1980b) and this is in keeping with their greater number of transferrin-binding sites. No clear explanation has yet emerged for any of these phenomena but they appear especially relevant to the interpretation of lymphocyte function and the expression of surface markers in those conditions where iron status is also disturbed.

Ferritin

Recent reviews deal with the structure and function of ferritin (Harrison et al, 1980; Bomford & Munro, 1980) and the clinical aspects of ferritin and its measurement in serum (Worwood, 1980). The spherical protein shell of ferritin contains 24 subunits of molecular weight about 19 000 giving a molecular weight for apoferritin of about 450 000. An electron density map at 0.6 nm resolution shows a hollow shell with internal and external diameter of 7 and 12 nm respectively (Hoare et al, 1975). The shell is penetrated by six channels along the molecular fourfold axes. These are square in cross-section, widening towards the inside from 0.9 to 1.2 nm. Each molecule can accommodate up to 4500 iron atoms in its central core in the form of ferric hydroxyphosphate. This has a variable crystalline structure and is firmly attached to the protein (Massover & Cowley, 1975; Massover, 1978). The most recent crystallographic studies at 0.28 nm resolution (Banyard et al, 1978) show the helical structure of the subunits. The four approximately parallel helices form the wall of the shell and the smaller fifth E helices, which are perpendicular to the others, form the walls of the penetrating channels and may well be of importance in regulating iron uptake and release. While it has been suggested that there is free passage of iron through the channels with the rate depending on the dynamics of crystal formation within the molecule (Harrison et al, 1974) there is evidence that iron uptake is associated with the oxidation of Fe^{2+} to Fe^{3+} by ferritin itself (Bryce & Crichton, 1973) and that mobilisation is associated with reduction by reduced flavins (Sirivech et al, 1974; Jones et al, 1978).

The stimulation of ferritin synthesis by iron is a well recognised phenomenon and has been observed in intact animals, whole organs, tissue slices, cell cultures and cell-free systems (Harrison et al, 1980). Lee et al (1975) have used an immunofluorescent technique with an antibody to subunits and shown that in rat livers subunits are synthesised within 2 to 3 minutes and are detectable before ferritin or apoferritin is found. The response to iron stimulation is insensitive to actinomycin D and is presumably post-transcriptional but it is not known whether it acts by stimulating the attachment of RNA to polyribosomes, the translation of apoferritin subunits, chain release from polyribosomes or the assembly of subunits. Drysdale & Shafritz (1975) suggest that the effect is post-translational. A review of possible mechanisms for the control of synthesis are given by Bomford & Munro (1980) and it should be noted that in certain circumstances such as experimental inflammation (Konijn & Hershko, 1977) stimulation of ferritin synthesis is not necessarily dependent on iron.

It has long been known that ferritin from different organs may differ on electrophoresis but evidence, arising largely from isoelectric focusing, has suggested a microheterogeneity of ferritin from single organs. A number of isoferritins have been found in most human tissues and several of these are common to most tissues. Drysdale (1977) has postulated that this heterogeneity arises through the existence of two types of subunit which are present in different proportions in the different proteins, an H subunit which predominates in the acidic isoferritins and has a molecular weight of 21 000 and an L subunit predominating in the more basic isoferritins, with a molecular weight of 19 000. This explanation has not received universal acceptance though it is supported by biosynthetic studies in a cell free system (Arosio et al, 1978) and immunological and functional differences between isoferritins (Wagstaff et al, 1978).

Clinical interest in ferritin has been stimulated by studies of the circulating protein (Jacobs & Worwood, 1975) which is usually present in serum at concentrations of 20 to 300 μg/litre. The concentration is directly related to body iron stores in normal subjects (Walters et al, 1973). It is reduced in iron deficiency and increased to levels as high as 25 000 μg/litre in patients with iron overload. An abnormal amount is released into the circulation following liver damage (Prieto et al, 1975) and in inflammatory conditions such as rheumatoid arthritis when increased serum ferritin may be associated with a low serum iron concentration. Increased serum ferritin concentrations are found in a wide variety of malignant states including carcinoma of the breast,

Hodgkins disease and leukaemia. Increased synthesis of the protein has been shown in leukaemic cells (White et al, 1974) and in mononuclear cells of patients with Hodgkins disease (Sarcione et al, 1977) but no clinical value has yet been found for any of these phenomena. Drysdale & Singer (1974) showed that HeLa cells and placental tissue have an acidic isoferritin in common and suggested that this could be a specific carcinofetal antigen. Similar 'carcinofetal' ferritins were found in mammary and pancreatic carcinoma (Marcus & Zinberg, 1974), hepatoma (Alpert, 1975) and acute leukaemia (Cragg et al, 1977). However, a detailed study of tissue and serum ferritin in patients with a wide variety of malignant conditions using specific immunoradiometric assays for acidic (HeLa) and basic (spleen) isoferritins did not indicate any specific diagnostic value for the assay in these disorders (Jones et al, 1980).

A detailed review of the physiology, biochemistry and clinical aspects of serum ferritin has been provided by Worwood (1980). The heterogeneity of serum ferritin has been shown to be due largely to glycosylation (Worwood et al, 1979) and studies in a large series of thalassaemic patients with transfusional iron overload shows that much of the large amounts of the circulating protein are related to tissue damage rather than simple iron loading (Worwood et al, 1980). A simple relationship between serum ferritin concentration and iron stores cannot be assumed when ferritin concentrations exceed 4000 μg/l or in patients who have received more than 100 units of transfused blood.

The main clinical use of serum ferritin measurements at the present time is in the evaluation of increased or decreased iron stores. It has no place at present in the investigation of leukaemia or other malignant disease.

Intracellular iron metabolism

The regulation of iron uptake by cells and the pathways followed by iron from the cell membrane to the sites where iron proteins are synthesised are not well understood. In the red cell the main terminal point of this pathway is within the mitochondria where the iron is incorporated into haem through the action of haem synthetase. Iron uptake by cells appears to be related to the requirements for haem synthesis. Iron deficient erythroblasts have an increased avidity for iron (May et al, 1980) and the same is true for iron deficient liver (Morton & Tavill, 1975), iron deficient intestinal epithelium (Howard & Jacobs, 1972) and iron deficient lymphocytes (Summers & Jacobs, 1976).

Although ferritin is present in the cytoplasm of all mammalian cells and may behave as an intermediate compound (Fielding & Speyer, 1974) it seems likely that iron which has crossed the cell membrane and has been released from transferrin enters a labile intermediate pool from which it is available for haem synthesis, the activation of iron enzymes, for incorporation into ferritin or for return to extracellular transferrin (Jacobs, 1977; Romslo, 1980). Enlargement of this pool probably stimulates the synthesis of ferritin protein and it is probably also a major source of iron chelated by agents such as desferrioxamine. Iron probably enters this transit pool not only from transferrin but also from endogenous haem breakdown and the mobilisation of ferritin iron. Evidence for the occurrence of such a transit pool has been obtained for reticuloendothelial cells, red cell precursors, cultured Chang cells and liver but details of the pathway of iron from transferrin to the mitochondrion are unknown. Our knowledge of iron uptake by the mitochondrion has been summarised by Romslo (1980).

Systemic effects of iron deficiency

In a state of negative iron balance there is progressive depletion of iron in all tissues. In the earlier stages iron is gradually mobilised from storage compounds to meet the needs for haemoglobin synthesis and other metabolic activities until no further stores remain. This stage has been called 'prelatent' iron deficiency and has been characterised by the absence of stainable iron in the bone marrow, increased iron absorption but no decrease in either serum iron or haemoglobin concentration. The quantitation of iron stores by estimating serum ferritin concentration has limited the value of this diagnostic label. When further iron depletion results in a fall in serum iron concentration there may still be no interference with erythropoiesis and a state of so called 'latent' iron deficiency results (Dagg et al, 1971). In the third stage of iron depletion a reduction in iron supply to the bone marrow leads to iron deficient erythropoiesis and the appearance of iron deficiency anaemia.

A wide range of non-erythroid tissue abnormalities have been described both in iron deficient patients and in experimental animals (Dallman, 1974; Beutler & Fairbanks, 1980). It is generally assumed that these result from the defective synthesis of tissue iron enzymes though no clear biochemical relationship to morphological and functional changes has been demonstrated. The total iron content of these tissue compounds is probably no more than 50 mg in an adult male compared to 2.5 to 3.0 g in the form of haemoglobin and perhaps 0.5 to 1.5 g in storage forms but the degree of complexity of the metabolic pathways involved may partly explain the relative lack of clinical studies. There is some suggestion that the long debated symptoms of iron deficient patients may be related to metabolic changes. The compensatory mechanism within red cells leading to decreased oxygen affinity in response to mild anaemia results in normal oxygen delivery to the tissues of iron deficient patients until their haemoglobin concentration falls to below 10 g/dl. This may well be adequate in patients at rest but on exercise small decreases in haemoglobin concentration within the 'normal range' may lead to impaired physical work capacity (Viteri & Torun, 1974). Hjelm & Wadman (1974) suggest that symptoms may be related to the effectiveness of intra-erythrocytic adaptive changes. Studies in Indonesia, where severe iron deficiency is common, have shown a relationship between haemoglobin concentration and productivity in agricultural workers (Basta et al, 1979). A similar study in Sri Lanka, (Ohira et al, 1979) showed that treatment with parenteral iron-dextran resulted in improved work capacity within 4 days, which could not be totally accounted for by rise in haemoglobin concentration.

A wide variety of isolated iron-enzyme defects have been described in iron deficient tissues (Dallman, 1974, Beutler & Fairbanks, 1980) and in rats profound physical abnormalities due to iron deficiency have been demonstrated. Simultaneous studies of a range of activities in the myocardium (Blayney et al, 1976) and liver (Bailey-Wood et al, 1975) of iron deficient rats has shown considerable differences between different tissues and between enzymes in the same tissue. There was widespread depletion of myocardial cytochromes and impaired activity throughout the electron transport pathway while in the liver only succinic-cytochrome C reductase activity was affected. Microsomal cytochrome P-450 was quite unaffected by iron deficiency. An unexpected early change in the liver was a reduction of enzyme activity in the pentose phosphate shunt. Finch et al (1976) have shown that work performance in iron deficient rats increases five fold after 3 days administration of iron even though the haemoglobin concentration remains unchanged. Conversely increasing the haemoglobin concentration by transfusion alone did not increase work performance. The change in activity was not related to concentrations of cytochromes or myoglobin but appeared to be associated with a change in a glycerophosphate mediated phosphorylation. Siimes et al (1980) have shown that when dietary iron deficiency of increasing severity is induced in rats, the cytochrome C content of muscle falls in parallel with the fall in haemoglobin concentration but myoglobin concentration falls only at more severe degrees of deficiency. Severe iron deficiency in weanling rats results in a deficit of brain iron which persists into adult life and cannot be rectified by subsequent therapy (Dallman et al, 1975). Youdim & Green (1977) found marked behavioural changes in iron deficient rats which were reversed on treatment with iron and suggested that these might be related to an abnormality in monoamine neurotransmission. Behavioural changes in iron deficient infants and children have also been described. (Pollitt & Leibel, 1976; Oski & Honig, 1978) but there is some debate regarding their significance (Pollitt et al, 1979).

Marked structural changes have been shown in the hepatic and myocardial mitochondria of iron deficient rats (Dallman, 1974). In both cases the organelles are enlarged and translucent and it is suggested that mitochondrial enlargement accounts for much of the cardiac hypertrophy of iron deficiency. Peripheral blood lymphocytes in iron deficiency anaemia show mitochondrial swelling, vacuolation and rupture of cristae (Jarvis & Jacobs, 1974). In some cases there may be rupture of the outer membrane. Similar changes are seen in bone marrow cells (Dallman, 1974).

Most microorganisms obtain soluble iron from their environment by secreting chelating agents know as siderochromes (Neilands, 1980) and there is good evidence that iron plays a part in determining pathogenicity and virulence of infecting organisms. Transferrin deprives these organisms of the iron they require but this is abolished by saturation with iron (Sussman, 1974). Weinberg (1974) has assembled much evidence that hyperferraemia whether due to disease or to iron therapy is associated with an increased incidence of infection and that hypoferraemia may be protective but these views are not entirely in keeping with a widespread clinical impression especially amongst pediatricians, that infants and children with iron deficiency anaemia tend to have increased incidence of infections. This impression has been supported by a study of Chicago children by Andelman & Sered (1966) who showed that iron supplementation of the diet resulted in. control of iron deficiency anaemia together with a significant reduction in respiratory infections. Cantwell (1972) showed a similar effect of parenteral iron given to Maoria infants. No such effect of iron was found in a well-nourished population (Burman, 1972). Patients with iron deficiency anaemia may have an abundance of unsaturated transferrin to act as a bacteriostatic agent but they also have impaired cellular defence mechanisms. Joynson et al (1972) demonstrated defective lymphocyte transformation and reduced production of macrophage migration inhibition factor (MIF) after antigenic stimulation. The latter was associated with negative skin sensitivity to the appropriate antigen. MIF production returned to normal rapidly after iron therapy and in some cases was associated with Mantoux conversion from negative to positive. Similar results have been overserved by Chandra and Saraya (1975) and Macdougal et al (1975), both of whom also confirmed the earlier observation (Chandra, 1973) of reduced bactericidal activity of polymorphs from iron deficient patients. These phenomena, which were also found in latent iron deficiency (Macdougal et al, 1975), were all reversed by iron therapy. It seems likely that the normal physiological state is associated with optimum defences against bacterial infection. Weinberg (1974) has noted that orally administered iron is not effective in promoting systemic infection and it is almost impossible to fully saturate circulating transferrin by this route. There are no studies showing bacteraemia or septicaemia in animals given oral iron. The US Committee on Nutrition (1978) conclude that iron deficiency increases the risk of infection, depending on its severity and, possibly on whether it is nutritional in origin.

IRON OVERLOAD

Primary idiopathic haemochromatosis

Sheldon's review of this condition in 1935 presented a clinical picture of the disease that has required no essential amendment (Powell & Halliday, 1980). His view that the disease results from an inborn error of metabolism has now been substantiated though the nature of the lesion remains unknown. Recent work has greatly clarified our knowledge of the mode of inheritance which has been obscured in the past by the late development of the clinical disorder, the influence of other factors such as alcohol, expression of the disease and inconsistency regarding diagnostic criteria. Simon et al (1976) showed that patients had a significantly higher frequency of HLA-A3 and HLA-B14 antigens than a control population and later showed that the haemochromatosis gene is closely linked with the HLA loci on chromosome 6 (Simon et al, 1977). Subsequent studies from Utah (Edwards et al, 1977; Cartwright et al, 1979), Ontario (Lloyd et al, 1978) and Rennes (Beaumont et al, 1979) have confirmed this observation. Its importance is that the haemochromatosis gene can be traced through a family without waiting, sometimes many years, for pathological manifestations to emerge. Those family members having the same HLA haplotype as the propositus can be considered at risk, though the precise HLA antigens involved may differ in different families.

Within families, unaffected members, heterozygotes and homozygotes defined on the basis of HLA typing are found to have normal, raised and greatly increased values for transferrin saturation, serum ferritin and liver non-haem iron (Cartwright et al, 1979; Beaumont et al, 1979). The terms dominant and recessive no longer seem appropriate in considering the inheritance of this disorder. While homozygotes show severe iron overload, heterozygotes may have minor degrees of overload which may give rise to symptoms only if other factors increase the tendency to loading. From the practical point of view of detecting early signs of the disease in members of an affected family, the combined determination of serum ferritin and transferrin saturation is indicated. In those who are too young for any manifestations to be obvious, homozygotes should be retested regularly to prevent the occurrence of severe overload, those considered heterozygous should be warned of the possible ill-effects of alcohol and iron therapy and should also be retested periodically. Those relatives whose HLA genotype is entirely different from the propositus can be considered to be at very low risk.

Some uncertainty exists regarding the prevalence of idiopathic haemochromatosis (IH). Scheinberg (1973) estimated that it occurred no more than once in 10 000 individuals but more recent studies suggest a homozygote frequency of three per thousand in Utah (Cartwright et al, 1979) and one in four hundred in Brittany (Beaumont et al, 1979). Olsson et al (1978) found 5 per cent of normal men between 30 and 39 years old to have a high serum iron concentration and of these 2 per cent also had an increased serum ferritin concentration.

The classic clinical picture of primary haemochromatosis represents the end-point of a process in which a genetically determined excessive iron absorption over many years results in the gradual accumulation of parenchymal iron and subsequent tissue damage. In such cases iron absorption is normal or only slightly increased but as the iron load is removed by venesection, absorption again increases until it is well above the normal range. Iron absorption is inversely proportional to body iron load both in normal subjects and in those with haemochromatosis (Walters et al, 1975) though in the latter case it is higher than normal at any given iron load. If patients are allowed to reaccumulate iron after the completion of venesection, absorption again falls and as a small amount of the excess iron may be excreted into the gut, equilibrium may be achieved at very high loads.

A number of hypotheses have been proposed to account for the development of iron overload in this condition but none have been associated with any evidence for a primary biochemical lesion. Many authors have suggested that the abnormally high iron absorption is the primary abnormality, possibly due to factors in the gastrointestinal lumen or within the intestinal epithelial cell. The older evidence for various luminal abnormalities has not been confirmed (Jacobs, 1970) and no new evidence has emerged. Crosby, (1963) showed that jejunal biopsies from patients with IH did not contain the normal F bodies, which are membrane-bound accumulations of ferritin, and suggested that failure of ferritin synthesis at this site, or failure to incorporate iron, could lead to uncontrolled absorption. Beamish et al (1974) showed that patients with haemochromatosis who have normal iron stores following treatment by venesection or whose disease is in an early stage of development are characterised by normal serum ferritin concentration together with an abnormally high concentration of serum iron and a greatly increased pool of chelatable iron in the body. The occurrence of such an imbalance in the small intestinal epithelium could result in an inappropriately high iron absorption due to failure to sequestrate iron as ferritin at this site with a consequent increased amount remaining in the labile pool, available for serosal transfer. Walters et al (1975) found that in haemochromatotic patients at various stages of iron loading there was a close correlation between the chelatable iron: ferritin ratio and iron absorption. More recently Cox & Peters (1978) have shown that iron uptake by human duodenal mucosa in vitro was higher in iron loaded patients with IH than was appropriate in relation to control subjects. They suggested that a primary abnormality of a cellular iron carrier resulted in an increased affinity of the carrier for iron. However, this hypothesis assumes a failure of the cells to sequestrate iron as ferritin if it is to account for increased absorption.

The inappropriately low serum ferritin concentration in early, presymptomatic haemochromatosis has been confirmed (Wands et al, 1976; Edwards et al, 1977), though this is not universally observed (Halliday et al, 1977). This phenomenon can be explained either by a failure of ferritin synthesis or a failure to incorporate iron, though neither have been convincingly demonstrated. Cook & Finch (1975) also noted high concentrations of serum iron in four patients with normal levels of serum ferritin but showed that a fall in serum iron could be induced by restricting the dietary iron to less than 2 mg daily. They concluded that the early rise in serum iron concentration is due to an abnormality of iron absorption alone rather than a generalised metabolic defect.

Attention has recently focussed on the imbalance of iron deposition between hepatic parenchymal cells and reticuloendothelial cells during the early stages of iron loading in IH. Valberg et al (1975) noted that excess haemosiderin appears to be deposited predominantly and preferentially in hepatic parenchymal storage sites until the later stages of the disease and discussed five possible reasons for this. (1) When transferrin saturation is high, iron absorbed from the gastrointestinal tract is deposited in the liver on its first passage through the portal system. (2) It is the result of liver disease. (3) There is an increased affinity of the hepatic cells for iron. (4) There is a primary abnormality of the reticuloendothetical cell resulting in failure to retain iron. (5) There is an increased deposition of circulating ferritin in hepatocytes. The same histological distribution of iron was observed by Ross et al (1975) who placed emphasis on a hypothetical failure of the RE cells to retain iron and by Brink et al (1976) who felt that the pathogenesis of IH could be explained by a failure of both intestinal epithelial cells and RE cells to retain iron. Direct experimental observations in support of these various hypotheses are scanty, though the observations of Pollycove et al (1971) are of interest. They showed that patients with IH, even when rendered iron deficient by venesection, show an increased uptake of injected transferrin-bound radioiron to the liver compared to control subjects. This finding has been confirmed by Batey et al (1978) who suggest a cellular abnormality of hepatic iron absorption.

It seems likely that the diagnosis of IH will be made more frequently during the presymptomatic stage in the future and that careful monitoring of affected persons to prevent initial iron accumulation will avoid morbidity. It remains to be seen whether life expectancy is normal in such subjects. Bomford & Williams (1976) have shown that in severely affected patients venesection therapy results in 66 per cent survival after 5 years and 32 per cent survival after ten years compared with 18 per cent and 6 per cent respectively for untreated patients. The control of diabetes was improved in 28 per cent of those with diabetes mellitus. However there was a striking mortality from hepatoma and other neoplasms which was not improved by therapy. We do not know the reason for this, nor whether this will be true for patients who have never suffered from iron overload.

Transfusion siderosis
Patients with chronic aplastic anaemia or homozygous β-thalassaemia often receive repeated blood transfusion and for many of them this may be the only effective treatment. If this regime is prolonged the short-term benefits are gradually overshadowed by the effects of iron overload. The liver and spleen become grossly siderotic and although the total amount of iron deposited in the heart is relatively small, myocardial damage is a major factor in determining prognosis. Buja & Roberts (1971) described 19 patients who had cardiac iron deposits following multiple transfusions. Extensive siderosis was the rule in patients receiving more than 100 units of blood. The deposits were always more extensive in the ventricular myocar-

dium than in the atria and were noted in the contractile cells rather than the conducting system. Five of these patients had chronic congestive cardiac failure, and atrial iron deposits were associated with supraventricular arrhythmias. There is little evidence regarding the ultrastructural effects due to myocardial iron toxicity though Sanyal et al (1975) report widespread damage including disruption of mitochondria and disappearance of myofibrils.

Risdon et al (1975) have studied the relationship between iron load and hepatic fibrosis in biopsy samples taken from patients with homozygous β-thalassaemia during a high transfusion regime. The rate of iron accumulation in the liver depended on whether the patient was receiving continuous chelation therapy. The severity of fibrosis was related both to age and to liver iron concentration. A reduction in liver iron concentration by treatment with desferrioxamine was associated with failure of fibrosis to progress even though the amount of iron remaining was still grossly excessive. It is possible to speculate that fibrosis may be stimulated by 'chelatable' iron rather than the more stable storage iron compounds and Hunt et al (1979) have shown that desferrioxamine can inhibit collagen synthesis by cultured fibroblasts. The clinical consequences have been reviewed by Hoffbrand (1980).

In recent years an attempt has been made to prevent iron accumulation by the use of desferrioxamine, but although the iron load can be reduced by a regime of daily injections over a prolonged period (Barry et al, 1974) serum ferritin concentrations remain 40 to 100 times normal. The need to administer desferrioxamine daily by intramuscular injection together with the virtual impossibility of preventing iron accumulating to toxic levels has stimulated the investigation of continuous sub-cutaneous infusion of desferrioxamine (Propper et al, 1976; Hussain et al, 1977) or of newer chelating agents. Most of the compounds that have been studied are microbial products (Neilands, 1980) and these have been investigated in vitro, in vivo using the hypertransfused rat as an experimental model (Grady et al, 1976) and in cell culture using Chang cells (White et al, 1976). Many of the compounds are either hydroxa-mates, like desferrioxamine, or derivatives of 2,3-dihydroxybenzoic acid (2,3-DHB), like enterochelin (Neilands, 1980). A variety of other substances such as tropolones, semicarbazones, hydrazones and analogues of EDTA have been investigated but while a few promising chelators have been proposed for potential therapeutic use none has yet proved superior to desferrioxamine (Jacobs, 1979).

The new drugs under investigation at the present time fall into three groups. Firstly, improved agents for parenteral administration, of which rhodotorulic acid is an example. Secondly, there are iron chelators for oral administration of which cholyhydroxamic acid and isoniazidpryridoxal hydrazone (Hoy et al, 1979) seem possible candidates. Thirdly, there is the possibility that depot preparations of desferrioxamine or polymeric hydroxamic acids (Winston & Kirchner, 1976) might be of value for parenteral use so that prolonged action can be obtained without the need for continuous infusion. None of the more experimental approaches to iron chelation therapy such as the use of liposomes, combination therapy or drug entrapment in red cell ghosts has yet proved to be a practical answer to the problem of iron overload. At present, treatment of transfusional iron overload must be directed to preventing iron accumulation by all possible means. Negative iron balance can be achieved by the continuous infusion of desferrioxamine whatever the level of iron loading and in transfusion dependent thalassaemics overload may be entirely prevented by early introduction of regular chelation therapy (Pippard et al, 1978). The major problem here is patient compliance. The maintainance of a high haemoglobin concentration reduces erythropoietic activity (Cavill et al, 1978), plasma iron turnover (Propper et al, 1980) and iron absorption (de Alarcon et al, 1979). Theoretically the availability of dietary iron might be reduced by the exclusion of meat from the diet and an increased intake of foods with a high content of phytate, phosphate or tannin, but dietary iron is a relatively minor source of iron loading.

Pathology of iron overload

This subject has been reviewed by Richter (1978) and Jacobs (1980).

Ultrastructural changes

Iron loading is associated with increased ferritin synthesis in all cells. Ferritin is the predominant iron storage compound under normal conditions and haemosiderin tends to appear in iron loaded states. The latter is a relatively amorphous condensation of electron dense iron particles consisting mainly of ferric hydroxide and probably derived from a conglomeration of iron cores after the degradation of ferritin protein. In a cell culture model of iron overload Jacobs et al (1978) showed that a 50 fold increase in iron content can be induced in Chang cells. Most of the intracellular iron is seen to be membrane-bound bodies on electron microscopy. With increasing concentrations of iron the intracellular ferritin concentration rises to a plateau level about 6 to 10 times normal. The concentration of non-haem, non-ferritin iron rises continuously with increased loading, nearly all of this being found in irregular, dense lysosomal accumulations.

The difficulty in the definition of haemosiderin and ferritin remains; although they are chemically and structurally dissimilar, there are undoubtedly intermediate compounds between the two. There is no doubt regarding the identity of pure ferritin either on biochemical or electron microscopic examination (Harrison et al, 1980) or of the insoluable aggregates with a high iron/protein ratio called haemosiderin, but between the two are a range of ferritin polymers, membrane-bound accumulations of ferritin, ferritin accumulations with a well-defined crystalline structure, and membranous bodies including ferritin, lipid, and pigment aggregates which defy simple analysis. Richter & Bessis (1965) have noted that natural haemosiderin is not a single unique substance and that when isolated from the tissues it represents an artifact which cannot be considered separately from its intracellular environment. However, when isolated in a test tube the iron components of ferritin and haemosiderin examined by X-ray diffraction, Mossbauer spectroscopy, and electron microscopy show a similar atomic structure but a slightly smaller particle size in the case of haemosiderin (Fischbach et al, 1971). These results suggest that haemosiderin is formed by the denaturation and proteolytic cleavage of ferritin, leaving a slightly small iron core, presumably because some of the iron is lost during the process. Closely packed ferritin molecules seen on electron microscopy have a 50 Å gap between each iron core because of the 25 Å thickness of each protein shell. In haemosiderin the iron cores sit more closely together because of protein loss, and the compound might almost be defined as one where the distance between the 70 Å iron cores is less than 50 Å.

The factors controlling haemosiderin formation are unknown. Ferritin degradation may be simply related to close packing, possibly to polymer formation, or possibly to enzymatic attack following incorporation into lysosomes. Recent observations on iron loaded Chang cells suggest that iron rich ferritin molecules may undergo a conformational change that alters their surface properties and predisposes them to lysosomal processing (Hoy & Jacobs, 1981). Starch gel electrophoresis of purified ferritin gives rise to a number of bands representing monomers, dimers and trimers. Oligomers containing up to five molecules have been seen on electron microscopy by Williams & Harrison (1968) and according to these authors cannot be dissociated except under conditions leading to disaggregation of subunits. The intercore distances are slightly less than 50 Å in some cases, and although this could result from a technical artifact it is consistent with some degree of condensation of the protein shells. The appearance of ferritin polymers in extracts prepared by different techniques from different tissues suggests that they probably exist within cells in vivo. Lee & Richter (1976) have suggested that the concentration of ferritin may be a major factor in polymerisation, association or dissociation being reversible according to the conditions in solution, and this may be relevant to the molecular packing that occurs in cytoplasmic vesicles. Powell and co-workers (1974) reported an abnormal isoferritin distribution in idiopathic haemochromatosis, but later found a similar pattern in other iron storage disorders (Powell et al, 1975). Wagstaff et al (1978) found no significant deviation from normal in transfusional siderosis but Bomford et al (1980) comparing six control subjects with five patients having idiopathic haemochromatosis found the latter to have a predominance of acidic isoferritins with increasing levels of iron storage. They suggested that this might be due to preferential synthesis or retarded degradation of acidic isoferritins in iron loaded states.

The ability of cells to synthesize ferritin as a response to iron forms part of a protective mechanism, any excess of intracellular iron being sequestered in a nontoxic form. Variations in the synthetic capacity of different tissues is, to some extent, matched by their capacity to take up iron. The low level of ferritin synthesis in polymorphonuclear leukocytes and lymphocytes (Summers et al, 1975) does not lead to iron toxicity, since their iron uptake is also low. Mononuclear phagocytes which have an obligatory iron load due to their role in haemoglobin catabolism have a high synthetic capacity for ferritin (Summers et al, 1975). Long-term experiments with Chang cells in culture show that exposure to high iron concentrations leads to the appearance of ferritin scattered in the cytoplasm followed by membrane-bound accumulations of ferritin, some of which appear to be lysosomal, and later by the occurrence of membrane-bound masses of amorphous electron-dense deposits (Jacobs et al, 1978). These processes do not appear to interfere with the cells normal activities or multiplication. When there is a continuous process of ferritin synthesis this is balanced by its conversion into haemosiderin.

It has been suggested that iron overload is easily produced in the liver because its considerable capacity to synthesize ferritin cannot be matched by its ability to process the product in secondary lysosomes prior to excretion. Instead the lysosomal accumulation of ferritin behaves as a sump that gradually converts the protein to haemosiderin, which then remains in situ (Trump et al, 1973). Although in the early experiments of Goldberg & Smith (1960) high doses of parenteral iron resulted in increased activity of hepatic lysosomal enzymes, recent studies have shown that it is possible to iron load rats with no liver abnormality except a massive lysosomal accumulation of iron granules (Arborgh et al, 1974). Similar lysosomal accumulations can be found in the pancreatic acini (Pechet, 1969) and the greatly increased density of such organelles aids their isolation from tissues (Glaumann et al, 1975). When cell death occurs in experimental iron overload the microscopic picture may show no specific changes. In addition to the inevitable secondary lysosomes containing amorphous electron dense debris, remains of partly digested organelles, and the contents of the cell sap, there will be degenerate organelles in the cytoplasm with widespread evidence of membrane damage, myelin whorls, lipid droplets, and residual bodies. The precise mechanism of death is not obvious at the visual level.

There are not many ultrastructural studies of human tissue from patients with iron overload. Sanyal et al (1975) have examined the myocardium of a child dying of transfusional overload and found iron deposited around the nuclei of muscle cells or diffusely throughout the cytoplasm. Iron was invariably found within the nuclei and mitochondria, a surprising difference from the experimental studies. In addition there was thought to be an increase in mitochondrial numbers and some myofibril fragmentation. In one case however, mitochondria were thought to be decreased (Arnett et al, 1975).

The most satisfactory ultrastructural study of iron overload in human liver is that of Iancu and Neustein (1977), who have examined biopsy material from ten patients with homozygous thalassaemia and transfusion siderosis. They found practically no ferritin molecules in any other cellular compartments apart from the cell sap and lysosomes. Beyond infancy the density of cell sap ferritin does not increase, but the number of iron loaded lysosomes increases with age until in the most severely affected cases they displace most of the normal cell components. Haemosiderin is considered to be present when the individual electron-dense ferritin cores and their surrounding protein shells can no longer be defined, a state found only within lysosomes. Many of the hepatocyte lysosomes contain fat droplets, myelin bodies, and peculiar lamellar structures which often have ferritin molecules arranged in linear patterns along the membranes.

In idiopathic haemochromatosis Ross et al (1975) have shown the ferruginous bodies within hepatic cells to be close to bile canaliculi, suggesting an excretory process. Both diffuse cytoplasmic ferritin and dense membrane-bound accumulations of iron are found in gastric mucosal cells in idiopathic haemochromatosis (Zeitoun & Lamblin, 1967). The dense ferritin bodies found in the jejunal epithelium of Bantu patients with dietary siderosis appear to be lysosomes (Theron & Mekel, 1971).

Mechanisms of toxicity
Acute iron toxicity following the oral ingestion of large amounts of iron salts has catastrophic effects due partly to the direct corrosive effect of iron salts on the gut and the subsequent problems of shock and partly to the direct toxicity of large amounts of ionic iron absorbed from the intestines. Reissmann & Coleman (1955) reported marked lactic and citric acidosis prior to circulatory collapse and suggested that iron is toxic to the Krebs cycle enzymes. Other studies have shown liver cell necrosis preceded by mitochondrial swelling and the formation of intracristal granules (Witzleben, 1966; Ganote & Nahara, 1973). In chronic iron toxicity due to paren-chymal overload it is unlikely that free ionic iron is present in the body but a number of iron compounds may be found in excess. Increased transferrin-bound iron is not

itself toxic, but it is associated with an increased uptake by tissue cells (Jandl & Katz, 1963; Bailey-Wood et al, 1975)

Recent studies of cultured rat kidney cells suggest that iron uptake is maximal in the G_1 phase of the cell cycle (Fernandez-Pol et al, 1978). In states of extreme loading circulating iron may be found attached to other plasma proteins from which it is easily detached and may play an important role in tissue iron deposition and toxicity (Hershko et al, 1978). A similar phenomenon is found in congenital atransferrinaemia (Lynch et al, 1974). It has been suggested that circulating low molecular weight complexes also occur normally (Sarkar, 1970), but this has not been confirmed. Increased intracellular iron is present either as labile iron complexes, ferritin, or ferritin derivatives. It is possible that some of the insoluble amorphous deposits may not be derived from ferritin; in the case of mitochondrial loading ferritin has never been clearly identified. The labile intermediate iron pool is normally in equilibrium both with transferrin iron and ferritin iron and is likely to be increased in overload states. Although the chemical nature of this iron is not known, it appears to be a reactive low molecular weight complex (Jacobs, 1977), and an increase in this pool can be expected to interfere directly with cell metabolism.

Most accounts of iron toxicity point, directly or indirectly, to evidence of increased lipid peroxidation and consequent membrane damage (Jacobs, 1980). In iron loaded patients with thalassaemia major excess lipid peroxidation in erythrocytes is associated with reduced levels of vitamin E (Rachmilewitz et al, 1976). Peroxidation results in the destruction of sulfhydryl groups in a variety of compounds (Lewis & Wills, 1962). Mitochondrial membrane damage is associated with loss of components of the electron transport pathway and the inactivation of a number of other enzyme systems including parts of the Krebs cycle (Hunter et al, 1963; McKnight & Hunter, 1966). Mitochondrial ghosts produced by exposure to $10\,\mu M Fe_2$, show no respiratory control or coupled phosphorylation. Biochemical damage to suspensions of mitochondria is demonstrable at $1\,\mu M$ iron concentrations (McKnight et al, 1965).

Microsomal lipid peroxidation in rat liver appears to be dependent on a non-ferritin, non-haem iron component, and the process can be inhibited by iron chelators such as desferrioxamine (Wills, 1969). Increasing the inorganic iron content of the suspending medium increases the rate of lipid peroxidation up to maximum levels at $30\,\mu M$ iron. Ascorbic acid stimulates a marked increase in lipid peroxidation in liver, heart, and kidney. Ferritin is inactive in promoting the oxidation of fatty acids but it has a marked effect when ascorbic acid is present (Wills, 1966). The effect of ascorbate can be attributed to its ability to mobilize ferritin iron into a low molecular weight catalytic form and this should be noted in considering its therapeutic use in increasing the availability of iron for chelation or countering the effects of iron induced scurvy. In scorbutic subjects an intravenous injection of ascorbic acid has the invariable effect of increasing the plasma iron concentration by up to 300 per cent in a few hours (Bothwell et al, 1964), presumably through the mobilization of storage iron into the intracellular labile pool. More recently Roeser et al (1980) have demonstrated that in iron loaded guinea pigs raised serum ferritin concentration depends on adequate ascorbic acid status, implying a role for the vitamin in the mechanism of protein secretion.

Wills (1972) has shown that iron overload in rats is associated both with increased lipid peroxide formation in hepatic endoplasmic reticulum and impaired aminopyrine metabolism. This may be related to the loss of haem from cytochrome P-450 which has been demonstrated in vitro (de Matteis et al, 1977) and which does not appear to be due to the normal process of haem degradation. A number of metal ions, including iron, may play a part in reducing the activity of microsomal drug metabolising enzymes. They act partly by reduction of ALA synthetase activity and partly through increasing haem oxygenase activity (Maines & Kappas, 1977a; Ibrahim et al, 1979). The effect varies in different organs, is potentiated by SH blocking agents and neutralised by reducing agents such as cysteine (Maines & Kappas 1977b). Iron may also act directly on glutathione or enzymes depending on free SH groups.

Lysosomal abnormalities in experimental iron overload are well recognised (Arborgh et al, 1974; Goldberg & Smith, 1960; Pechet, 1969). Peters & Seymour (1976) have shown that lysosomal enzymes are increased in liver biopsy specimens from patients with both primary and secondary overload. The lysosomes appear to be abnormally fragile, having both a low latency and a low sedimentable β-glucosaminidase activity. It is tempting to consider that the degraded ferritin and amorphous iron deposits physically damage the organelle with intracellular release of its enzymes. An alternative explanation for lysosome-mediated cell damage is the gradual solubilisation of its iron deposits at a relatively low pH with the release of chemically reactive iron stimulating lipid peroxidation both of the lysosomal membrane and beyond. Jauregui et al (1975) exposed HeLa cell cultures to a high concentration (500 μg/per ml) of ferrous sulphate and found that a rapid increase in cell ferritin was associated with a marked decrease in cell multiplication after 12 hours and an increased cell death within 24 hours. This was associated with accumulation of iron in lysosomal vesicles. The experiments of Jacobs et al (1978) show that lower concentrations of iron (50 μg per ml), cause cell death in Chang cell cultures but are no longer toxic if the cells are first exposed to a non-toxic concentration (10 μg per ml) which stimulates ferritin synthesis and lysosomal iron loading, both of which appear to behave as protective mechanisms. We still have relatively little precise information about the metabolic abnormalities occurring in iron overload and our knowledge of the mechanisms of iron toxicity remains scanty.

REFERENCES

Aisen P, Leibman A 1968 Biochemical and Biophysical Research Communications 32 220: 15
Aisen P, Leibman A 1973 Biochimica et Biophysica Acta 304: 797
Aisen P, 1974 British Journal of Haematology 26 159
Aisen P 1980 In: (eds) Jacobs A and Worwood M Iron in Biochemistry and Medicine II. Academic Press, London and New York
Åkeson A, Biork G, Simon R 1968 Acta Medica Scandinavica 183: 307
Alpert E, Isselbacher K J, Drysdale J W 1973 Lancet 1: 43
Alpert E, 1975 Cancer Research 35: 1505
Andelman M B, Sered B R 1966 American Journal of Diseases of Childhood 111: 45
Arborgh B A M, Glaumann H, Ericsson J L E 1974 Laboratory Investigation 30: 664
Arnett E N, Nienhuis A W, Henry W L, Ferrans V J, Redwood D R, Roberts W C 1975 American Heart Journal 90: 777
Arosio P, Adelman T F, Drysdale J W 1978 Journal of Biological Chemistry 253: 4451
Awai M, Chipman B, Brown E B 1975a Journal of Laboratory and Clinical Medicine 85: 769
Awai M, Chipman B, Brown E B 1975b Journal of Laboratory and Clinical Medicine 85: 785
Bailey-Wood R, Blayney L M, Muir J R, Jacobs A 1975 British Journal of Experimental Pathology 56: 193
Bailey-Wood R, White G P, Jacobs A 1975 British Journal of Experimental Pathology 56: 358
Banyard S, Stammers D K, Harrison P M 1978 Nature 271: 282
Barnes R, Connelly J L, Jones O T G 1972 Biochemical Journal 128: 1043

Barry M, Flynn D M, Letsky E A, Risdon R A 1974 British Medical Journal 2: 16
Basta S S, Soekirman M S, Karyadi D, Scrimshaw N S 1979 3: 916
Batey R G, Pettit J E, Nicholas A W, Sherlock S, Hoffbrand A V 1978 75: 856
Beamish M R, Walker R, Miller F, Jacobs A, Williams R, British Journal of Haematology 27: 219
Beaumont C, Simon M, Fauchet R, Hespel J P, Brisso T P, Genetet B, Bourel M 1979 New England
    Journal of Medicine 301: 169
Bennett R M, Kokcinski T 1979 Clinical Science 57: 453
Beutler E, Fairbanks V F 1980 In: (eds) Jacobs A, Worwood M Iron in Biochemistry and Medicine II.
    Academic Press, London and New York
Beuzard Y, Rodvien R, London I M 1973 Proceedings of the National Academy of Science 70: 1022
Blayney L, Bailey-Wood R, Jacobs A, Henderson A, Muir J 1976 Circulation Research 39: 744
Bomford A, Bullock F, Williams R 1980 (in press)
Bomford A B, Munro H N 1980 In: (eds) Jacobs A and Worwood M Iron in Biochemistry and Medicine II.
    Academic Press, London and New York
Bomford A, Williams R 1976 Quarterly Journal of Medicine 45: 616
Bothwell T H, Bradlow B A, Jacobs P, Keeley K, Cramer S, Seftel H C, Zail S 1964 British Journal of
    Haematology 10: 50
Brink B, Disler P, Lynch S, Jacobs P, Charlton R, Bothwell T 1976 Journal of Laboratory and Clinical
    Medicine 88: 725
Brock J H, Arzabe F R, Richardon N E, Deverson E V 1978 Biochemical Journal 171: 73
Brown E B 1975 In (ed) Crichton R R Protein of Iron Storage and Transport in Biochemistry and Medicine.
    North Holland, Amsterdam
Broxmeyer H E, Smithyman A, Eger R R, Meyers P A, De Sousa M 1978 Journal of Experimental
    Medicine 148: 1052
Broxmeyer H E 1979 Journal of Clinical Investigation 64: 1717
Broxmeyer H E, De Souza M, Smithyman A, Ralph P, Hamilton J, Kurland J I, Bognacki J 1980 Blood
    55: 324
Broxmeyer J E, Ralph P, Bognacki J, Kincade P W, De Souza M 1980 Journal of Immunology (in press)
Bryce C F A, Crichton R R 1973 Biochemical Journal 133: 301
Buchanan W M 1971 Journal of Clinical Pathology 24: 328
Buja L M, Roberts W C 1971 American Journal of Medicine 51: 209
Bullen J J, Rogers H J, Griffiths D, 1972 British Medical Journal 1: 69
Bullen J J, Armstrong J A 1979 Immunology 36: 781
Burman D 1972 Archives of Disease in Childhood 47: 261
Cantwell R J 1972 Clinical Paediatrics 11: 443
Cartwright G E, Edwards C Q, Kravitz K, Skolnick M, Amos D B, Johnson A, Buskjaer L 1979 New
    England Journal of Medicine 301: 175
Cavill I, Ricketts C 1974 In: (eds) Jacobs A and Worwood M Iron in Biochemistry and Medicine. Academic
    Press, London and New York
Cavill I, Ricketts C, Jacobs A, Letsky E 1978 New England Journal of Medicine 298: 8 776
Chandra R K 1973 Archives of Diseases in Childhood 48: 864–866
Chandra R K, Saraya A K 1975 Journal of Paediatrics 86: 899
Cook J D, Finch C A 1975 Clinical Research 23: 402 A
Cox T M, Peters T J 1978 Lancet 1: 123
Cragg S J, Jacobs A, Parry D H, Wagstaff M, Worwood M 1977 British Journal of Cancer 35: 635
Crosby W H 1963 Blood 22: 441
Dagg J H, Cumming R L C, Goldberg A 1971 In (eds) Goldberg A and Brain M C Recent Advances in
    Haematology. Churchill-Livingstone, Edinburgh
Dallman P 1974 In (eds) Jacob A and Worwood M Iron in Biochemistry and Medicine. Academic Press,
    London and New York
Dallman P R, Siimes M A, Manies E C 1975 British Journal of Haematology 31: 209
de Alarcon P A, Donovan M A, Forbes G B, Landau S E, Stockman J A 1979 New England Journal of
    Medicine 300: 5
de Matteis F, Gibbs A H, Unseld A, 1977 Biochemical Journal 168: 417
de Matteis F, 1980 In (eds) Jacob A and Worwood M Iron in Biochemistry and Medicine II. Academic
    Press, London and New York
Drysdale J W, Singer R M 1974 Cancer Research 44: 3352
Drysdale J W, Shafritz D A1975 Biochimica et Biophysica Acta 383: 97
Drysdale J W, 1977 In (ed) Fitzsimmons D W Iron metabolism, North Holland. Amsterdam.
Edwards C Q, Carroll M, Bray P, Cartwright G E 1977 New England Journal of Medicine 297: 7
Egyed A, May A, Jacobs A 1980 Biochemica et Biophysica Acta 629: 391
Fernandez-Pol J A, Klos D, Donati R N 1978 Cell Biology International Reports 2: 433

Fielding J, Speyer B V 1974 Biochimica et Biophysica Acta 363: 387
Finch C A, Miller L R, Inamdar A R, Person R, Seiler K, Mackler B 1976 Journal of Clinical Investigation 58: 447
Fischbach F A, Gregory D W, Harrison P M et al 1971 Journal of Ultra structural research 37: 495
Fletcher J, Huehns E R 1967 Nature 215: 584 W23
Ganote C E, Nahara G 1973 Laboratory Investigation 28: 426
Glaumann N H, Jansson H, Arborgh B et al 1975 Journal of Cell Biology 67: 887
Goldberg L, Smith J P 1960 American Journal of Pathology 36: 125
Gorinsky B, Horsburgh C, Lindley P R, Moss D S, Parker M, Watson J L 1979 Nature 5727: 157
Grady R W, Graziano J H, Akers H A, Cerami A 1976 Journal of Pharmacology and Experimental Therapeutics 196: 478–485
Hall D O, Cammack R, Rao K 1974 In (eds) Jacobs A and Worwood M Iron in Biochemistry and Medicine. Academic Press, London and New York
Halliday J W, Russo A M, Cowlishaw J L, Powell L W 1977 Lancet 2: 621
Harris D C, Aisen P, 1975a Nature 257: 821
Harris D C, Aisen P 1975b Biochemistry 14: 262
Harrison P M, Hoare R F, Hoy T G, Macara I G 1974 In (eds) Jacobs A and Worwood M Iron in Biochemistry and Medicine. Academic Press, London and New York
Harrison P M, Clegg G A, May K 1980 In: (eds) Jacobs A and Worwood M Iron in Biochemistry and Medicine II. Academic Press, London and New York
Hershko C, Karsai A, Eylon L, Isak G, 1970 Blood 36: 321
Hershko C, Graham G, Bates G W, Rachmilewitz E A, 1978 British Journal of Haematology 40: 255–263
Hjelm M, Wadman B, 1974 Clinics in Haematology 3: 689
Hoare R J, Harrison P M, Hoy T G 1975 Nature 255: 653
Hoensch H, Woo C H, Raffin S B, Schmid R 1976 Gastroenterology 70: 1063
Hoffbrand A V, Broitman S A 1969 Proceedings of the Society for Experimental Biology and Medicine 130: 595
Hoffbrand A V, Ganeshaguru K, Hooton J W L, Tattersall M H N 1976 British Journal of Haematology 33: 517
Hoffbrand A V 1980 In (eds) Jacobs A and Worwood M Iron in Biochemistry and Medicine II. Academic Press, London and New York
Howard J, Jacobs A 1972 British Journal of Haematology 23: 595
Hoy R, Humphrys J, Jacobs A, Williams A 1979 British Journal of Haematology 43: 443
Hoy T G, Jacobs A 1981 Biochemical Journal 193: 87
Hu H-Y Y, Gardner J, Aisen P, 1977 Science 197: 559
Hunt J, Richards R J, Harwood R, Jacobs A 1979 British Journal of Haematology 41: 69–76
Hunter F E, Gebicki J M, Hoffstein P E, Weinstein J, Scott A 1963 Journal of Biological Chemistry 238: 828
Hussain M A M, Flynn D M, Green N, Hoffbrand A V 1977 Lancet 1: 977
Iancu T C, Neustein H B 1977 British Journal of Haematology 37: 527
Ibrahim N G, Hoffstein S T, Friedman M L, 1979 Biochemical Journal 180: 257
Jacobs A, Miller F, Worwood M, Beamish M R, Wardrop C A 1972 British Medical Journal IV: 206
Jacobs A 1977a Seminars in Haematology 14: 89
Jacobs A 1977b In: (ed) Fitzsimmons D W Iron Metabolism Ciba Foundation Symposium No 51
Jacobs A, White G P, Tait G H 1977 Biochemical and Biophysical Research Communications 74: 1626
Jacobs A, Hoy T, Humphrys J, Perera P 1978 British Journal of Experimental Pathology 59: 489
Jacobs A 1979 British Journal of Haematology 43: 1
Jacobs A 1980 In: (eds) Jacobs A and Worwood M Iron in Biochemistry and Medicine II. Academic Press, London and New York
Jacobs A, Worwood M 1980 Iron in Biochemistry and Medicine II. Academic Press, London and New York
Jandl J H, Inman J K, Simmons R L, Allen D W 1959 Journal of Clinical Investigation 38: 161
Jarvis J H, Jacobs A 1974 Journal of Clinical Pathology 27: 973–979
Jauregui II O, Bradford W D, Arstila A U, Kinney T D, Trump B P 1975 American Journal of Pathology 80: 33
Jones B M, Worwood M, Jacobs A 1980 Clinica Chimica Acta 106: 203
Jones T, Spencer R, Walsh C 1978 Biochemistry 17: 4011–4017
Joynson D H M, Jacobs A, Murray-Walker D, Dolby A E 1972 Lancet 2: 1058–1059
Kailis S G, Morgan E H 1974 British Journal of Haematology 28: 37
Kapadia A, De Souza M, Markenson A L, Miller D R, Good R A, Gupta S 1980 British Journal of Haematology 45: 405
Konijn A M, Hershko C 1977 British Journal of Haematology 37: 7

Lane R S 1966 British Journal of Haematology 12: 249
Lee J C K, Lee S S C, Schlesinger K J, Richter G W (1975) American Journal of Pathology 80: 235
Lee S S C, Richter G W 1976 Biochemistry 15: 65
Leibman A, Aisen P 1977 Biochemistry 16: 1268
Lemberg R, Barratt J 1973 Cytochromes London, Academic Press
Lewis S E, Wills E D 1962 Biochemical Pharmacology 11: 901
Loh T T, Yeung Y G, Yeung D 1977 Biochimica et Biophysica Acta 471: 118
Lynch S R, Lipschitz D A, Bothwell T H, Charlton R W 1974 In: (eds) Jacobs A and Worwood M Iron in
    Biochemistry and Medicine. Academic Press, London and New York
Macdonald R A, MacSween R N M, Pechet G S 1969 Laboratory Investigation 21: 236–245
Macdougal L G, Anderson R, McNab G M, Katz J 1975 Journal of Paediatrics 86: 833–843
MacGillivray R T A, Brew K 1975 Science 190: 1306
MacGillivray R T A, Mendez E, Brew K 1977 In: (eds) Brown E B, Aisen P, Fielding J, and Crichtoh R R
    Proteins of Iron Metabolism. Grune and Stratton
Maines M D, Kappas A 1977a Clinical Pharmacology and Therapeutics 22: 780
Maines M D, Kappas A 1977b Science 198: 1215
Malmquist J, Hansen N E, Carle H 1978 Scandinavian Journal of Haematology 21: 5
Marcus D L, Ibrahim N G, Gruenspecht N, Freedman M L 1980 Biochimica et Biophysica Acta 607: 136
Marcus D M, Zinberg N 1974 Archives of Biochemistry and Biophysics 162: 493
Mason D Y, Taylor C R 1978 Journal of Clinical Pathology 31: 316
Masson P 1970 La Lactoferrine Editions Arscia, Brussels
Massover W H, Cowley J M, 1975 In: (ed) Crichton R R Proteins of Iron Stores and Transport in
    Biochemistry and Medicine. North Holland, Amsterdam
Massover W H 1978 Journal of Molecular Biology 123: 721
Mathews M B, Hunt T, Brayley A 1973 Proceedings of the National Academy of Science 70: 1022
Matzner Y, Hershko C, Polliack A, Konijn A M, Izak G 1979 British Journal of Haematology 42: 345
May A, De Souza P, Jacobs A 1980 British Journal of Haematology 46: 329
McKnight R C, Hunter F E, Oehlert W H 1965 Journal of Biological Chemistry 240: 3439
McKnight R C, Hunter F E 1966 Journal of Biological Chemistry 241: 2757
Moore K E, Dominic J A 1971 Federation Proceedings 30: 859–870
Morgan E H, Appleton T C 1969 Nature 223: 1371
Morgan E H 1974 In: (eds) Jacobs A and Worwood M Iron in Biochemistry and Medicine. Academic Press,
    London and New York
Morton A G, Tavill A S 1977 British Journal of Haematology 36: 383
Neilands J B, 1980 In: (eds) Jacobs A and Worwood M Iron in Biochemistry and Medicine II. Academic
    Press, London and New York
Nicholls P, Elliott W B 1974 In: (eds) Jacobs A and Worwood M Iron in Biochemistry and Medicine.
    Academic Press, London and New York
Nishiya K, De Souza M, Tsoi E, Bognacki J J, de Harven E 1980a Cellular Immunology 53: 71
Nishiya K, Chiao J W, De Souza M 1980b British Journal of Haematology 46: 235
Nunez M T, Glass J, Fischer S, Lavidor L M, Lenk E M, Robinson S H 1977 British Journal of
    Haematology 36: 519–526
Ohira Y, Edgerton V R, Gardner G W, Senewiratne B, Barnard R J, Simpson T R 1979 British Journal of
    Haematology 41: 365
Olsson K S, Heedman P A, Staugard F 1978 Journal of the American Medical Association 239: 1999
O'Shea M J, Kershenobich D, Tavill A S 1973 British Journal of Haematology 25: 707–714
Oski F A, Honig A S 1978 Journal of Paediatrics 92: 21
Pechet G S 1969 Laboratory Investigation 20: 119
Peschle C, Jori G P, Marone G, Condorelli M 1974 Blood 44: 353
Phillips J L, Azari P 1975 Cellular Immunology 15: 94–99
Pippard M J, Letsky E A, Callender S T, Weatherall D J 1978 Lancet 1 1178
Pollitt E, Leibel R L 1976 Journal of Paediatrics 88: 372
Pollitt E, Greenfield D, Leibel R 1979 Infant behaviour and development 2: 235
Pollycove M, Fawwaz R A, Winchell H S 1971 Journal of Nuclear Medicine 12: 28–30
Ponka P, Neuwrit J, Borova J, Fuchs O 1977 In: (ed) Fitzsimmons D W Iron Metabolism. North Holland,
    Amsterdam
Pootrakul P, Christensen A, Josephson B, Finch C A 1977 Blood 49: 957
Powell L W, Alpert E, Isselbacher K J et al 1974 Nature 250: 333
Powell L W, Alpert E, Isselbacher K J, Drysdale J W 1975 British Journal of Haematology 30: 47
Powell L W, Halliday J W 1980 In: (eds) Jacobs A and Worwood M Iron in Biochemistry and Medicine II.
    Academic Press, London and New York
Princiotto J V, Zapolski E J 1975 Nature 255: 87

Prockop D J 1971 Federation Proceedings 30: 984–990
Propper R D, Shurin S B, Nathan D G 1976 New England Journal of Medicine 294: 1421
Propper R D, Button L N, Nathan D G 1980 Blood 55: 55
Rabinowitz M, Waxman H S 1965 Nature 206: 897–900
Rachmilewitz E A, Lubin B H, Shohet S B 1976 Blood 47: 495
Reissmann K R, Coleman T J 1955 Blood 10: 46
Richter G W, Bessis M C 1965 Blood 25: 370
Richter G W 1978 American Journal of Pathology 91: 363
Risdon R A, Barry M, Flynn D M 1975 Journal of Pathology 116: 83
Robbins E, Pederson T 1970 Proceedings in the National Academy of Sciences 66: 1244
Roeser H P, Halliday J W, Sizemore P J, Nikles A, Willgoss D, 1980 British Journal of Haematology (in press)
Romslo I 1980 In: (eds) Jacobs A and Worwood M Iron in Biochemistry and Medicine II. Academic Press, London and New York
Ross C E, Muir W A, Ng A B P, Graham R C, Kellermeyer R W 1975 American Journal of Clinical Pathology 63: 179
Sanyal S K, Johnson W, Jayalakshmamna B, Green A A 1975 Paediatrics 55: 336
Sarcione E J, Smalley J R, Lema M J, Stutzman L 1977 International Journal of Cancer 20: 339
Sarkar B 1970 Canadian Journal of Biochemistry 48: 1339
Scheinberg H 1973 Archives of Internal Medicine 132: 126
Siimes M A, Refino C, Dallman P R 1980 American Journal of Clinical Nutrition 33: 570
Simon M, Bourel M, Fauchet R, Genetet B 1976 Gut: 17: 332
Simon M, Bourel M, Genetet B, Fauchet R 1977 New England Journal of Medicine 297: 1017
Sirivech S, Frieden E, Osaki S 1974 Biochemical Journal 143: 311
Sly D A, Grohlic D, Bezkorovainy A 1975 Biochimica et Biophysica Acta 385: 36
Soltys H D, Brody J I 1970 Journal of Laboratory and Clinical Medicine 75: 250
Spik G, Mazurier J 1977 In: (eds) Brown E B, Aisen P, Fielding J, Crichton R R Proteins of Iron Metabolism Grune and Stratton.
Sullivan A L, Grasso J A, Weintraub L R 1976 Blood 47: 133
Sullivan A L, Weintraub L R 1978 Blood 52: 436
Summers M, White G, Jacobs A 1975 British Journal of Haematology 30: 425
Summers M R, Jacobs A 1976 British Journal of Haematology 34: 221
Sussman M 1974 In: (eds) Jacobs A, Worwood M Iron in Biochemistry and Medicine. Academic Press, London and New York
Tavill A S, Kershenobich D 1972 In: Protides of the Biological Fluids. Pergamon Press, Oxford
Theron J J, Mekel R C P M 1971 British Journal of Haematology 21: 165
Trump B F, Valigorski J M, Arstila A U, Mergner W J, Kinney T D 1973 American Journal of Pathology 72: 295
US Committee on Nutrition 1978 Pediatrics 62: 246
Valberg L S, Simon B, Manley I P N, Corbett W E, Ludwig J 1975 Journal of Laboratory and Clinical Medicine 86: 479
Van Bockxmeer R, Morgan E H 1979 Biochimica et Biophysica Acta 584: 76
Van Snick J L, Masson P L, Heremans J F (1975) Journal of Experimental Medicine 140: 1068
Van Snick J L, Markowitz B, Masson P L 1977 Journal of Experimental Medicine 146: 817
Viteri F E, Torun B 1974 Clinics in Haematology 3: 609
Wagstaff M, Worwood M, Jacobs A 1978 Biochemical Journal 173: 969
Walters G O, Miller F M, Worwood M 1973 Journal of Clinical Pathology 26: 770
Walters G O, Jacobs A, Worwood M, Trevett D, Thompson W, 1975 Gut 16: 188
Wands J R, Rowe J A, Mezey S E, Waterberry L A, Wright J R, Halliday J W, Isselbacher K J, Powell L W 1976 New England Journal of Medicine 294: 302
Weinberg E D 1974 Science 184: 952
Wenn R V, Williams J 1968 Biochemical Journal 108: 69
White G P, Worwood M, Parry D H, Jacobs A 1974 Nature 250: 584
White G P, Bailey-Wood R, Jacobs A 1976 Clinical Science and Molecular Medicine 50: 145
White G P, Jacobs A, Grady R W, Cerami A 1976 British Journal of Haematology 33: 487–496
Williams J 1980 Personal Communications
Williams J, Moreton K 1980 Biochemical Journal 185: 483
Williams M A, Harrison P M 1968 Biochemical Journal 110: 265
Wills E D 1966 Biochemical Journal 99: 667
Wills E D 1969 Biochemical Journal 113: 325
Wills E D 1972 Biochemical Pharmacology 21: 239
Winston A, Kirchner D 1976 Polymer Preprints 17: 294–299

Witzleben C L 1966 American Journal of Pathology 49: 1053
Worwood M, Cragg S J, Wagstaff M, Jacobs A 1979 Clinical Science 56: 83
Worwood M 1980 In: (eds) Jacobs A and Worwood M Iron in Biochemistry and Medicine II. Academic Press, London and New York
Worwood M, Cragg S J, Jacobs A, McLaren C, Ricketts C, Economidou J 1980 British Journal of Haematology (in press)
Wrigglesworth J M, Baum H 1980 In: (eds) Jacobs A, Worwood M Iron Biochemistry and Medicine II. Academic Press, London and New York
Youdim M B H, Woods H F, Mitchell B, Grahame-Smith D G, Callender S 1975 Clinical Science and Molecular Medicine 48: 289
Youdim M B H, Green A R 1977 In: (ed) Fitzsimmons D Iron Metabolism. North Holland, Amsterdam
Zeitoun P, Lambing A 1967 Zeitoun P, Lambing A 1967 Scandinavian Journal of Gastroenterology 2: 222

2. Megaloblastic anaemia

A V Hoffbrand   R G Wickremasinghe

The last major review of the megaloblastic anaemias in this series was in 1971. Since then, Chanarin (1979) and an issue of Clinics in Haematology (Hoffbrand, 1976) have reviewed all aspects of the subject and monographs on pernicious anaemia (Kass, 1976), vitamin B_{12} (Babior, 1975; Zagalak & Friedrich, 1979) and on folic acid (Botez & Reynolds, 1979) have appeared as well as extensive reviews of various aspects of the field (Allen, 1975; Hoffbrand, 1975; Herbert, 1980; Chanarin, 1980). Although the main principles of investigation and therapy in megaloblastic anaemia have not changed substantially over the last decade, there have been major advances in the understanding of the metabolism, transport and interrelations of vitamin B_{12} and folate and of the mechanism by which their deficiency or altered metabolism impairs DNA synthesis. Recent observations suggest that, like the anaemia, vitamin B_{12} neuropathy may be due to a primary disturbance of the homocysteine-methionine reaction. The present review deals with these major advances in biochemical knowledge in the megaloblastic anaemias as well as covering some other selected topics in this field where it appears to the authors substantial new knowledge has accumulated.

BIOCHEMICAL BASIS OF MEGALOBLASTIC ANAEMIA

The concept that megaloblastic anaemia is due to unbalanced nucleic acid synthesis with impaired DNA replication but normal RNA synthesis originated over 30 years ago. This has been supported in many subsequent studies and advances in knowledge of how normal mammalian DNA is replicated have been accompanied by a more detailed understanding of the nature of the DNA defect in megaloblastic anaemia.

Normal human DNA replication

Human chromosomes replicate in a semi-conservative fashion, i.e. each new daughter chromosome is synthesised using one parent chromosome as a template. The bases in the parent chromosome, the purines adenine (A) and guanine (G) and the pyrimidines, thymine (T) and cytosine (C) are used to form 'base pairs' with appropriate bases in the new daughter DNA strand (A-T, G-C, T-A and C-G respectively). The backbone of each DNA strand is made up of alternating sugar (deoxyribose) and phosphate groups and the bases form links or rungs between two strands in the double helix. The phosphate groups link up carbons 3' and 5' of adjacent sugar moieties. A new strand of DNA is synthesised mainly by an enzyme α-DNA polymerase which uses as substrates four deoxyribonucleoside triphosphates (dNTP), dATP, dGTP, dTTP and dCTP (Fig. 2.1). The base, one phosphate group and the sugar moiety are incorporated into DNA and two of the three phosphate groups are lost from each nucleotide.

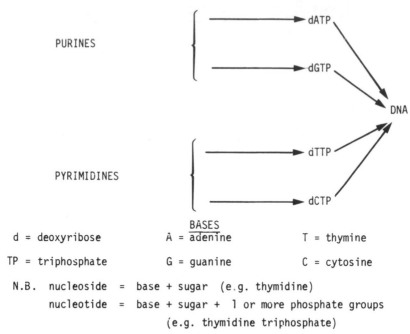

Fig. 2.1   The four deoxyribonucleoside triphosphates (dNTP) precursors of DNA.

Replication of the full length of the DNA molecule that comprises the circular chromosome of bacteria commences at an unique point, the replication origin. At this point separation of the two parental DNA strands occurs, with the formation of two replication forks. The forks move in opposite directions, away from the origin, with sequential insertion of new DNA bases in the two growing strands of each fork. In bacteria e.g. E. coli, replication proceeds in this manner with the insertion of 16 000 new bases per minute, at a speed of 5μm/minute. During mammalian DNA replication, however, the replication fork moves more slowly, at 0.8μm/minute in early S to 2.8μm/minute in late S (Weissbach, 1979). It would take approximately 30 days for a single replication fork to move from one end of the human chromosome to the other, whereas the 'S' phase of the cell cycle during which all the new DNA is synthesised lasts about eight hours. In order to achieve this speed DNA replication begins at multiple 'origins' along the chromosome. These are points at which the two parent strands separate; new DNA is then synthesised out from each origin on both parent strands and in both directions (Fig. 2.2). The distance between two adjacent origins is called a 'replicon' and the new daughter chromosomes are formed by fusion of the short pieces of new DNA (50 000 to 300 000 base pairs) synthesised in each replicon. A second enzyme, a DNA ligase joins up adjacent newly synthesised DNA strands. It is estimated that a total of 10 000 replicons are growing simultaneously in mammalian chromosome replication in a single cell. Not all the replicons originate new DNA synthesis simultaneously, however, but the exact explanation why some replicate earlier than others is unknown. Chromosome connections with the nuclear membrane are not now thought to be important but an intranuclear protein skeleton appears to incorporate the sites of DNA replication (Pardoll et al, 1980).

DNA IS SYNTHESIZED IN REPLICATING UNITS (REPLICONS)

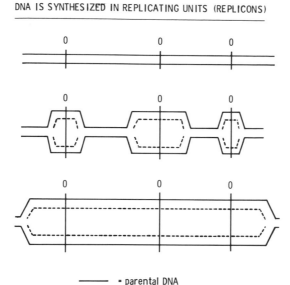

——— = parental DNA

- - - - - = newly synthesized DNA

O = origin

Fig. 2.2 Human DNA is synthesised in replicons.

Because of the characteristics of the α-DNA polymerase, the main replicative enzyme, there are two additional requirements for new DNA synthesis to proceed. First, the enzyme cannot initiate new DNA synthesis without the presence of a 'primer' with a free 3'OH end on the sugar on which the enzyme can commence DNA synthesis (Fig. 2.3). An RNA primer, approximately 10 bases long is first synthesised, new DNA is synthesised from this and the RNA primer is subsequently excised and the gap then filled with DNA. It is uncertain whether or not a separate DNA polymerase is involved in this gap-filling process. Second, the α-DNA polymerase can only synthesise in one direction along the DNA strand, in the 5' to 3' direction according to the sugar (deoxyribose)-phosphate linkages. Since the two parent DNA strands are orientated in opposite directions, the two new strands are also synthesised in opposite directions. Moreover, synthesis on each new strand is bidirectional from the replication origins. Thus, half the new DNA on both strands must ultimately be synthesised in the 3' to 5' direction. In order to do this, small (Okazaki) pieces, approximately 200 bases long are synthesised discontinuously back (in the 5' to 3' direction) from the replication fork, each with its own RNA primer. These small pieces are joined together (after excision of the RNA primer and gap filling) by a second enzyme, DNA ligase which is also probably the one responsible for linking up adjacent replicon sized pieces of DNA. Whether or not Okazaki piece formation also occurs in that half of new DNA being synthesised in the 5' to 3' direction or this synthesis is continuous is not yet established for human DNA replication.

Lesion in megaloblastic anaemia
In a series of experiments, defects in all these aspects of DNA replication have been

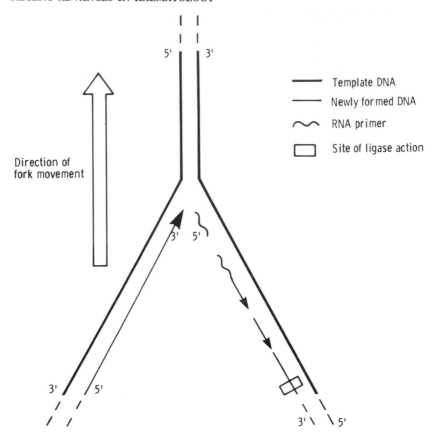

Fig. 2.3   The replication fork of human DNA synthesis. 5′,3′ refers to the carbon atoms on the deoxyribose moieties to which intervening phosphate groups are linked.

shown in the cells of patients with untreated megaloblastic anaemia. Using a caesium-chloride gradient separation technique with bromodeoxyuridine density labelling, Wickremasinghe & Hoffbrand (1980a) found that the average rate of replication fork movement is approximately 50 per cent slower in lymphocytes from patients with untreated megaloblastic anaemia compared to control cells. Joining of Okazaki pieces was measured by following formation of double stranded DNA from partially single stranded DNA in replicating lymphocytes, using a chromatographic technique on BND cellulose. Untreated megaloblastic cells were found to convert new DNA to fully double stranded DNA at a slower rate than control vitamin-replete cells (Wickremasinghe & Hoffbrand, 1980b). An earlier study using an alkaline-sucrose gradient technique had shown that the growth of the new DNA to large, chromosomal sized pieces was also slower in megaloblastic compared to control cells (Wickremasinghe & Hoffbrand, 1979). The DNA that is formed, however, is of normal base composition.

All these defects of DNA replication in megaloblastic anaemia can be reproduced by exposure of lymphocytes to antimetabolite drugs such as methotrexate which inhibits dihydrofolate reductase and thus thymidylate synthesis and so deprives the cells of one of the four immediate DNA precursors, dTTP, or to hydroxyurea which inhibits ribonucleotide reductase and decreases dATP and dGTP supply for DNA synthesis (Wickremasinghe & Hoffbrand, 1979, 1980a and b). Moreover, these drugs are known to cause megaloblastic changes in the bone marrow when administered in vivo. It therefore seems probable that vitamin B_{12} or folate deficiency also cause the DNA replication defects by reducing supply of a precursor. The α-DNA polymerase itself is present in normal or even increased amounts in megaloblastic cells, since Hooton & Hoffbrand (1977) showed that nuclei isolated from megaloblastic cells incorporated more dNTP into new DNA once these were provided in excess amounts than did control nuclei. The greater incorporation than normal suggests that megaloblasts have more replicating units opened but not completed than normal cells and that the α-DNA polymerase itself is present in normal or increased concentration.

Why the megaloblast is large and how the characteristic chromatin pattern develops is not completely clear. Slowing of DNA synthesis in a temperature sensitive mutant mouse cell line causes changes in the morphological and chromosome appearances closely resembling those of megaloblasts (Dardick et al, 1978). The cell and nuclear volume increase with dispersal of condensed chromatin and dissociation of nuclear and cytoplasmic maturation.

The longer 'S' phase in megaloblastic cells probably allows greater RNA and protein synthesis to occur. The unwinding and particularly the rewinding of the DNA double helix may be impaired and asynchronous due to the slower rate of DNA synthesis. Moreover, in some cells the slower rate of synthesis may lead to chromosome breakages due to mechanical or enzyme forces at single-stranded regions which remain for longer periods than normal. Many of the bone marrow cells may never completely join up their newly synthesised DNA pieces and these cells will die without completing the 'S' phase, accounting for ineffective haemopoiesis.

Evidence for impaired thymidylate synthesis: the deoxyuridine suppression test
In view of the solid evidence that megaloblastosis arises through lack of one or other of the dNTP DNA precursors, the abnormal deoxyuridine (dU) suppression test in megaloblasts (see below) and the known role of folate as its 5, 10 methylene-tetrahydrofolate coenzyme in thymidylate synthesis, it was a surprising finding that the concentration of dTTP in megaloblastic cells is raised (Hoffbrand et al, 1974). It is known that the concentrations of the four dNTPs rise substantially in proliferating compared to resting cells (Tattersall et al, 1975). All four dNTPs were indeed found to be raised (between two or three times on average) in megaloblastic compared to normoblastic marrow cells (Hoffbrand et al, 1974). All four dNTP concentrations including that of dTTP were, however, comparable between megaloblastic marrow cells and primitive marrow cells from patients with untreated acute myeloblastic leukaemia. The concentration of dTTP was also not selectively in PHA-stimulated megaloblastic lymphocytes compared with control cells.

Despite the normal low or raised dTTP concentration in megaloblastic cells, however, newer evidence does confirm that megaloblastic anaemia due to folate or vitamin B_{12} deficiency arises because of impaired synthesis of thymidylate (dTMP) and thus of dTTP (Fig. 2.4). The evidence for reduced synthesis of dTMP in megaloblastic cells and the explanation why the overall cell dTTP concentration is unexpectedly normal or raised is therefore considered next.

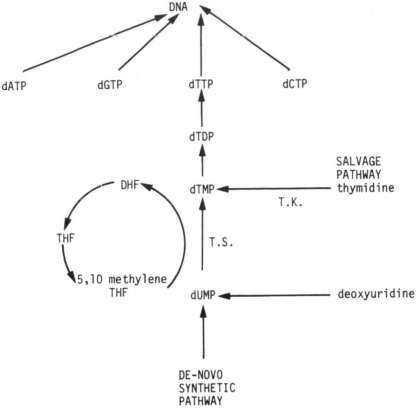

Fig. 2.4   The 'de novo' and 'salvage' pathways of synthesis of thymine nucleotides.

MP = mono- ⎫	TS = thymidylate synthetase
DP = di- ⎬ phosphate	TK = thymidine kinase
TP = tri- ⎭	DHF = dihydrofolate
	THF = tetrahydrofolate

The evidence for impaired thymidylate (dTMP) synthesis is largely based on the deoxyuridine (dU) suppression test which shows a clear difference between normoblastic and megaloblastic cells. Deoxyuridine has been found to inhibit uptake of radioactive thymidine into DNA in normoblasts to a greater extent than it inhibits this uptake in megaloblasts. In the concentrations usually used, thymidine incorporation into DNA of normal cells is reduced by dU to less than 10 per cent of the value without additional dU, but its incorporation is reduced by dU to a lesser extent (to between 10 and 40 per cent) in megaloblastic cells. The suggested explanation for this difference is the block in the de novo synthetic pathway of synthesis of thymidine monophosphate (dTMP) from deoxyuridine monophosphate (dUMP) in megaloblasts (Fig. 2.4). It is thought that in megaloblasts, dU is unable to cause a substantial build up of thymine nucleotides, particularly of dTTP which will feed-back inhibit thymidine kinase, the enzyme responsible for 'salvage' of labelled thymidine into the cell. The concentration of thymidine kinase itself is increased in megaloblasts compared to normoblasts (Hooton & Hoffbrand, 1976; Ellims et al, 1979). The action of dU in inhibiting ^{3}H-thymidine uptake is obviously complicated since Ganeshaguru

& Hoffbrand (1978) did not find a consistent difference in dTTP accumulation between normoblastic and megaloblastic cells with added dU, while Pelliniemi & Beck (1980) found that dU inhibits uptake of ^{3}H-thymidine into normal cells when thymidylate synthetase is totally inhibited by 5-fluorouracil, implying a direct inhibitory action of dU or its phosphorylated derivatives on thymidine kinase.

Although Wickramasinghe & Saunders (1980) could not detect an absolute difference in the incorporation of labelled dU itself into the DNA of normoblastic or megaloblastic marrow cells, Taheri et al (1981a) more recently have shown that labelled dU accumulates as dUMP in megaloblastic cells while in the same cells treated with folinic acid the label is rapidly incorporated into DNA thus directly confirming a block in thymidylate synthesis in megaloblasts. Labelled dU incorporation into DNA was found to be as sensitive as the dU suppression test for detecting the supposed block in thymidylate synthesis in megaloblasts and analysing which folate or B_{12} compound corrected this in individual cases. Van der Weyden (1979) rather surprisingly found no decrease in dU incorporation into DNA in megaloblastic marrows compared to similar cells with appropriate vitamins added. The different concentrations of dU added may partially explain the difference in their results.

Compartmentalisation and degradation of thymine nucleotides
In order to explain the normal dTTP concentration in megaloblastic cells despite the overwhelming evidence summarised above for impaired thymidylate synthesis in B_{12} or folate deficient megaloblastic cells, Taheri et al (1981b) have suggested that the thymine nucleotides (dTMP, dTDP and dTTP) are functionally compartmentalised in human cells, only a small proportion of the overall total cell thymine nucleotides being present in small but high concentration pools at the DNA replication fork, the major fractions being present at lower concentrations in larger pools not available for DNA synthesis and probably used for DNA repair or destined for degradation (Fig. 2.5). Such compartmentalisation of DNA precursor nucleotide pools has been shown by deoxyribonucleotide pool kinetics in T_4-phage infected bacteria (Reddy &

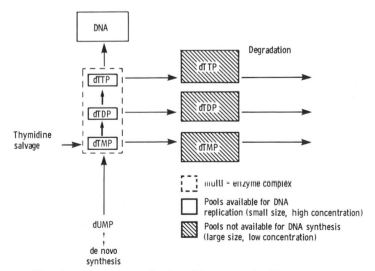

Fig. 2.5   Proposed functional compartmentalisation of thymine nucleotides.

Mathews, 1978; Mathews et al, 1978) and in Chinese hamster cells (Reddy & Pardee, 1980). The precise nature of the compartmentation, whether physical or only functional is not certain. Taheri et al (1981b) postulate that the degradative pool (which accounts for the bulk of the overall cell dTTP pool) remains normal in megaloblastic cells because reduced input is balanced by reduced degradation. There is, however, they suggest, reduced supply of dTTP at the replication fork. Thymidylate synthetase has been shown to be part of the multi-enzyme complex which forms at the replication fork during the 'S' phase (Reddy & Pardee, 1980). This complex normally ensures that high concentrations of the dNTP are available for new DNA synthesis throughout the 'S' phase of the cell.

ROLE OF VITAMIN B_{12} IN DNA SYNTHESIS

Most workers now agree that B_{12} is concerned in provision of the correct folate coenzyme for thymidylate synthetase but the exact mechanism for this remains controversial. The apoenzyme itself is present in normal or increased amounts (Sakamoto et al, 1975). The most widely accepted view is that B_{12} through its involvement in conversion of homocysteine to methionine is required in the metabolism of 5-methyltetrahydrofolate (methyl THF) a monoglutamate form of folate to tetrahydrofolate (THF) and so to all other folate compounds including the polyglutamate forms, the intracellular coenzyme folate compounds. In B_{12} deficiency, it is supposed that cells become depleted of THF, a substrate, in contrast to methyl THF, for folate polyglutamate synthesis and so for folate coenzyme formation (see reviews Hoffbrand, 1975; Das & Herbert, 1976).

Methyl THF is the form of folate to which dietary folates are first converted by the small intestine (Chanarin & Perry, 1969), and which circulates in plasma, cerebrospinal and other body fluids and which enters all body cells. Methyl THF accumulates in plasma but not in cells in B_{12} deficiency probably because, as a monoglutamate form of folate, it readily diffuses from cells unless it is converted to the larger polyglutamate forms (Fig. 2.6). B_{12} deficient cells all show a lower folate content than corresponding normal cells and this is due to reduced folate polyglutamate formation.

Observations that methyl THF may be metabolised by reactions other than the homocysteine-methionine pathway (including possibly for amine synthesis in the brain, Pearson & Turner, 1975) do not necessarily detract from the methylfolate 'trap' hypothesis (Das & Herbert, 1976) since the Km values for other reactions at neutral pH do not suggest a substantial escape route (more than 1 per cent) for methyl THF. Reduced formation of S-adenosyl methionine (SAM), a compound which inhibits reduction of 5,10 methylene THF to methyl THF is thought to aggravate the 'pile up' of folates in the methyl THF form in B_{12} deficiency (Shane et al, 1977) (Fig. 2.6) (see p. 34).

Studies of polyglutamate synthesis in B_{12} deficient human lymphocytes (Lavoie et al, 1974) and in nitrous oxide treated rats (McGing et al, 1978; Lumb et al, 1980) confirm that B_{12} deficiency or inactivation does not interfere with folate polyglutamate synthesis from all folate substrates since polyglutamate synthesis from both folic acid and 5-formyl THF is unimpaired in B_{12} deficiency or with B_{12} inactivation. Studies with the dU suppression test have also shown that forms of folate other than

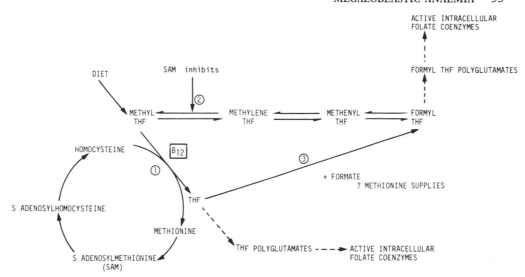

Fig. 2.6   Possible roles of vitamin $B_{12}(B_{12})$ in folate coenzyme synthesis.
(1)   reduced supply of THF from methyl-THF; THF is a substrate for folate polyglutamate synthesis.
(2)   diminished cell concentration of SAM allows greater accumulation of folate as methyl-THF
(3)   provision of formate group (via methionine) to form the correct substrate (formyl THF) for synthesis of
      folate polyglutamate derivatives. Lack of formate may also indirectly cause a shortage of the 1-carbon
      units needed for thymidylate synthesis.

methyl THF e.g. folic acid or formyl THF (folinic acid) correct the test in B_{12} deficiency, folinic acid being both an excellent substrate for polyglutamate formation (Hoffbrand et al, 1976) and an excellent compound for correcting the dU test in both folate and B_{12} deficiency (Zittoun et al, 1978; Gangeshaguru & Hoffbrand, 1978; Deacon et al, 1980a and b).

On the other hand, Perry et al (1979) have shown that in nitrous oxide (N_2O) treated rats, not only methyl THF but also THF cannot be converted to polyglutamate forms, whereas 5-formyl-, 10-formyl- and 5,10 methylene-THF are converted to polyglutamate forms normally in the presence of nitrous oxide and thus of B_{12} inactivation. Deacon et al (1980a) also found that formyl folates corrected the dU suppression test in nitrous oxide treated rats more effectively than did THF and these workers have found a similar spectrum of folate compounds which correct the test in B_{12} deficient human cells (Deacon et al, 1980b). The failure of THF to correct the test as well as formyl THF in human B_{12} deficiency and in rats with N_2O inactivation of B_{12} and the failure of THF to act as a substrate for folate polyglutamate synthesis after N_2O exposure in rats are not consistent with the methyl-folate trap concept. These observations have therefore led Chanarin et al (1980) to suggest that formyl THF and not THF is the correct substrate for folate polyglutamate synthesis and that B_{12} is concerned with the provision of the formyl rather than THF component of formyl THF. Failure of formylation of THF it is supposed, may be due to shortage of intracellular methionine. Recent in vitro studies, however, suggest THF is a satisfactory substrate for folate polyglutamate synthesis in mammalian cells (Moran & Colman, 1980).

Earlier observations on the effect of methionine on folate coenzyme formation in B_{12} deficiency are conflicting. Waxman et al (1969) found that methionine aggravated and homocysteine alleviated the defect in dU suppression in B_{12} deficiency. On the other hand, methionine reduces high excretion of forminoglutamic acid (FIGLU), aminoimadazole carboxamide and formate in B_{12} deficient rats, increasing the proportion of formylated to methylated folates and the proportion of polyglutamate folates (Shin et al, 1975). Krebs et al (1976) noted an accelerating effect of methionine on the conversion of formate to CO_2. SAM (S-adenosyl methionine) inhibits reduction of the 5,10 methylene THF to 5-methyl THF (Shane et al, 1977). Krebs et al proposed that a reduction of cell methionine concentration (as caused by B_{12} deficiency) lowers cell SAM concentration and this decreases the reduction of formyl THF to CO_2 and THF by increasing cell methyl THF and lowering cell 5,10-methylene THF concentration (Fig. 2.6). Methionine increases the cell concentrations of both formyl THF and THF relative to methyl THF in livers of B_{12} deficient rats (Shane et al, 1977). Thus, the beneficial effect of methionine on folate metabolism in B_{12} deficient rats does not discriminate between lack of THF or lack of formyl THF or lack of both being the main lesion in folate metabolism caused by B_{12} deficiency.

The results on whether or not the THF can by-pass the block in folate metabolism in B_{12} deficiency await confirmation. Our preliminary results confirm the observations of Deacon et al (1980a) that THF at low concentration corrects the dU suppression defect in B_{12} deficiency less well than it does in folate deficient human bone marrow and also show that THF relieves the block in dU incorporation into DNA less well than formyl THF in B_{12} deficient cells (Taheri et al, 1981a). In view of the instability of THF, however, the exact interpretation of these findings is uncertain.

Lumb et al (1980) have found no accumulation of methyl THF in the liver cells of rats exposed to N_2O and only a transient accumulation of its polyglutamate derivatives and concluded there is no 'methylfolate trap'. However, since transport of methyl THF into cells is impaired in B_{12} deficient (and presumably also in N_2O exposed cells), methyl THF in the monoglutamate form may accumulate in serum rather than inside cells from which it readily diffuses. Moreover, the essential feature of the 'methylfolate trap' hypothesis is reduced formation of THF rather than a persistent accumulation of methyl THF in B_{12} deficiency.

In conclusion, it seems possible that there may be a triple effect on folate coenzyme synthesis due to a block in homocysteine-methionine conversion in B_{12} deficiency:
1. Reduced supply of THF from methyl THF.
2. A lowered cell level of S-adenosylmethionine which results in the equilibrium between methyl- and methenyl-THF being pushed in the direction of methyl-THF and away from methenyl- and therefore formyl-THF.
3. Reduced formylation of THF, possibly due to intracellular shortage of methionine. This awaits further confirmation.

Whatever the exact mechanism, the end-result is failure of folate polyglutamate and hence of folate coenzyme formation because of lack of provision of the correct folate substrate. There is, therefore, failure of all folate mediated reactions including thymidylate synthesis in B_{12} deficiency.

Vitamin B_{12} neuropathy
B_{12} neuropathy may also be related to the block in the homocysteine-methionine reaction. The folate independent but B_{12} dependent reaction methylmalonyl (MM)

CoA mutase, although impaired when the coenzyme ado-B_{12} is deficient, is unlikely to be the fundamental lesion in B_{12} deficient neuropathy. Three lines of evidence point to this conclusion:

1. Babies born with methylmalonic aciduria due to lack of the apoenzyme methyl-malonyl CoA mutase or due to a selective failure of synthesis of ado-B_{12}, do not show a neuropathy resembling that due to B_{12} deficiency.

2. Children with TCII deficiency may develop a neuropathy identical with that due to B_{12} deficiency but do not show methylmalonic aciduria (Burman et al, 1979, Hoffbrand et al, 1981).

3. Prolonged N_2O exposure in monkeys causes a neuropathy identical to that due to lack of B_{12} but no methylmalonic aciduria occurs (Dinn et al, 1978).

B_{12} neuropathy is possibly due to a block in the homocysteine-methionine reaction, which has been shown to be impaired in the brains of N_2O exposed rats (Deacon et al, 1980c). Lack of THF, however, does not seem to be a major factor. Recent observations suggest that it may be the lack of SAM which is responsible. Cycloleucine, which inhibits conversion of methionine to SAM, causes a neuropathy in rats (Jacobsen et al, 1973). Moreover, methionine feeding to monkeys treated with N_2O protects from the neuropathy (Dinn et al, 1980). It may be that lack of SAM which is needed for methylation reactions in lipid synthesis in the brain is the cause of the myelin degeneration in B_{12} deficiency. Methyl THF itself has been shown to inhibit kainic acid receptors in rat brain (Ruck et al, 1980). Although kainic acid is a potent neuronal depolarising agent, it is difficult to imagine that accumulation of methyl THF could cause demyelination on the basis of this action.

Although neuropathies have been described in folate deficient patients, it is still uncertain whether or not folate deficiency is a cause of organic nervous damage. The recent study of Shovron et al (1980) has shown that affective disorders occurred in 19 (56 per cent) of 34 patients with folate deficiency compared with only 10 (20 per cent) of 50 patients with B_{12} deficiency whereas a peripheral neuropathy occurred in 40 per cent of the B_{12} deficient patients and 18 per cent of those with folate deficiency. It was not shown, however, whether the organic mental changes (present in 27 per cent) or peripheral neuropathy in folate deficiency was actually a result rather than association of the deficiency. It is clear, however, that the folate antagonist methotrexate can cause severe brain damage. Folate deficiency has been associated with decreased brain 5-hydroxytryptamine synthesis in man and rat (Botez et al, 1979) but this is unlikely to be relevant to organic brain damage.

If the neuropathy of B_{12} deficiency is due to SAM deficiency, why does folate deficiency not cause a similar neuropathy since folate is also required for SAM synthesis (Fig. 2.6)? Cerebrospinal fluid folate concentration is three times that in serum, and so folate deficiency may not lead to severe intracellular folate deficiency in the brain and thus to a block in intracellular methionine and SAM synthesis whereas the intracellular block in homocysteine-methionine conversion caused by B_{12} deficiency might cause such a block in SAM synthesis even in the presence of adequate folate supply. However, it remains unclear why folate therapy should exaggerate the effect of B_{12} deficiency on the brain in some patients and further studies in this area are awaited.

B_{12} as ado-B_{12} is also required for the interconversion of α-leucine and β-leucine via the enzyme leucine 2, 3 aminomutase (Poston, 1976). In untreated pernicious anaemia the serum concentration of β-leucine is increased while that of α-leucine is decreased (Poston, 1980). It seems unlikely that these amino acid changes could be related to the neuropathy in view of the ado-B_{12} requirement for this reaction and the development of severe neuropathy due to N_2O in monkeys without any evidence of ado-B_{12} deficiency.

Megaloblastic anaemia not due to vitamin B_{12} or folate deficiency

Disturbances of B_{12} metabolism (e.g. congenital TCII deficiency or nitrous oxide administration) or of folate metabolism, (e.g. congenital deficiency of folate requiring enzymes or methotrexate administration) cause megaloblastic anaemia by inhibiting supply of the correct folate coenzyme for thymidylate synthesis. For instance, a rapid fall in cell dTTP concentration occurs when cells are exposed to methotrexate. All other causes of megaloblastic anaemia where the biochemical lesion has been established also interfere with DNA synthesis at one or other point. Drugs may cause megaloblastic anaemia without interfering with folate or B_{12} metabolism and they usually do this by interfering with supply of one or other dNTP e.g. 5-fluorouracil inhibits thymidylate synthesis, hydroxyurea inhibits ribonucleotide reductase and impairs supply of both dATP and dGTP. Cytosine arabinoside inhibits DNA polymerase activity directly by competing with dCTP for binding to the enzyme. Drugs which inhibit mitosis (e.g. vincristine) or alkylate DNA (e.g. chlorambucil, cyclophosphamide or busulphan) do not cause megaloblastic anaemia.

The inherited metabolic abnormality orotic aciduria in which two consecutive enzymes orotidylic phosphorylase and orotidine decarboxylase involved in conversion of orotic acid to uridylate (UMP) from which both pyrimidine DNA precursors, dTTP and dCTP are ultimately formed, causes megaloblastic anaemia responsive to uridine which bypasses the block. Less well established is megaloblastic anaemia responding to adenine in the Lesch-Nyhan syndrome in which purine synthesis is impaired. The site of the DNA synthesis defect in the acquired megaloblastic change seen in erythroleukaemia and primary acquired sideroblastic anaemia remains unknown. The dU suppression test is normal excluding thymidylate synthesis as the site. It is also unclear how alcohol directly inhibits DNA synthesis to cause megaloblastosis. Ganeshaguru & Hoffbrand (1978) showed alcohol causes a consistent rise in dATP in human cells but the exact enzyme inhibited was not pin-pointed.

Where macrocytosis occurs with a normoblastic marrow, it is presumed that a DNA replicative defect is not present. Enlargement of the cell may arise from increase in cell membrane, early release of the cell from the marrow and possibly from reduced number of cell divisions during erythropoiesis. These are some of the possible mechanisms for non-megaloblastic macrocytic cells.

Plasma vitamin B_{12} binding proteins

Transcobalamins I and III

These glycoproteins (approximately 33 per cent sugar by weight) with slightly different sugar moieties (M.W. 56 to 58 000) are closely related to the 'R' B_{12} binding proteins (or 'cobalothins') present in other body fluids (saliva, gastric juice, milk etc.). TCI binds most of the B_{12} in plasma in a one-to-one molecular relation. The source of these proteins is thought to be granulocytes and possibly other tissues. There is some evidence that TCI is synthesised mainly by earlier cells e.g. myelocytes while TCIII is synthesised mostly by mature neutrophils (Zittoun et al, 1975a). Kolhouse & Allen (1977) propose that one function of the R binders is to bind potentially toxic B_{12} analogues which may be absorbed from food or from bacterial synthesis in the intestine (Brandt et al, 1979) and to transport these analogues to the liver for excretion in bile, the liver cells having receptors for the sialic acid portion of the glycoprotein. Some but not all B_{12} analogues, depending on the degree of difference from the B_{12} structure bind to intrinsic factor (IF). Congenital absence of TCI has been found to cause no clinical abnormality other than a low serum B_{12} level. Raised TCI concentrations are found in serum associated with high B_{12} levels in myeloproliferative diseases and have also been observed with a variety of tumours e.g. hepatoma, carcinoma of the breast. Purification of the B_{12} binding protein in high concentration in the plasma of a patient with hepato-cellular carcinoma showed this to have the same amino-acid composition of other purified R-type binding proteins, differences in sialic acid and fucose content accounting for differences in electrophoretic mobility from purified milk and saliva R-proteins (Burger et al, 1975).

Raised TCIII levels, sometimes, but not invariably associated with raised B_{12} levels are more often found in benign increase in leucocytes e.g. chronic inflammatory bowel disease and also in polycythaemia rubra vera but in many patients with both benign and malignant increase in granulocytes, both TCI and III are increased.

Transcobalamin II

This polypeptide is essential to transport B_{12} into bone marrow cells, placenta, brain and other tissues. Its binding of B_{12}, like that of IF seems to be much more specific for 'true' B_{12} compared with TCI and III. The TCII receptor on human placenta has been partly purified and found to bind in the presence of calcium ions holoTCII (TCII-B_{12} complex) twice more firmly than apo-TCII (free TCII) (Seligmann & Allen, 1978). The receptor is a glycoprotein of MW approximately 50 000. TCII-B_{12} complex is thought to enter liver cells by pinocytosis with subsequent lysosomal digestion of TCII and transfer of B_{12} largely into mitochondria (Pletsch & Coffey, 1971). A similar uptake process has been shown in cultured fibroblasts and rat kidney cells. In other cells, however, uptake may be by a non-pincytotic mechanism. TCII normally is largely desaturated in plasma. Synthesis occurs in multiple organs including the liver, macrophages (Gilbert & Weinred, 1976; Rachmilewitz et al, 1978) and the ileum (Rotherberg et al, 1978; Chanarin et al, 1978). Following bone marrow transplantation, the TCII iso-protein pattern of the recipient partly conforms to that of the donor, consistent with the concept that macrophages are an important source (Fräter-Schroder et al, 1980).

Congenital absence of TCII has now been described in several infants who present at about six weeks of age with severe megaloblastic anaemia and normal serum B_{12} and folate levels (Hakami et al, 1971) The anaemia responds well to massive injections of hydroxocobalamin, e.g. 1000 μg three times weekly which presumably cause sufficient B_{12} to enter cells by passive transfer. The failure of B_{12} absorption in all the children suggest a direct role for TCII in B_{12} absorption. Two children in whom the correct diagnosis was not made in infancy have developed B_{12} neuropathy implying a direct role for TCII in providing the brain with B_{12} although whether this is via the cerebrospinal fluid or bloodstream is uncertain. TCII like vitamin B_{12} is present in normal CSF although both are in low concentrations compared to plasma. More recently Haurani et al (1980) have described a patient, a female of 34 with abnormal TCII (TCII Cardeza) which could bind B_{12} but did not facilitate its entry to cells. Seligman et al (1980) have also reported a baby born with TCII that did not bind B_{12}.

Raised TCII levels have been described in acute monoblastic leukaemia by Zittoun et al (1975b), in Gaucher's disease (Gilbert & Weinred, 1976) and in autoimmune diseases. Indeed it has been proposed that the serum TCII concentration can be used to monitor the progress of some widespread inflammatory diseases (Fräter-Schroder et al, 1978). The serum B_{12} level itself is not usually raised in these diseases.

Five isoproteins of TCII have been described (Fräter-Schroder et al, 1979). These are inherited in two alleles from each parent so that four possible patterns may occur in any set of siblings. As yet there is no evidence for a functional difference between these isoproteins.

Assay of serum vitamin B_{12}

In most reported studies, the radioassays of B_{12} in serum have given higher results both in patients with B_{12} deficiency and in normal subjects, than the microbiological assays, e.g. with E. gracilis or L. Leichmannii (Mollin et al, 1980). The discrepancy is particularly marked with certain sera, e.g. some patients following partial gastrectomy. A number of explanations for the discrepancy have been suggested. The presence in serum of 'pseudo-vitamin B_{12}' compounds or B_{12} analogues which compete with B_{12} for R-B_{12} binding proteins but do not attach to pure IF and do not support growth of the microbiological assay organisms appears the most likely explanation (Kolhouse et al, 1978). Cooper & Whitehead (1978) found false normal serum B_{12} levels in 10 per cent of untreated pernicious anaemia patients using a radioassay. Although this is a higher discrepancy rate than in most other series, it has led to attempts to improve the radioassays either by using only pure IF as the binding protein or by 'blocking' binding of pseudo-vitamin B_{12} compounds to the 'R' protein used in the assays by adding a pseudo-B_{12} compound (cobinamide) to the 'R' protein to block binding sites other than those for 'true' B_{12}. Results with these modified radioassays are awaited but preliminary reports suggest that they give results more closely comparable with those of the microbiological assays (Kubasik et al, 1980).

Nitrous oxide (N_2O) inactivation of vitamin B_{12}

The observation by Amess et al (1977) that subjects exposed for prolonged periods to N_2O show megaloblastic marrow changes with abnormal dU suppression corrected by B_{12} has led to widespread interest in this phenomenon, both because of the clinical implications as well as because of the possibility of using exposure to N_2O as a method of producing a block of B_{12} metabolism in experimental animals or in tissue culture (see earlier). It is now clear that N_2O oxidises the cobalt atom in B_{12} from the fully reduced Cob (I) form found in methylcobalamin to the Cob (III) state. The homocysteine-methionine reaction (methionine synthetase) is blocked in marrow, brain and other tissues (Chanarin, 1980). On the other hand, ado-B_{12} is unaffected and methylmalonic acid excretion is not increased (Deacon et al, 1978). DNA synthesis is inhibited (Cullen et al, 1979) and an abnormal dU blocking occurs in 24 hours in humans but takes several days after discontinuing N_2O exposure to correct spontaneously in vivo. Although both rats and monkeys develop an abnormal dU blocking reaction after N_2O exposure, megaloblastic anaemia does not occur in these species even after many months of exposure. The monkey, but not rats or mice, does, however, develop a neuropathy clinically and pathologically indistinguishable from sub-acute combined degeneration of the cord (see earlier). A peripheral neuropathy and myelopathy resembling that of B_{12} deficiency has also been described in dentists chronically exposed to nitrous oxide (Layzer, 1978; Gutman et al, 1979).

Vitamin B_{12} absorption and malabsorption

Intrinsic factor (IF) mediated attachment of B_{12} to the ileal brush border microvillus membrane is now well-studied. The ileal receptor appears to be a macromolecule lipoprotein with a MW over one million, relatively easily detached by sonication (Katz & Cooper, 1974). Human ileal mucosa contains $0.3–4.9 \times 10^{12}$ receptor molecules per gram of mucosa. Each receptor consists of two subunits, one facing in, the other out (Kouvonen & Gräsbeck, 1981). Earlier work suggested that newly absorbed B_{12} enters the mitochondria of the ileal enterocyte but recent studies show lysosomal localisation implying absorption by a pinocytotic mechanism (Jenkins et al, 1981). This would parallel observations of lysosomal localisation, both of TCII-B_{12} taken up by liver cells and of B_{12} reabsorbed by renal tubular cells. It would also help to explain the association of proteinuria and specific malabsorption of B_{12} implying a lysosomal defect in both renal tubular epithelium and in ileal enterocytes. As yet, however, it is uncertain whether or not IF or a portion of it gains entry to the ileal cell and if so whether to lysosomes or mitochondria.

The major role of IF has been established for many years and children with congenital lack of IF or a congenitally abnormal IF have been found to have severe malabsorption of B_{12}. More recently the role of other proteins in B_{12} absorption has become apparent. There is now evidence that TCII has an active role in carrying B_{12} out of the ileal cell (see earlier). In addition the role of pancreatic secretion has been clarified.

Role of the pancreas

Chronic pancreatitis and cystic fibrosis are associated with malabsorption of B_{12} and pancreatic secretion is known to enhance B_{12} absorption; several mechanisms have been proposed. One idea was that the secretion helped to maintain the ileal pH and calcium ion concentration optimal. However, both trypsin and bicarbonate have been found to improve the absorption. More recently, Allen et al (1978) proposed that pancreatic enzymes including trypsin digest R binder secreted in gastric juice which competes with IF for newly released food B_{12} even at the low pH of gastric juice. B_{12} bound to R binder is unavailable for absorption whereas free IF is present in the small intestinal lumen and is capable of binding B_{12} released from R binder by pancreatic secretion (Kapadia et al, 1976).

Absorption of food-bound vitamin B_{12}

B_{12} absorption tests are usually carried out with labelled crystalline cyanocobalamin in aqueous solution, the subject being fasting. Doscherholmen and colleagues have produced evidence that in some clinical situations e.g. atrophic gastritis, and after partial gastrectomy, absorption of crystalline vitamin B_{12} may be normal but absorption of food-B_{12} is impaired and this may correlate with the clinical status.

They proposed the use of an ovalbumin-bound B_{12} absorption test (Doscherholmen et al, 1976). As yet, however, there is no widespread use of food-bound B_{12} absorption tests since the more usual and convenient tests remains reliable at separating pernicious anaemia from normal.

FOLATE

Absorption
All ingested natural folate compounds are converted in the intestinal lumen and mucosa to a monoglutamate form 5-methyl THF. Full reduction and methylation occurs in the duodenal or jejunal cell but the exact site of deconjugation of the polyglutamate forms to the monoglutamate remain uncertain. The failure of folate compounds with more than three glutamates to enter marrow cells and the intra-lysosomal localisation of folate conjugase (pteroyl – or folate – polyglutamate hydrolase, the enzyme responsible for deconjugation) suggests that deconjugation to the triglutamate form, at least, occurs in the gut lumen if the folate is to be absorbed from the higher polyglutamate derivatives. On the other hand, Halsted (1979) suggests initial deconjugation occurs close to the surface of the epithelial cell by means of a second folate conjugase with a pH optimum near neutral and localised at the brush border (Reisenauer et al, 1977). This remains unproven.

Serum folate assay
A number of radioassays of serum and red cell folate have been introduced, particularly by commercial manufacturers (Dawson et al, 1980). These use labelled pteroylglutamic acid or labelled methyl THF to compete with serum folate for the binder – lactoglobulin or crude milk protein. The results, in general, correlate reasonably well with L. casei assay and do not give consistently higher answers which have been found with some of the radio-B_{12} assays compared with microbiologic assays (Jones et al, 1979). It is not yet clear, however, how reliable are the radioassays for serum folate and particularly for red cell folate.

Folate transport

Folate binding proteins
Specific folate binders have been detected in a number of body fluids and cells including serum, bile, milk, saliva, normal and leukaemic leucocytes, intestinal epithelial cell and kidney brush border membranes, gastrointestinal carcinoma and liver cells (Rothenberg & DaCosta, 1976; McHugh & Chong, 1979). In general, they bind unreduced folates e.g. pteroylglutamic acid more tightly than reduced, physiological folates. Moreover, they do not promote folate uptake by bone marrow cells or placenta and are glycoproteins which take folates in serum preferentially to liver cells, for storage or for excretion in the bile (Fernandez-Costa & Metz, 1979; Rubinoff et al, 1980). Their main role in serum may therefore be to assist in the excretion of unwanted oxidised folates and folate breakdown products. Only a tiny proportion of endogenous serum folate is bound to this protein. Folate in serum is about two-thirds loosely attached to albumin and possibly α-macroglobulins and one-third is free. In milk, the protein may facilitate folate uptake by intestinal cells (Colman et al, 1981).

The intracellular folate binders (Corrocher et al, 1974; Zamierowski & Wagner, 1977) may help to keep folates inside cells. Rothenberg and DaCosta (1976) have also postulated that by binding intracellular folates they may have a role in controlling the rates of different folate reactions e.g. in DNA synthesis where the preferential binding of dihydrofolate (DHF) compared to tetrahydrofolate, could impair reutilisation of DHF and hence impair thymidylate synthesis.

Separate mechanisms exist for transport of reduced and non-reduced folates into cells (Huennekens et al, 1979). Transport of reduced compounds whether into isolated hepatic cells, reticulocytes, marrow cells, PHA-stimulated lymphocytes or through the choroid plexus is active, energy-dependent and carrier-mediated but independent of folate-binding protein in the medium. The transport process is shared by methotrexate, inhibited by mercurials and by a rise in cell cyclic AMP. It is several times greater than transport of non-reduced folic acid itself, which based on substrate competition studies appears to have a separate transport system in all cells tested.

A familial defect of folate transport has been described in a family in which aplastic anaemia with some megaloblastic changes was the main haematological abnormality in the propositus (Branda et al, 1978). In the propositus, folate therapy was associated with haematological improvement but red cell folate remained low and a transport defect of folate into cells was shown to be present.

Folate catabolism

In the rat, folate catabolism has been shown to occur via splitting of the C_9-N_{10} bond with the formation of aminobenzoylglutamate and various pteridines which are excreted in the urine (Murphy et al, 1976). Kelly et al (1979) have shown that the anticonvulsant diphenylhydantoin increases the excretion of isotopically-labelled folate in the mouse and this is consistent with the hypothesis that anticonvulsant drugs induce enzymes involved in folate catabolism and that this is the mechanism for folate deficiency in patients receiving anticonvulsant drug therapy.

REFERENCES

Allen R H 1975 Human vitamin B_{12} transport proteins. In: (ed) Brown E B Progress in Hematology 10. Grune & Stratton, New York pp 57–84
Allen R H, Seetheram B, Allen N C, Podell E R, Alpers D H 1978 Journal of Clinical Investigation 61: 1628–1634
Ames J A L, Burman J F, Rees G M, Nancekievill D G, Mollin D L 1978 Lancet II: 339–342
Babior B M (ed) 1975 Cobalamin: Biochemistry and pathophysiology. Wiley, New York
Botez M I, Reynolds E H (eds) 1979 Folic acid in neurology, psychiatry and internal medicine. Raven Press, New York
Botez M I, Young S N, Bachevalier J, Gauthier S 1979 Nature 278: 182–183
Branda R F, Moldow C F, MacArthur J R, Wintrobe M M, Anthony B K, Jacob H S 1978 New England Journal of Medicine 298: 469–475
Brandt L J, Goldberg L, Bernstein L H, Greenberg G 1979 Clinical Nutrition 32: 1832–1836
Burger R L, Waxman S, Gilbert H S, Mehlman C S, Allen R H 1975 The Journal of Clinical Investigation 56: 1262–1270
Burman J F, Mollin D L, Sourial N A, Sladden R A 1979 British Journal of Haematology 43: 27–38
Chanarin I 1979 The megaloblastic anaemias (Second Edition) Blackwell Scientific Publications, Oxford
Chanarin I 1980 Journal of Clinical Pathology (in press)
Chanarin I, Deacon R, Lumb M, Perry J 1980 Lancet ii: 505–508
Chanarin I, Muir M, Hughes A, Hoffbrand A V 1978 British Medical Journal 1: 1453–1455
Colman N, Hettiarachchy N, Herbert V 1981 Science 211: 1427–1428
Cooper B A, Whitehead V M 1978 New England Journal of Medicine 299: 816–818
Corrocher R, De Sandre G, Pacor M L, Hoffbrand A V 1974 Clinical Science and Molecular Medicine, 46: 551–554

Cullen M H, Rees G M, Nancekievill D G, Ames J A L 1979 British Journal of Haematology 42: 527–534
Dardick I, Sheinin R, Setterfield G 1978 British Journal of Haematology 39, 483–490
Das K C, Herbert V 1976 Clinics in Haematology 5: 697–725
Dawson D W, Delamore I W, Fish D, Flaherty T A, Gowenlock A H, Hunt L P, Hyde K, MacIver J E, Thornton J A, Waters H M 1980 Journal of Clinical Pathology 33: 234–242
Deacon R, Chanarin I, Perry J, Lumb M 1980a Biochemical and Biophysical Research Communications 93: 516–520
Deacon R, Chanarin I, Perry J, Lumb M 1980b British Journal of Haematology 46: 523–528
Deacon R, Lumb M, Perry J, Chanarin I, Minty B, Halsey M J, Nunn J F 1978 Lancet ii: 1023–1024
Deacon R, Lumb M, Perry J, Chanarin I, Minty B, Halsey M J, Nunn J F 1980c European Journal of Biochemistry 104: 419–422
Dinn J J, McCann S, Wilson P, Reed B, Weir D, Scott J 1978 Lancet ii: 1154
Dinn J J, Weir D G, McCann S, Reed B, Wilson P, Scott J M 1980 Irish Journal of Medical Science 149, 1–4
Doscherholmen A, McMahon J, Ripley D 1976 British Journal of Haematology 33: 261–272
Ellims P H, Jayman R J, Van Der Weyden M B 1979 Biochemical and Biophysical Research Communications 89: 103–107
Ellims P H, Hayman R J, Van Der Weyden M B 1979 Biochemical and Biophysical Research Communications 89 103–107
Folic Acid 1977 Biochemistry and physiology in relation to the human nutrition requirements. National Academy of Science, Washington
Fernandez-Costa F, Metz J 1979 British Journal of Haematology 41: 335–342
Fräter-Schroder M, Grob P J, Hitzig W H, Kenny A B 1978 Lancet ii: 238–239
Fräter-Schroder M, Hitzig W H, Butler R 1979 Blood 53: 193–203
Fräter-Schroder M, Nissen C, Amur J, Hitzig W H 1980 Blood 56: 560–563
Ganeshaguru K, Hoffbrand A V 1978 British Journal of Haematology 40: 29–41
Gilbert H S, Weinred N 1976 New England Journal of Medicine 295: 1096–1101
Gutman L, Farrell B, Crosby T W, Johnson D 1979 Journal of the American Dental Association 98: 58–59
Hakami N, Neiman P E, Canellos G P, Lazerson J 1971 New England Journal of Medicine 285: 1163–1170
Halsted C H 1979 American Journal of Clinical Nutrition 32: 846–855
Haurani F I, Hall C A, Rubin R 1979 The Journal of Clinical Investigation 64: 1253–1259
Herbert V 1980 Seminars in Hematology Vols I & II: 1–176
Hoffbrand A V (ed) 1976 Clinics in Haematology Vol 5 No 3: 471–769
Hoffbrand A V 1975 In: (ed) Brown E B Progress in Hematology 9: 85–105
Hoffbrand A V, Ganeshaguru K, Lavoie A, Tattersall M H N, Tripp E 1974 Nature 248: 602–604
Hoffbrand A V, Tripp E, Lavoie A 1976 Clinical Science and Molecular Medicine 50: 51–68
Hoffbrand A V, Tripp E, Jackson B F A, Luck W 1981 New England Journal of Medicine (in press)
Hooton J W L, Hoffbrand A V 1977 Biochimica Biophysica Acta 477: 250–263
Huennekens F M, Vitols K S, Henderson G B 19 Advances in Enzymology and Related Areas of Molecular Biology 47: 313–346
Jacobson W, Gandy G, Sidman R L 1973 Journal of Pathology 109: p xiii
Jenkins W J, Empson R, Jewell D P, Taylor K B 1981 Gut (in press)
Jones P, Grace C S, Rozenberg M C 1979 Pathology 11: 45–52
Kapadia C R, Mathan V I, Baker S J 1976 Gastroenterology 70: 704–706
Kass L 1976 Pernicious anemia. Vol. VII In: Major problems in internal medicine. Saunders, Philadelphia
Katz M, Cooper B A 1974 British Journal of Haematology 26: 569–579
Kelly D, Weir D, Reed B, Scott J 1979 Journal of Clinical Investigation 64: 1089–1096
Kolhouse J H, Allen R H 1977 Journal of Clinical Investigation 60: 1381–1392
Kolhouse J F, Kondo H, Allen N C, Podell E, Allen R H 1978 New England Journal of Medicine 299: 785–792
Krebs H A, Hems R, Tyler B 1976 Biochemical Journal 158: 341–353
Kubasik N P, Ricotta M, Sine H E 1980 Clinical Chemistry 25: 598–600
Kouvonen I, Gräsbeck R 1981 Journal of Biological Chemistry 256: 154–158
Lavoie A, Tripp E, Hoffbrand A V 1974 Clinical Science & Molecular Medicine 47: 617–630
Layzer R B 1978 Lancet ii: 1227–1230
Lumb M, Deacon R, Perry J, Chanarin I, Minty B, Halsey M J, Nunn J F 1980 Biochemical Journal 186: 933–936
McGing P, Reed B, Weir D G, Scott, J M 1978 Biochemical Biophysical Research Communication 82: 540–546
McHugh M, Cheng Yun-Chi 1979 Journal of Biological Chemistry 254: 11312–11318
Mathews C K, North T W, Reddy G P V 1978 Advances in Enzyme Regulation 17: 133–156

Mollin D L, Hoffbrand A V, Ward P G, Lewis S M 1980 Journal of Clinical Pathology 33: 243–248
Moran R G, Colman P D 1980 Proceedings of the American Association for Cancer Research 21: 25 (Abstract)
Murphy M, Keating M, Boyle P, Weir D G, Scott J M 1976 Biochemical and Biophysical Research Communications 71: 1017–1024
Pardoll D M, Vogelstein B, Coffey D S 1980 Cell 19: 527–536
Pearson A G M, Turner A J 1975 Nature 258: 173–174
Pelliniemi T-T, Beck W S 1980 Journal of Clinical Investigation 65: 449–460
Perry J, Chanarin I, Deacon R, Lumb M 1979 Biochemical and Biophysical Research Communications 91: 678–684
Pletsch Q A, Coffey J W 1971 Journal of Biological Chemistry 246: 4619–4629
Poston J M 1976 Journal of Biological Chemistry 251: 1859–1863
Poston J M 1980 Journal of Biological Chemistry (in press)
Rachmilewitz B, Rachmilewitz M, Chaouat M, Schlesinger M 1978 Blood 52: 1089–1908
Reddy G P V, Matthews C K 1978 Journal of Biological Chemistry 253: 3461–3467
Reddy G P V, Pardee A B 1980 Proceedings of the National Academy of Science 77: 3312–3316
Reisenauer A M, Krumdieck C L, Halsted C H 1977 Science 198: 196–197
Rothenberg S P, Da Costa M 1976 Clinics in Haematology 5: 569–587
Rothenberg S P, Weiss J P, Cotter R 1978 British Journal of Haematology 40: 401–414
Rubinoff M, Abramson R, Schreiber C, Waxman S 1980 British Journal of Haematology (in press)
Ruck A, Kramer S, Metz J, Prennan M J W 1980 Nature 287 852–853
Sakamoto S, Niina M, Takaku F 1975 Blood 46: 699–704
Seligman P A, Allen R H 1978 Journal of Biological Chemistry 253: 1766–1772
Seligman P A, Steiner L L, Allen R H 1980 New England Journal of Medicine 303: 1209–1212
Shane B, Watson J E, Stokstad E L R 1977 Biochimica and Biophysica Acta 497: 241–252
Shin Y S, Buehring K U, Stokstad E L R 1975 Molecular Cell Biochemistry 9: 97–108
Shovron S D, Carney M W P, Chanarin I, Reynolds E H 1980 British Medical Journal 281: 1036–1038
Taheri R, Wickremasinghe R G, Hoffbrand A V 1981a Biochemical Journal 196: 451–461
Taheri R, Wichremasinghe R G, Hoffbrand A V 1981b Biochemical Journal 196: 225–235
Taheri M R, Wickremasinghe R G, Hoffbrand A V 1981c British Journal of Haematology 47: 628
Tattersall M H N, Lavoie A, Ganeshaguru K, Tripp E, Hoffbrand A V European Journal of Clinical Investigation 5: 191–202
Thenen S W, Stokstad E L R 1973 Journal of Nutrition 103: 363–370
Van Der Weyden M B 1979 Scandinavian Journal of Haematology 23: 37–42
Waxman S, Metz J, Herbert V 1969 Journal of Clinical Investigation 48: 284–289
Weissbach A 1979 Archives of Biochemistry and Biophysics 198: 386–396
Wickramasinghe S N, Saunders J E 1980 Acta Haematologica 63: 196–203
Wickremasinghe R G, Hoffbrand A V 1979 Biochimica Biophysica Acta 563: 46–58
Wickremasinghe R G, Hoffbrand A V 1980a Journal of Clinical Investigation 65: 26–36
Wickremasinghe R G, Hoffbrand A V 1980b Biochemica et Biophysica Acta 607: 411–419
Zagalak B, Friedrick W (ed) 1979 Vitamin B_{12}. Walter de Gruyter, Berlin
Zamierowski M M, Wagner C 1977 The Journal of Biological Chemistry 252: 933–938
Zittoun J, Marquet J, Zittoun R 1975 British Journal of Haematology 31: 299–310
Zittoun J, Marquet J, Zittoun R 1978 Blood 51: 119–128
Zittoun J, Zittoun R, Marquet J, Sultan C 1975b British Journal of Haematology 31: 287–298

ADDENDUM

Recent work by Scott, Dinn, Wilson and Weir (Lancet, 1981, ii: 334–337) has clearly shown that feeding methionine to monkeys exposed to nitrous oxide protects them from the development of a neuropathy closely resembling sub-acute combined degeneration. They suggest that B_{12} neuropathy is due to methionine deficiency and this is secondary to failure of remethylation of homocysteine to methionine. Jacobsen and co-workers (J Pathology, 1973, 109: xii and J Physiology, 1973, 223: 1–3) had earlier proposed that lack of methionine and of S-adenosylmethionine (SAM) caused defective transmethylation of the myelin of the CNS leading to the neuropathy.

Scott and co-workers suggest that the neuropathy does not occur in folate deficiency because the lower level of methionine leads to a lower cell level of SAM and this causes adaptation of the relevant enzymes (particularly 5,10 methylene-THF reductase) to direct folate towards the form (methyl-THF) needed for methionine synthesis and away from the forms needed in DNA synthesis. This adaptation which also occurs in B_{12} deficiency fails because the methionine synthetase step is blocked. Moreover, as suggested earlier in this chapter, the high CSF folate may help to protect the brain against the effects of folate deficiency.

Folic acid therapy in vitamin B_{12} deficient patients, it is suggested (Scott & Weir, Lancet, 1981, ii: 337–340), aggravates methionine deficiency in the brain by diverting methionine towards protein synthesis by increasing cell divisions in the bone marrow and elsewhere.

Megaloblastic anaemia in kwashiorkor with normal serum vitamin B_{12} and folate level is, they propose, due to lack of methionine with consequent lack of the homocysteine necessary for utilisation of methyl-THF.

Their hypothesis is an important expansion of the methyl-folate trap hypothesis, which they suggest might be termed the 'methyl-folate trap process'. They regard the hypothesis that methionine must be degraded to formate and subsequently resynthesised to methionine for folate to be incorporated into cells (see earlier in this chapter) as improbable since this would result in no net gain of methionine.

3. The molecular genetics of haemoglobin — the thalassaemias

D J Weatherall

Since the last volume of Recent Advances in Haematology spectacular progress has been made in the human haemoglobin field. This has resulted from the development of new techniques for examining the fine structure of the haemoglobin genes and hence for more detailed analysis of genetic disorders of haemoglobin synthesis, particularly the thalassaemias and related conditions.

In this short review I shall concentrate on these new developments, particularly the molecular genetics of the thalassaemias. Readers who wish to obtain a more extensive account of other aspects of the abnormal haemoglobin field are referred to several recent reviews and monographs which deal with the subject in greater breadth (Bunn et al, 1977; Weatherall & Clegg, 1979; Huehns, 1981).

Before outlining our present understanding of the molecular genetics of human haemoglobin it is worth digressing briefly to describe some of the new techniques which have been applied to analysis of the haemoglobin genome.

Recently developed methods for analysing the human haemoglobin genes

The analysis of the fine structure of the haemoglobin genes has been made possible by the further development of the techniques of nucleic acid hybridisation, and, most recently, by the application of recombinant DNA technology to the problem (Maniatis, 1980).

In the early 1960s it was found that the two strands of native DNA can be dissociated and reassociated in vitro by heating and subsequent cooling. These reannealing reactions are highly specific. A few years later an enzyme called reverse transcriptase was discovered in certain RNA tumour viruses which is capable of synthesising a DNA molecule from an RNA template (Temin & Mizutani, 1970; Baltimore, 1970). Hence, using globin messenger RNA as a template, it is possible to synthesise a DNA copy (cDNA) with a nucleotide sequence exactly complementary to that of its template, i.e. a copy which is identical to the sequence of one of the two strands of DNA from which the messenger RNA was originally transcribed. Furthermore, if the cDNA is radioactively labelled it can be used as a highly sensitive hybridisation probe for testing for the presence of complementary sequences in genomic DNA or, indeed, in total cellular RNA. Because of the precise specificity of the molecular hybridisation reaction, and because it is possible to synthesise highly radioactive cDNA copies, such cDNA probes can be used for detecting one or two copies of any particular globin gene among the many million genes which make up the human genome. Techniques have been developed using soluble hybridisation methods which are capable of measuring the number of globin genes and of determining the relative amounts of α and β globin messenger RNA in reticulocytes and bone marrow cells.

Although the techniques of soluble hybridisation give some extremely important information about the haemoglobin genes, they have the disadvantage that they only provide quantitative data about the numbers of globin gene sequences present in DNA but provide no information about the actual arrangement of the globin genes along the chromosome. However, in the early 1970s two further important advances were made. The first was the discovery of restriction endonucleases i.e. enzymes which are produced by bacteria and which cut DNA at very precise sequences (Nathans & Smith, 1972). A whole variety of these enzymes have been isolated, each of which is highly specific for a particular DNA sequence. Thus, if DNA is treated with one or more restriction enzyme, it is cut into many smaller pieces which can then be separated by agarose gel electrophoresis into classes of different sizes. In 1975 Southern introduced a method of hybridisation in which one of the components of the reaction, i.e. the DNA under study, is immobilised on a cellulose nitrate filter. He showed that it is possible to transfer DNA fractions from agarose gel electrophoresis onto these filters and hence they can then be assayed for the presence of specific genes using radioactive cDNAs under stringent hybridisation conditions. The DNA fractions containing the globin genes, or parts of them, can then be visualised by radioautography of the gels. Hence by analysing normal human DNA with several restriction enzymes separately, or by using them in combination, a series of overlapping DNA fragments are produced which can then be aligned to give an indication of their physical arrangement in the original DNA. Using this approach detailed restriction enzyme maps of the human haemoglobin genes have been obtained (reviewed by Proudfoot et al, 1980).

The most recent technological advances in this field have followed the use of recombinant DNA methodology (Maniatis, 1980). One of the main difficulties in producing pure cDNA probes is obtaining a sufficient quantity of pure α, β and γ globin messenger RNA to act as a suitable template for their production. Recently it has become possible to clone a chosen DNA sequence in bacterial plasmids. The latter are small circular pieces of DNA which are found in the cytoplasm of various bacteria and which replicate independently from the bacterial DNA. It is now possible to restrict suitably sized pieces of human DNA, insert them into plasmids, and provided that the plasmid carries a gene which confers a selective advantage to the bacteria for a chosen growth media, to develop clones containing the appropriate DNA fractions, e.g. those containing particular globin genes. Indeed whole libraries of cloned DNA fragments representing the entire human genome have become available for study (Maniatis et al, 1978; Lawn et al, 1978). In this way it has been possible to obtain pure α, β and γ globin gene probes together with probes developed from adjacent areas of the genome in the relatively large quantities required for detailed analysis of the structure of the human haemoglobin genes. The same technology has been used for producing sufficient quantities of relatively pure genes to enable their base sequence to be determined in detail.

In describing the fine structure of the globin genes it is now usual to define the restriction enzyme sites by the name of the particular enzyme, e.g. Hpa, Hinde, Eco R1, etc., and to define the sizes of the restriction fragments in kilobases i.e. 1000 bases or 1 kb.

The structure and genetic control of the human haemoglobins
The structure and organisation of genetic control of the normal human haemoglobins

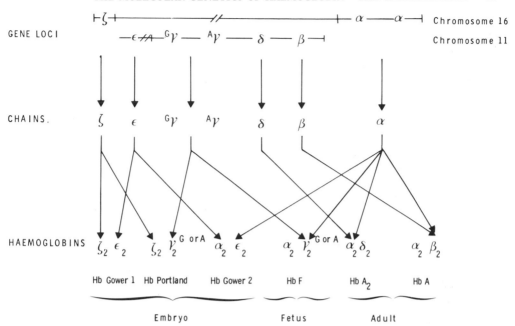

Fig. 3.1   The organisation of the genetic control of the human embryonic, fetal and adult haemoglobins.

is summarised in Figure 3.1. They all have a tetrameric structure. Adult and fetal haemoglobins have α chains associated with β chains (Hb A, $\alpha_2\beta_2$), δ chains (Hb A$_2$, $\alpha_2\delta_2$) or γ chains (Hb F, $\alpha_2\gamma_2$). In embryonic life ζ chains combine with γ chains (Hb Portland, $\zeta_2\gamma_2$) or ε chains (Hb Gower 1, $\zeta_2\varepsilon_2$) and α and ε chains combine to form Hb Gower 2 ($\alpha_2\varepsilon_2$). The ζ and ε chains are the embryonic counterparts of the adult α and β, γ or δ chains respectively. Haemoglobin F shows further heterogeneity. There are two varieties of γ chain which differ in their amino acid composition at position 136 where they contain either glycine or alanine (Schroeder et al, 1968). Those γ chains which contain glycine at position 136 are called $^G\gamma$ chains and those which contain alanine at this position are called $^A\gamma$ chains. The $^G\gamma$ and $^A\gamma$ chains are products of separate loci. Thus during normal human development the ζ and ε genes are activated first, followed by the α and γ genes in the fetus and then just before birth by the δ and β genes. The way in which this beautifully synchronised series of changes in haemoglobin production during development is regulated is completely unknown.

From information obtained from pedigree analysis (see Weatherall & Clegg, 1981) it has been known for some time that the α and non-α globin genes are on different chromosomes. Furthermore, these studies suggested that there are two α globin genes per haploid genome and that the non-α globin genes lie in a linked cluster in the order $^G\gamma$-$^A\gamma$-δ-β. These observations have been confirmed recently by the application of restriction endonuclease analysis to the determination of the fine structure of the globin genes and of their relationship to each other. Furthermore, somatic cell fusion analysis using human and mouse fibroblasts under conditions in which it has been possible to obtain hybrid cell lines devoid of various human chromosomes has provided unequivocal evidence that the linked α globin genes are on chromosome 16 and the $\gamma\delta\beta$ gene cluster is on chromosome 11 (Deisseroth et al, 1977, 1978).

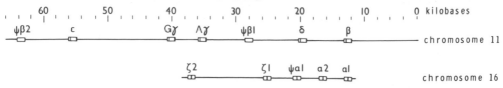

Fig. 3.2   The structure of the α and non-α globin gene clusters. The top line shows the relative positions of the five functional β-like globin genes and the two β-like pseudogenes. The bottom line shows the four functional α-like globin genes and the α globin non-functional pseudogene. The direction of transcription of the two gene clusters is indicated by the arrow.

Complete maps of the α and non-α globin gene clusters have been obtained recently (Fig. 3.2). Detailed references to this work are given by Proudfoot et al (1980). The linked α genes lie 'upstream' from an inactive α globin locus ($\psi\alpha$) and two ζ chain loci. The linked δ and β loci are separated from the $^{G}\gamma$ and $^{A}\gamma$ loci by 13.9 kb which contain a β-like gene called $\psi\beta 1$. The ε loci lie 13.3 kb to the left of the γ loci. The loci designated $\psi\alpha$, $\psi\beta 1$ and $\psi\beta 2$ are pseudogenes i.e. they have sequence homology with the α and β genes but have mutations that prevent their expression. Possibly they represent evolutionary remnants of what may have been functional loci.

An unexpected outcome of these mapping studies has been that the haemoglobin genes, and for that matter most other mammalian genes that have been analysed in this way to date, have one or more non-coding inserts or intervening sequences (introns) at the same position along their length. Thus the β, γ, δ and ε genes each contain two inserts of 122 to 130 and 850 to 900 base pairs between codons 30 and 31 and 104 and 105 respectively. Similar though smaller non-coding segments occur in the mouse and human α globin genes.

The fact that the globin genes contain non-coding inserts means that the processing of globin messenger RNA is an extremely complex mechanism. The primary gene transcripts are large RNA molecules which contain the intervening sequences and these have to be excised and the remaining three pieces of globin messenger RNA (exons) 'spliced' together before the definitive messenger RNA molecule is delivered to the cell cytoplasm. There is little overall homology in the nucleotide sequences of the inserts apart from the splicing regions where the coding and non-coding sequences join. Their function is uncertain although there is evidence that their integrity is required for the normal transcription of messenger RNA.

The complete sequences of the five non-α globin genes, i.e. ε, $^{G}\gamma$, $^{A}\gamma$, δ and β have now been determined and compared with those of other mammals. Some interesting homologies have been observed. At the 5' (upstream) sides of the β genes there are two blocks of sequence homology which are present in analogous positions in many eukaryotic genes. The first is AT-rich (A = adenine; T = thymine), a sequence originally found in the histone gene cluster of *Drosophilia* and called the Hogness box. The second region of homology called the CCAAT box (C = cystosine) is found about 70 base pairs to the 5' end of the gene. These regions may be involved in transcription initiation or RNA processing, or both. Another interesting result of these structural studies is that in the gene clusters there are non-globin repeat sequences, some of which are reiterated up to 300 000 times in the total human genome. Their function is unknown.

As well as providing a wealth of information about the fine structure of the normal human haemoglobin genes these new techniques are starting to clarify the molecular basis of many of the common genetic disorders of haemoglobin synthesis, particularly the thalassaemias. Furthermore, they have provided some promising areas of research into the antenatal diagnosis of some of these disorders.

The genetic disorders of haemoglobin synthesis
The genetic disorders of haemoglobin synthesis fall into four general categories although there is considerable overlap between them. First there are the structural haemoglobin variants, most of which have single amino acid substitutions in one or other of the globin chains; in a few cases they result from either a deletion or an insertion of one or more amino acids. Whether or not these structural changes produce any clinical disability depends on the type of amino acid substitution and its site in the molecule. Although many of them are harmless some, because they alter the configuration, function or stability of the haemoglobin molecule, result in clinical disorders of varying importance. It is not possible to cover these here and the reader is referred to several recent reviews of these conditions which include the sickle cell syndromes (Huehns, 1981), haemoglobin C and E disease (Huehns, 1981), the genetic methaemoglobinaemias and polycythaemias (Bellingham, 1976), and the unstable haemoglobin disorders (White, 1976).

The second and largest group of genetic disorders of haemoglobin synthesis are the thalassaemias which are all characterised by a reduced rate of production of one or more of the globin chains of haemoglobin, leading to globin chain imbalance (Weatherall & Clegg, 1981). The third group is made up of structural haemoglobin variants which are synthesised at a reduced rate and hence give rise to the same clinical phenotypes as the thalassaemias. Finally, there is the heterogeneous group of conditions characterised by persistent fetal haemoglobin synthesis after the neonatal period in the absence of major haematological abnormalities which are known collectively as 'hereditary persistence of fetal haemoglobin (HPFH)'.

Clearly then, there are many different kinds of genetic disorder of haemoglobin synthesis which can produce the clinical phenotype of thalassaemia. We shall discuss some of them in the following sections.

General classification of the thalassaemias
The thalassaemias can be defined as a group of genetic disorders of haemoglobin synthesis characterised by a reduced rate of production of one or more of the globin chains of haemoglobin leading to imbalanced globin chain synthesis. They can be classified into the α, β, $\delta\beta$, δ and $\gamma\delta\beta$ thalassaemias (Tables 3.1 and 3.2). Although the conditions which are categorised as HPFH are separated from the thalassaemias, at least some of them should probably be classified as mild forms of thalassaemia. It was suggested recently that HPFH can be divided into the pancellular forms i.e. conditions in which the haemoglobin F is relatively homogeneously distributed among the red cells, and heterocellular forms in which the haemoglobin F is heterogeneously distributed among the red cells (Boyer et al, 1977). There is increasing evidence that pancellular HPFH is a very well compensated form of $\delta\beta$ thalassaemia and we shall discuss this condition with the $\delta\beta$ thalassaemias in a later section. The heterocellular HPFHs are less thoroughly characterised but what little is known about them suggests that they are perhaps the best candidates that we have for

Table 3.1 The β thalassaemias. Each group is undoubtedly heterogeneous at the molecular level

Type	Homozygote	Heterozygote	Molecular defect
β°	Thal major No Hb A ~98% Hb F	Thal minor ~5% Hb A_2	Heterogeneous Some undefined β globin gene deletion Premature chain termination
β^+ (Mediterranean)	Thal major ~10–20% Hb A ~70–80% Hb F	Thal minor ~5% Hb A_2	?mRNA processing defect in some cases
β^+ (Negro)	Thal intermedia ~30–50% Hb F ~50–70% Hb A	Thal minor ~5% Hb A_2	?mRNA processing defect in some cases
Normal Hb A_2 (type 1) ('silent')	Mild thal intermedia 10–30% Hb F Elevated Hb A_2 level	Minor red cell changes Normal Hb A_2 level	Not defined
Normal Hb A_2 (type 2)	Not described	Thal minor Normal Hb A_2 level	Not defined

Table 3.2(A) and (B) General classification of the α thalassaemias
(A) Genetic determinants

Designation	Haplotype	Heterozygous state	Homozygous state
α thal 1*	$--/$	α° Thalassaemia 5–10% Hb Bart's at birth Low MCH and MCV	Hb Bart's hydrops
Dysfunctional α thal‡	$-\alpha^\circ$	?As above	May not be viable
α thal 2*	$-\alpha/$	α^+ Thalassaemia 0–2% Hb Bart's at birth Minimal haematological change	As for heterozygous α thal 1
Non deletion α thal†	$\underline{\alpha\alpha}/$	May be similar to above but haematological changes may be more severe	Hb H disease in some cases
Hb Constant Spring (CS) α 142 Gln	UAA→CAA	0–2% Hb Bart's at birth 0.5–1% Hb CS	Phenotype more severe than heterozygous α thal 1 5–6% Hb CS
Hb Icaria α 142 Lys	UAA→AAA	As for Hb CS 0.5–1% Hb Icaria	?
Hb Koya Dora α 142 Ser	UAA→UCA	As for Hb CS 0.5–1% Hb Koya Dora	?
Hb Seal Rock α 142 Glu	UAA→GAA	As for Hb CS 0.5–1% Hb Seal Rock	?

(B) Genetic interactions

Interaction	Genotype	Disorder
α thal 1/α thal 2	$--/-\alpha$	Hb H disease
α thal 1/non-deletion α thal	$--/\underline{\alpha\alpha}$	Hb H disease
Non-deletion α thal/non-deletion α thal	$\underline{\alpha\alpha}/\underline{\alpha\alpha}$	Hb H disease
Dysfunctional α thal/α thal 2	$-\alpha^\circ/-\alpha$ (2.6 kb)	Hb H disease
α thal 1/Hb CS	$--/\alpha\alpha^{CS}$	Hb H disease
α thal 1/Hb Q	$--/-\alpha^{Q}$	Hb Q–H disease
α thal 1/Hb G(Phil)	$--/-\alpha^{G}$	Hb G–H disease
α thal 1/Hb Hasharon	$--/-\alpha^{Hash}$	Hb Hasharon–H disease

*The terms α thalassaemia 1 and 2 are used in the phenotypic sense as in the original genetic analysis of the Oriental α thalassaemias.
†Several different non-deletion α thalassaemias are known. A full explanation of the different types of α thalassaemia determinant and their interactions is given in appropriate sections of this chapter.
‡Now known to be partial deletions of α globin genes.

regulatory gene mutations; even in their homozygous states they bear no resemblance to the thalassaemia syndromes (Weatherall et al, 1975; Wood et al, 1979).

THE α THALASSAEMIAS

One of the major difficulties in reviewing recent advances in the α thalassaemia field is that the vast amount of information about these conditions which has been derived recently from restriction endonuclease mapping analysis has left us in the unfortunate position of not having an adequate nomenclature to describe many of the genetic determinants for these disorders. Thus at the time of writing this review it is extremely difficult to classify the α thalassaemias or indeed to discuss them at all!

At the phenotypic level the α thalassaemias can be recognised by several well defined clinical disorders (Weatherall & Clegg, 1981). These include the haemoglobin Bart's hydrops syndrome, haemoglobin H disease and two different carrier states, the more severe and easily recognisable form, α thalassaemia 1 or $\alpha°$ thalassaemia, and the more or less 'silent' carrier state, α thalassaemia 2 or α^+ thalassaemia. The homozygous state for α thalassaemia 1 produces the haemoglobin Bart's hydrops syndrome and the compound heterozygous state for α thalassaemia 1 and 2 results in haemoglobin H disease.

The terms α thalassaemia 1 and 2 are unsatisfactory but because they are so firmly established in the literature I shall continue to use them in this article. Alpha thalassaemia 1 is better called $\alpha°$ thalassaemia since it is used to describe an α thalassaemia determinant which results in the complete absence of output from the α globin genes on chromosome 16. Alpha thalassaemia 2 should really be called α^+ thalassaemia since it is associated with a reduced output of α chains.

During the last two years it has become apparent that both α thalassaemia 1 and 2 are caused by a very heterogeneous series of molecular defects. It follows, therefore, that the main clinical disorders which result from the interaction of these determinants, i.e. the haemoglobin Bart's hydrops syndrome and haemoglobin H disease, are themselves very heterogeneous at the molecular level. Unfortunately, much of this information has been obtained so recently that it has not yet been possible to determine whether the different genetic interactions which produce these conditions are associated with distinguishable clinical phenotypes.

The α thalassaemia 1 determinants

The heterozygous state for α thalassaemia 1 is usually easy to recognise. The haematological changes are very similar to those of heterozygous β thalassaemia with significantly reduced MCH and MCV values. The α/β chain synthesis ratio is significantly reduced in the 0.6–0.7 region and the α/β globin messenger RNA ratios are clearly distinguishable from normals or α thalassaemia 2 heterozygotes (Hunt et al, 1980).

Using the techniques of soluble cDNA/DNA hybridisation it was found that the α thalassaemia 1 determinant results from the loss of both of the linked α chain genes on chromosome 16 (Ottolenghi et al, 1974; Taylor et al, 1974). Quite recently, using restriction endonuclease analysis of the DNA of homozygotes for α thalassaemia 1 or from individuals with haemoglobin H disease it has been possible to examine the extent of these deletions. These studies indicate that there is a remarkable heterogeneity of the defects which result in the α thalassaemia 1 phenotype; to date at least four different sized deletions have been identified.

As mentioned earlier, the two α genes are linked to two ζ genes with an inactive α locus, the $\varphi\alpha$ gene, in between (Lauer et al, 1980). The deletion which causes the α thalassaemia 1 phenotype in Thai patients involves both the α globin genes but leaves both ζ genes intact. On the other hand in a Greek infant with the Hb Bart's hydrops syndrome a deletion of about 17.4 kb was found which involved both α globin genes, the $\varphi\alpha$ gene and the $3'$ ζ globin gene. Since this infant was producing significant amounts of haemoglobin Portland ($\zeta_2\gamma_2$) these observations provide direct evidence that the 5′ ζ globin genes are functional (Pressley et al, 1980b; Kattamis et al, 1980). A similar deletion has been found in a Cypriot case of haemoglobin Bart's hydrops fetalis (Sophocleus et al, 1981). A third variety of deletion has been found in a Greek patient with haemoglobin H disease (Pressley et al, 1980a). This appears to involve the loss of a piece of the α globin genes about 5.2 kb in length. It starts within the 3′ (right hand) gene and extends downstream to involve the 5′ gene but not the two ζ genes (Fig. 3.3).

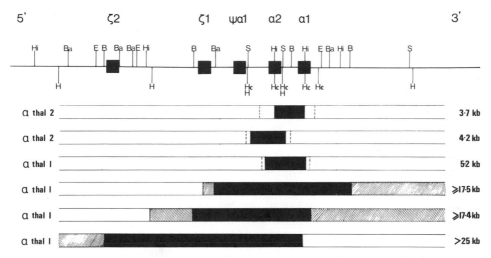

Fig. 3.3 The different deletions responsible for various forms of α thalassaemia 1 and α thalassaemia 2.

A further type of genetic determinant which produces the α thalassaemia 1 phenotype was first described by Orkin et al (1979b). When DNA is digested with the restriction enzyme Eco R1 the α genes are normally found on a fragment 22.2 kb in length. An α thalassaemia 1 determinant was found in several individuals with haemoglobin H disease which gave a fragment 2.6 kb in length. More recently Orkin & Michelson (1980) have isolated this fragment, cloned it in an appropriate phage, and then sequenced the DNA of the fraction purified in this way. They find that it contains part of a single α globin gene which appears to start at codon 57. Further analysis indicates that this particular α thalassaemia determinant has arisen by a large deletion involving all of the 3′ α globin gene and part of the 5′ α globin gene up to codon 57. Judging by the size of the original fragment obtained by Eco R1 digestion this must be a very extensive deletion, probably involving both the ζ globin genes. If this is the case then homozygotes for this determinant would not be able to synthesise any embryonic haemoglobin.

It seems likely that these different sized deletions of the α globin genes (Fig. 3.3) have resulted from unequal crossing over as occurred, for example, to produce the Lepore haemoglobins (Pressley et al, 1980b). The finding of haemoglobin Portland ($\zeta_2\gamma_2$) in infants with the haemoglobin Bart's hydrops syndrome who are homozygous for some of these determinants is of great interest. Since haemoglobin Bart's is physiologically useless it seems likely that these infants are able to survive to term by using haemoglobin Portland as an oxygen carrier. During normal fetal development haemoglobin Portland synthesis ceases in early fetal life. In the presence of these different deletions of the α globin gene cluster, there is persistent embryonic haemoglobin (i.e. ζ chain) synthesis. The situation seems closely analagous to that observed with deletions of the δ and β chain gene cluster which cause HPFH (see later section). It follows, therefore, that deletions which, as well as involving the α globin genes, involve both ζ globin genes will be incompatible with fetal survival. It will be interesting to determine whether infants homozygous for the Greek type of α thalassaemia 1 determinant in which one of the two ζ genes is deleted are less viable, i.e. are stillborn earlier in gestation, than those with the Oriental type of the disease in which both ζ genes are intact (Kattamis et al, 1980). Recent work suggests that the 3'3 ζ globin gene is a pseudogene (Dr N Proudfoot, personal communication, 1981) and hence homozygotes for the Greek deletion may not be phenotypically different from those with the Oriental deletion.

The α thalassaemia 2 determinants

In 1975 Kan and his colleagues, using the technique of soluble hybridisation, provided evidence that individuals with haemoglobin H disease were missing three out of the normal four α globin genes (Kan et al, 1975a). Since it had already been demonstrated that all the genes are deleted in the haemoglobin Bart's hydrops syndrome, and since haemoglobin H disease was thought to result from the compound heterozygous state for α thalassaemia 1 and 2, this indicated that the α thalassaemia 2 determinant must result from the loss of one of the linked pair of α globin genes per haploid genome. This observation has been confirmed by gene mapping analysis.

If the normal α globin gene haplotype (i.e. gene complement on a single chromosome) is written $\alpha\alpha$, the deletion form of α thalassaemia 2 can be written $-\alpha$. Extensive studies in the Jamaican and American Negro populations (Higgs et al, 1979; Dozy et al, 1979b) and some Mediterranean and Oriental populations (Orkin et al, 1979b; Kan et al, 1979) have indicated that the form of α thalassaemia 2 which results from a single α gene deletion is widespread. Studies in American Negroes (Dozy et al, 1979b) and in Jamaicans (Higgs et al, 1980c) indicate that approximately 23 to 35 per cent of these populations are heterozygous for the deletion form of α thalassaemia 2 ($-\alpha$) and about 2 per cent are homozygous ($-\alpha/-\alpha$) for this determinant. These findings have cleared up the long standing question of the nature of α thalassaemia in Negroes. In such populations many individuals have been encountered who have the phenotype of the severe form of α thalassaemia (α thalassaemia 1) and yet haemoglobin H disease is extremely rare and the haemoglobin Bart's hydrops syndrome has not been reported. It is now clear that individuals of African background who have the phenotype of α thalassaemia 1 are nearly always homozygous for the deletion form of α thalassaemia 2 ($-\alpha/-\alpha$), i.e. since the output of each of the α globin genes appears to be more or less equal (Hunt et al, 1980) the phenotypic expression of two α globin genes is the same whether they are both on one chromosome or on opposite pairs of homologous chromosomes, i.e. whether they have the genotype $-\alpha/-\alpha$ or $--/\alpha\alpha$.

Gene mapping analysis indicates that there is also heterogeneity in the molecular basis for the production of deletion forms of α thalassaemia 2. The commonest mechanism seems to have been unequal crossing over which has resulted in loss of parts of both the 5' and 3' α globin genes with the production of a single gene (Orkin

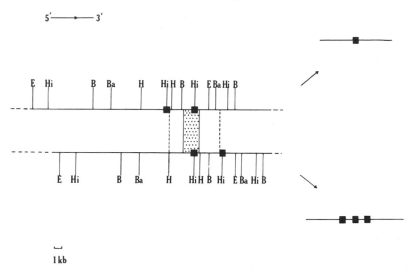

Fig. 3.4 The crossover event responsible for the production of the deletion form of α thalassaemia 2. The unequal crossing over gives rise to one chromosome with a single α chain locus and another with three α chain loci.

et al, 1979b; Phillips et al, 1979; Higgs et al, 1980c). However, a Chinese subject has been found with a different type of deletion which involves the 5' α globin gene (Embury et al, 1979). This deletion, which seems less common than the one mentioned above, has resulted from crossing over at a different site (Fig. 3.4). A consequence of unequal crossing over between mispaired α chain genes is that one of the chromosomes produced should have three α genes on it, just as the anti-Lepore chromosome has three non-α globin genes (Baglioni, 1962). Quite recently examples of the $\alpha\alpha\alpha$ haplotype have been discovered (Goossens et al, 1980; Higgs et al, 1980b). The clinical consequences of having five α globin genes, i.e. chromosomes with the arrangement $\alpha\alpha$ and $\alpha\alpha\alpha$, seem to be minimal. There are no haematological abnormalities and globin chain synthesis is almost balanced although it is clear that all five genes are expressed since there is an increased α/β globin messenger RNA ratio (Higgs et al, 1980b). Presumably the slight excess of α chains produced can be dealt with by the proteolytic enzymes of the red cell precursors. It is possible that this genotype may behave as a mild form of β thalassaemia (?silent β thalassaemia) and might interact with true β thalassaemia to produce a mild form of β thalassaemia intermedia.

Gene mapping analysis has also clarified some of the interactions between α thalassaemia and α chain haemoglobin variants. For instance, it has been found that at least one form of haemoglobin Q is due to a mutation on an α globin gene which is on a chromosome in which the other α chain locus is deleted ($-\alpha^Q$). Thus individuals who inherit this chromosome from one parent and an α thalassaemia 1 determinant from the other parent have haemoglobin Q-H disease ($-\alpha^Q/--$) in which the haemoglobin consists only of Q and H with no haemoglobin A (Lie-Injo et al, 1979; Higgs et al, 1980a).

Not all α thalassaemia 2 determinants result from gene deletions. Using soluble hybridisation techniques Kan et al (1977) reported a non-deletion form of α

thalassaemia 2 in a Chinese family. Non-deletion forms of α thalassaemia of this type have been found in many populations (Orkin et al, 1979b; Kan et al, 1979). It is becoming clear that there is considerable heterogeneity within this group of α thalassaemias. Thus although the non-deletion determinant described by Kan et al (1977) behaved phenotypically as an α thalassaemia 2, recent work by Pressley et al (1980c) in the Eastern Saudi Arabian population indicates that there is a non-deletion form of α thalassaemia which causes a greater deficiency of α chain production and which, in the homozygous state, produces typical haemoglobin H disease.

The phenotype of α thalassaemia 2 can also result from the inheritance of one of the α chain termination mutants such as haemoglobin Constant Spring (Weatherall & Clegg, 1975). This group of haemoglobin variants result from single base substitutions in the α chain termination codon so that instead of the α chains being 141 amino acid residues long they have an extra 30 residues at their C terminal ends due to 'read through' of α globin messenger RNA which is not normally translated. The reason for the grossly inefficient synthesis of these chain termination mutants appears to be instability of their messenger RNAs (Dr D M Hunt, unpublished data). Why the 'reading through' of normally untranslated α globin messenger RNA sequences causes this instability is not yet understood. This family of haemoglobin variants are all associated with the phenotype of α thalassaemia 2 and when inherited together with an α thalassaemia 1 gene produce haemoglobin H disease. The commonest variant in this group seems to be haemoglobin Constant Spring which occurs in approximately 3 per cent of the Thai population.

The relationship between genotype and phenotype in the α thalassaemias

It is clear from the preceding sections that the haemoglobin Bart's hydrops syndrome can result from the homozygous state for several different molecular forms of α thalassaemia 1. Similarly, haemoglobin H disease is very heterogeneous at the molecular level and can result from a whole series of different interactions between α thalassaemia 1 and the various forms of α thalassaemia 2 or α chain termination mutants or, indeed, can result from the homozygous state for the more severe non-deletion forms of α thalassaemia. It is too early to say whether the phenotypic expression of these different forms of haemoglobin H disease are different. Recent work in Thailand suggests that the haemoglobin H disease with haemoglobin Constant Spring is associated with a lower haemoglobin level than the form which results from α thalassaemia $1/\alpha$ thalassaemia 2 interactions. Furthermore, the homozygous state for haemoglobin Constant Spring is phenotypically more severe than that for α thalassaemia 2 (Wasi, personal communication, 1980).

It has long been apparent that it is extremely difficult to distinguish the different α thalassaemia carrier states at the phenotypic level (see Weatherall & Clegg, 1981). Indeed, it has been shown recently in studies of the Jamaican Negro population that there is a considerable overlap between the haematological findings and α/β globin chain synthesis ratios between individuals who are normal or heterozygous or homozygous for α thalassaemia 2 (Higgs et al, 1980c). However, the different α thalassaemia genotypes can be distinguished by measurement of α/β globin messenger RNA ratios (Hunt et al, 1980).

One of the most commonly used methods for assessing α thalassaemia gene frequencies has been the estimation of levels of haemoglobin Bart's in newborn infants. A recent study has analysed the relative levels of haemoglobin Bart's in Jamaican newborn infants in terms of their genotypes as determined by restriction endonuclease mapping (Higgs et al, 1980d). These studies indicate that, at least in this population, the homozygous state for α thalassaemia 2 is associated with haemoglobin Bart's levels ranging from 3 to 10 per cent. On the other hand only a small proportion of infants who are heterozygous for α thalassaemia 2 had elevated levels of haemoglobin Bart's. These findings confirm that increased amounts of haemoglobin Bart's at birth indicate the presence of an α thalassaemia gene but that an infant may be heterozygous for α thalassaemia 2 and show no detectable haemoglobin Bart's. Whether this is true of α thalassaemia in all racial groups is not yet known; certainly in earlier studies in Thailand the relatively frequency of α thalassaemia 2 as determined by haemoglobin Bart's levels at birth seemed to be compatible with the gene frequencies of α thalassaemia 1 and haemoglobin H disease in that population (Na-Nakorn & Wasi, 1970).

Acquired haemoglobin H disease
In the last few years there has been a renewal of interest in the early observation of White et al (1960) that cells containing haemoglobin H inclusions might occur occasionally in patients with leukaemia. There have now been several reports of the occurrence of an acquired form of haemoglobin H disease in elderly patients with unusual myeloproliferative disorders, usually but not always ending in acute leukaemia (Weatherall et al, 1978). This type of haemoglobin H disease differs from the genetic form in several ways. The blood films are dimorphic with both hypochromic and normochromic populations of red cells and in many cases the degree of defective α chain synthesis is much greater than in the genetic form of the disorder. Indeed there appears to be an almost complete shutdown of α chain production by the abnormal cell line. Despite this, the α globin genes are intact and the defect seems to be a non-deletion form of acquired α thalassaemia (Old et al, 1977; Weatherall et al, 1978). Although the molecular mechanism for this condition has not yet been worked out it is clear that it must be very unusual in that it cuts down the output of α chain production from both pairs of homologous chromosomes 16 and yet the globin genes are intact. It will be of great interest to determine the molecular basis for this condition not in the least because of the light it might throw on the mechanisms of leukaemic transformation.

THE β THALASSAEMIAS

The β thalassaemias show considerable heterogeneity. They can be broadly divided into β^+ thalassaemia in which there is some β chain synthesis and $\beta°$ thalassaemia in which there is a complete absence of β chain production. Recent work indicates that both forms of the condition are very heterogeneous at the molecular level.

β^+ thalassaemia
The homozygous state for β^+ thalassaemia usually produces a transfusion dependent form of thalassaemia major. However, this is not always the case and there is considerable clinical heterogeneity which almost certainly reflects a diversity of molecular forms of the condition. For example, in the severe Mediterranean form of

β^+ thalassaemia there is a very low level of β chain synthesis whereas in the milder Negro form there is considerably more β chain production. Evidence for the existence of several distinct forms of β^+ thalassaemia is reviewed by Weatherall & Clegg (1981).

Recently some progress has been made in establishing the molecular basis for the β^+ thalassaemias. Most of them are associated with a reduced output of β globin messenger RNA. At least in some cases this may result from a defect in processing of the nuclear messenger RNA precursor to its definitive cytoplasmic form (Nienhuis et al, 1977; Maquat et al, 1980). Maquat and her colleagues have speculated that the underlying genetic lesions are at splicing signal regions or within the introns of the β globin genes.

$\beta°$ thalassaemia

The homozygous state for $\beta°$ thalassaemia usually results in a transfusion dependent disorder although some patients with the disorder have the clinical phenotype of thalassaemia intermedia (Weatherall et al, 1980).

The $\beta°$ thalassaemias are very heterogeneous at the molecular level. In most cases globin gene mapping has shown no abnormality. An exception was found in DNA obtained from three Afro-Asians. Although these children appear to be homozygous for $\beta°$ thalassaemia, in fact they are compound heterozygotes for a $\beta°$ thalassaemia determinant associated with a normal β globin gene map and one in which there is an 0.6 kb deletion at the 3' end of the β gene (Orkin et al, 1979c; Flavell et al, 1979). More recently the β gene from one of these patients has been cloned and its structure determined. The 0.6 kb deletion has removed the terminal third of the large intervening sequence, the entire 3' coding block and about 150 base pairs past the end of the β globin gene (Orkin et al, 1980).

The technique of cDNA/mRNA hybridisation has also produced evidence for heterogeneity of the $\beta°$ thalassaemias. In some cases there appears to be no β globin messenger RNA transcribed (Forget et al, 1974, 1976a; Housman et al, 1974; Ottolenghi et al, 1975; Tolstoshev et al, 1976; Old et al, 1978; Benz et al, 1978), while in others some is detectable. Old et al (1978) and Benz et al (1978) analysed β globin messenger RNA in peripheral blood samples of $\beta°$ thalassaemics from a wide variety of racial groups. Three patterns were defined: (1) no β globin messenger RNA detectable, (2) significant amounts of apparently full-length but non-functional β messenger RNA, and (3) structurally abnormal β messenger RNA. Further analysis by Old et al (1978) showed that in one British $\beta°$ thalassaemia homozygote there was a full length β globin messenger RNA but that a hexanucleotide primer d(GCACCA), specific for the Met-Val-His coding sequence at the 5' end of the β globin messenger RNA, bound very inefficiently to the β thalassaemic messenger RNA as compared with normal RNA, suggesting a defect at or near the chain initiation site. In contrast β messenger RNA obtained from Saudi Arabian and Pakistani patients with $\beta°$ thalassaemia were shown to have abnormal 3' non-coding sequences, possibly involving a deletion or insertion of approximately 100 bases at the extreme 3' non-coding and coding sequences.

More recently Chang & Kan (1979) have determined the nucleotide sequence of the non-functional β messenger RNA from a Chinese patient with $\beta°$ thalassaemia. They have shown that the AAG codon for lysine at position $\beta17$ has changed to the chain termination codon UAG thus leading to premature chain termination with the production of a short 16 residue N-terminal fragment of the β chain. The same group went on to confirm these findings by translating the defective β globin messenger RNA in a cell-free system using a UAG tyrosine suppressor tRNA; full-length β globin genes were synthesised (Chang et al, 1979).

In addition to these cases of β° thalassaemia with non-functional β globin messenger RNA there are several reported cases in which β messenger RNA could be only detected in the nuclei of bone marrow cells (Comi et al, 1977). These observations suggest that some forms of β° thalassaemia may result from defects of processing β globin RNA precursor. Finally, there is the Ferrara form of β° thalassaemia in which it appears that β globin messenger RNA is present but β globin chain synthesis only occurs in the presence of a factor obtained from a soluble cell fraction from normal red cells (Conconi et al, 1972; Conconi & del Senno, 1974). This condition has not been found in any other racial group.

Clearly the β° thalassaemias are remarkably heterogeneous at the molecular level. It seems very likely that more nonsense mutations of the type described by Chang & Kan (1979) will be defined. As pointed out by Chang et al (1980) 25 different single base mutations in the β globin gene could result in termination codons. Thus, assay with suppressor tRNAs may be a useful screening method for detecting this type of lesion in β° thalassaemia.

Further diversity of the β thalassaemias

In the last two years some progress has been made in defining forms of the β thalassaemias in which there are normal haemoglobin A_2 levels in heterozygotes. In one type the haematological findings in carriers are normal and yet there is imbalanced globin chain synthesis; this determinant can interact with high haemoglobin A_2 β thalassaemia to produce a form of thalassaemia intermedia (Schwartz, 1969; Kattamis et al, 1979). In another variety the haematological changes in heterozygotes are indistinguishable from those of high haemoglobin A_2 β thalassaemia; this determinant interacts with the latter to produce a transfusion-dependent disorder (Kattamis et al, 1979). There is some evidence that the second variety of normal haemoglobin A_2 β thalassaemia may in fact represent the compound heterozygous state for both δ and β thalassaemia (Silvestroni et al, 1978). These varieties of β thalassaemia with normal haemoglobin A_2 levels are of considerable importance from the point of view of genetic counselling since haematologically they resemble the β thalassaemia carrier states.

There seem to be yet more distinct types of β thalassaemia. For a complete review the reader is referred to the monograph of Weatherall & Clegg (1981).

The $\delta\beta$ thalassaemias

The genetic disorders of δ and β chain synthesis include the haemoglobin Lepore syndromes, the $\delta\beta$ thalassaemias and some forms of hereditary persistence of fetal haemoglobin (HPFH). We will consider the latter group in a separate section.

The haemoglobin Lepore disorders have been reviewed recently (Efremov, 1978; Weatherall & Clegg, 1981). Haemoglobin Lepore consists of normal α chains combined with $\delta\beta$ chains which are the product of $\delta\beta$ genes which have arisen by unequal crossing over between the δ and β globin loci during meiosis (see Bank et al, 1980). The $\delta\beta$ fusion chains are inefficiently synthesised, at least in part because of instability of $\delta\beta$ globin messenger RNA (Wood et al, 1978). In the homozygous state, in which the haemoglobin consists of Lepore and F only, the clinical picture is similar to homozygous β thalassaemia although curiously some of the reported cases seem to have been forms of thalassaemia intermedia.

The $\delta\beta$ thalassaemias are classified according to the structure of the associated haemoblobin F into $^G\gamma$ and $^G\gamma^A\gamma$ varieties respectively. Homozygotes have a form of thalassaemia intermedia; only haemoglobin F is produced (Wood et al, 1979). It appears as though the $^G\gamma$ variety is slightly more severe in the homozygous state although the heterozygous carrier states for the two types are indistinguishable except by chemical analysis of the haemoglobin F.

Soluble hybridisation analysis of DNA prepared from $^G\gamma^A\gamma$ $\delta\beta$ thalassaemia homozygotes shows that there is a major deletion involving the δ and β globin genes although these studies suggest that at least part of the δ (or β) globin genes are still intact (Ottolenghi et al, 1976; Ramirez et al, 1976). These findings have been confirmed and extended by globin-gene mapping analysis which shows that $^G\gamma^A\gamma$ $\delta\beta$ thalassaemia results from a gene deletion which leaves the 5' end of the δ globin gene intact but extends right through the β globin gene and to some distance beyond its 3' end (Mears et al, 1978a, b; Ottolenghi et al, 1979; Fritsch et al, 1979; Bernards et al, 1979) (Fig. 3.5).

It is becoming increasingly clear that $^G\gamma$ $\delta\beta$ thalassaemia is heterogeneous at the molecular level (Fig. 3.5). In DNA from a Turkish $^G\gamma$ $\delta\beta$ thalassaemia homozygote it was found that there is a long deletion involving both δ and β globin genes together with the $^A\gamma$ gene (Fritsch et al, 1979; Orkin et al, 1979a). Recent work in the authors' laboratory indicates that the disorder can result from a major disruption of the γ-δ-β gene cluster arising from an inversion and two deletions (Jones et al, 1981).

γ-δ-β thalassaemia
Van der Ploeg et al (1980) have described a family in which studies of newborns and

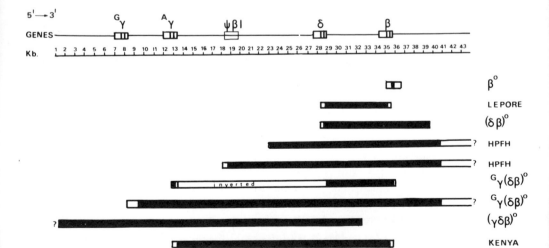

Fig. 3.5 The different deletions responsible for hereditary persistence of fetal haemoglobin (HPFH), the Lepore haemoglobins, $^G\gamma$ $\delta\beta$ thalassaemia, $^G\gamma^A\gamma$ $\delta\beta$ thalassaemia (($\delta\beta$)° thalassaemia), $\gamma\delta\beta$ thalassaemia and haemoglobin Kenya. The small deletion responsible for one form of β° thalassaemia is also shown.

their relatives provide evidence, ableit preliminary, that several individuals are heterozygous for a form of thalassaemia characterised by defective γ, δ and β chain synthesis. The condition results from an extensive deletion involving the γ and δ globin genes; the β gene and large segments of DNA which flank the 3' and 5' ends are intact. The particular interest of this finding is that a deletion some distance from the β gene appears to result in the suppression of its activity.

HEREDITARY PERSISTENCE OF FETAL HAEMOGLOBIN (HPFH)

This subject has been reviewed in detail recently (Wood et al, 1979; Bernards & Flavell, 1980; Weatherall & Clegg, 1981). The term HPFH describes a condition in which there is persistent haemoglobin F production in adult life in the absence of major haematological abnormalities. It was first defined in Negro and Greek populations. In the Negro type heterozygotes have between 15 and 30 per cent haemoglobin F and homozygotes have 100 per cent haemoglobin F, i.e. the HPFH determinant causes a complete absence of δ and β chain synthesis. The Greek form has not been observed in the homozygous state but heterozygotes have lower levels of haemoglobin F and there is indirect evidence that β chain (and possibly δ chain) synthesis is not entirely shut off on the chromosome carrying the HPFH determinant. These conditions can also be categorised according to the structure of the haemoglobin F. For example, most Negro types have both $^{G}\gamma$ and $^{A}\gamma$ chains although they are found at different ratios which appear to be genetically determined (see Huisman et al, 1974, 1975). The haemoglobin F in the Greek type has mainly $^{A}\gamma$ chains with about 10 per cent $^{G}\gamma$ chains (Clegg et al, 1979). The rarer forms of HPFH such as haemoglobin Kenya and $^{G}\gamma$ β^{+} HPFH are reviewed by Weatherall & Clegg (1981).

A characteristic of both the Negro and Greek forms of HPFH is that the haemoglobin F in heterozygotes is relatively uniformly distributed among the red cells. However, there is another type of HPFH in which the haemoglobin F level in heterozygotes are lower than are found in the Negro and Greek forms and it is heterogeneously distributed among the red cells. Hence Boyer et al (1977) suggested that HPFH should be divided into pancellular and heterocellular forms. In the only reported cases of homozygosity for heterocellular HPFH significant amounts of haemoglobin A and A$_2$ are present indicating that the genetic determinant for this condition does not cause a complete shutdown of δ and β chain synthesis (Weatherall et al, 1975).

Soluble hybridisation experiments using DNA from Negroes homozygous for $^{G}\gamma^{A}\gamma$ HPFH indicate that there is a major deletion involving the δ and β globin genes (Kan et al, 1975b; Ottolenghi et al, 1976; Ramirez et al, 1976; Forget et al, 1976b). Gene mapping analysis by Mears et al (1978b), Ottolenghi et al (1979), Fritsch et al (1979) and Tuan et al (1980) have shown that the $^{G}\gamma^{A}\gamma$ HPFH DNA contains neither 3' β sequences nor 5' β or δ sequences and that both δ and β globin genes are deleted; the excised region extends from 1 kb to the left of the δ gene to at least 4 kb to the right of the β gene. This form of HPFH is heterogeneous; the deletion studied by Tuan et al (1980) involves an additional 5 kb of the inter γ-δ flanking DNA as compared with that described by Fritsch et al (1979) and an even longer deletion is reported in another case by Bernards & Flavell (1980) (Fig. 3.5).

Recent studies by Tuan et al (1980), Bernards & Flavell (1980) and in the author's laboratory (Jones & Old, unpublished data) have shown that there is no abnormality of gene mapping of DNA obtained from individuals with the Greek form of HPFH or those homozygous for heterocellular HPFH. Whether these conditions result from a deletion which is too small to be seen by current mapping techniques, or whether they are caused by a more 'distant' regulatory mutation, remains to be seen.*

Lessons about the regulation of haemoglobin F production from $\delta\beta$ thalassaemia and HPFH

It is becoming clear that the pancellular HPFH is really a well compensated form of $\delta\beta$ thalassaemia. In all the homozygotes studied so far there have been low MCH and MCV values and imbalanced globin chain synthesis. The only difference between heterozygotes for pancellular HPFH and $\delta\beta$ thalassaemia is that in the former there are minimal haematological changes and the haemoglobin F is more or less uniformly distributed among the red cells whereas in the latter the red cells are poorly haemoglobinised and the haemoglobin F has a heterocellular distribution. Wood et al (1979) have suggested that these apparent differences may be artefactual and reflect the techniques used to determine the intercellular distribution of haemoglobin F, i.e. the only real difference between pancellular HPFH and $\delta\beta$ thalassaemia is in the amount of γ chain which is produced to compensate for the lack of δ and β chains. If this is correct, all these conditions can be regarded as a spectrum of disorders of δ and β chain production with varying levels of γ chain synthesis; at one end are the haemoglobin Lepore thalassaemias in which there is relatively little γ chain compensation while at the other end there are the Negro forms of $^G\gamma^A\gamma$ pancellular HPFH in which γ chain synthesis almost completely makes up for lack of δ and β chain production.

Has the detailed analysis of the various deletions which result in HPFH or $\delta\beta$ thalassaemia provided any insight into the regulation of γ and β chain synthesis during normal human development? It is beyond the scope of this review to more than briefly outline current ideas about human haemoglobin gene switching; they are covered in detail elsewhere (Nienhuis & Stamatoyannopoulos, 1978; Wood & Jones, 1980).

As mentioned earlier, the order of non-α globin genes on chromosome 11 is ε-$^G\gamma$-$^A\gamma$-δ-β. These genes are activated consecutively from the 5' (left hand) end during ontogeny. There is increasing evidence from both in vitro red cell colony work and from haemoglobin synthesis studies in fractionated erythroid precursors, that during erythroid maturation the γ globin genes are transcribed first, followed by the δ and β genes (see Stamatoyannopoulos et al, 1979; Comi et al, 1980; Wood & Jones, 1980). These observations, together with the fact that there is persistent γ chain synthesis associated with the deletions which produce $\delta\beta$ thalassaemia or pancellular HPFH, raise the question as to whether there are specific areas of the γ-δ-β gene cluster which are involved in the regulation of γ chain production during development. The fact that in some forms of Negro $^G\gamma^A\gamma$ HPFH the β and δ globin genes and their flanking regions are deleted, whereas in $^G\gamma^A\gamma$ $\delta\beta$ thalassaemia the 5' end of the δ globin gene is intact, suggest that there may be a 'regulation area' somewhere to the 5' flanking region of the δ globin gene (see Huisman et al, 1974; Bank et al, 1980; Tuan

---

* Recent restriction endonuclease analysis indicates that the genetic determinant for the British form of heterocellular HPFH is linked to the γ-δ-β gene complex (unpublished studies from the author's laboratory).

et al, 1980). Clearly, we need much more mapping data together with a careful correlation of the phenotypes which result from small deletions of this gene cluster. It is possible, of course, that a coherent story may not emerge; it may be that any major disruption of the γ-δ-β gene cluster will result in persistent activation of the γ chain genes.

ANTENATAL DIAGNOSIS OF HAEMOGLOBIN DISORDERS USING DNA ANALYSIS

Antenatal diagnosis of the β thalassaemias and sickle cell anaemia is currently carried out by fetal blood sampling followed by globin chain synthesis analysis (see Alter et al, 1980). This technique, while reliable, is still associated with a significant fetal loss and the laboratory procedures are relatively complex. Clearly it would be better if it were possible to diagnose these disorders by analysis of fetal DNA obtained from amniotic fluid cells. If sufficient DNA can be obtained, and if the fetus is at risk for a form of thalassaemia which is due to a gene deletion, it should be possible to determine whether it is homozygous for this condition. This approach has been used for the diagnosis of α thalassaemia and $\delta\beta$ thalassaemia in utero (Orkin et al, 1978; Dozy et al, 1979a). However, apart from the rare form of β° thalassaemia which is due to a partial β globin gene deletion, the majority of these disorders are associated with normal restriction enzyme maps and hence at the moment this approach has limited value.

However, it has been shown recently that there are polymorphisms of DNA sequences adjacent to the globin genes. For example, Kan & Dozy (1978a and b) discovered a polymorphism of the recognition site for the enzyme Hpa I which cleaves DNA at the sequence GTTAAC. When normal DNA is restricted with this enzyme the β globin genes are usually found on a DNA fragment about 7.6 kb long. However, in some individuals the DNA fragment containing the β globin genes is lengthened to 13 kb as a result of a mutation in the Hpa recognition site at the 3' side of the β globin gene. In the American Negro populations the variant 13 kb Hpa I fragment is very frequently associated with the sickle cell mutation (Kan & Dozy, 1978a and b; Kan et al, 1980b). This observation is of considerable anthropological interest and suggests that the sickle mutation in West Africa originated on a chromosome bearing the variant with the 13.0 kb Hpa I fragment. Interestingly this is not the case in East Africa or in the Middle East. It follows that it is possible to use this polymorphism for the antenatal diagnosis of sickle cell anaemia, at least in families of West African origin in which the mutation is on the chromosome containing the variant Hpa I site.

Another polymorphism of the DNA sequence close to the β globin gene has been found in Sardinia and promises to be useful for the antenatal diagnosis of β° thalassaemia in that population, at least in up to 30 per cent of cases (Kan et al, 1980a). Digestion of normal human DNA with the restriction enzyme Bam H1 splits the β globin gene into a 5' portion contained in a 1.8 kb fragment and a 3' portion with a 9.3 kb fragment. In some subjects variation in the nucleotide sequence affecting the site recognised by this enzyme on the 3' side of the β globin gene produces a fragment 22 kb in length which contains the 3' portion of the β globin gene. In Sardinians without β thalassaemia the frequency of the 9.3 kb fragment is 0.67 and that of the 22 kb fragment is 0.33. In contrast all the β° thalassaemia determinants in that population are associated exclusively with the 9.3 kb fragment. Thus it appears that the β thalassaemia lesion in Sardinians arose on a chromosome that had the polymorphism responsible for the 9.3 kb Bam H1 fragment. This observation can be used in the antenatal diagnosis of some cases of β° thalassaemia since if the 22.0 kb fragment is demonstrated it indicates that at least one normal β-globin-gene-carrying chromosome is present and excludes the β° thalassaemia lesion on that chromosome.

In some populations it has not yet been possible to find polymorphisms related to the β globin genes which might be applicable to this approach to antenatal diagnosis. However, it is early days and several groups are actively involved in further studies of this type. Another approach to this problem was reported recently by Little et al (1980) who used a polymorphism which occurs in the large intron of the $^G\gamma$ and/or $^A\gamma$ genes for the antenatal diagnosis of β thalassaemia. Since the γ and β genes are linked, and if family studies can determine whether the γ gene polymorphism is (or is not) on the same chromosome as the β thalassaemia determinant, this approach should be feasible.

Possibilities for correcting the genetic disorders of haemoglobin synthesis
Following these remarkable advances in the molecular genetics of human haemoglobin it is not surprising that in recent years thoughts have been turning to the possibility of replacing defective or missing globin genes.

Mammalian cells will accept foreign DNA although the process seems to be extremely inefficient. Furthermore, such DNA can be integrated into the chromosomes of the 'foreign' cells. Several methods have been used to try to improve the efficiency of methods for introducing DNA into recipient cells. For example the genes can be introduced into modified versions of certain DNA viruses such as SV40 or polyoma. If the gene is in the correct orientation and near a viral promotor site, RNA is made from the inserted gene as well as from the virus and sometimes genes inserted into these vectors can be properly transcribed, processed and translated. Another approach, in this case utilising a herpes virus, is to use the virus thymidine kinase (TK) gene as a selective marker for transformation of TK deficient cell lines by genes linked to fragments of virus DNA containing the TK gene. Indeed correct transcription and processing of rabbit globin genomic DNA linked to a cloned herpes TK gene has been demonstrated (see Mulligan & Berg, 1980).

Recently an extremely novel approach to the problem of obtaining selective proliferation of cells which have been treated with foreign DNA was described (Cline et al, 1980). These workers induced resistance to the drug methotrexate in bone marrow cells of mice by transformation in vitro with DNA from a drug-resistant cell line. The latter has many copies of the gene for dihydrofolate reductase (DHFR). The transformed cells were injected in vivo and haemopoietic cells expressing drug resistance were selected by drug treatment of the recipient animal. The transformed cells had elevated levels of dihydrofolate reductase and demonstrated a proliferative advantage over untransfused cells indicating successful gene transfer. The idea of conferring a selective resistance to a particular drug by genetic engineering is of great interest in several areas of haematology. In the present context it might be possible to transfer a globin gene together with genes for drug resistance and hence allow selective proliferation of a cell line in a recipient bone marrow by treating the patient with the appropriate drug after injection of the transformed marrow cells.

Of course, the difficulties in this field are immense. Bone marrow cells have to be transformed and the inserted genes have to be regulated in the same way as normal globin genes. Expression of globin genes in the wrong cell population or the production of imbalanced globin chain synthesis could be disastrous. Clearly, a method for obtaining preferential proliferation of a transformed stem cell line has to be worked out; a proliferative advantage later in the erythroid differentiation pathway would be useless. However, this field has moved so fast in the last few years that it is not inconceivable that by the time the next edition of this series is written such transformation experiments using human bone marrow will have been carried out successfully.

REFERENCES

Alter B P, Orkin S H, Forget B G, Nathan D G 1980 Annals of the New York Academy of Sciences 344: 151–164

Baglioni C 1962 Proceedings of the National Academy of Sciences of the United States of America 48: 1880–1886

Baltimore D 1970 Nature 226: 1209–1211

Bank A, Mears J G, Ramirez F 1980 Science 207: 486–493

Bellingham A J 1976 British Medical Bulletin 32: 234–238

Benz E J, Forget B G, Hillman D G, Cohen-Solal M, Pritchard J, Cavallesco C 1978 Cell 14: 229–312

Bernards R, Flavell R A 1980 Nucleic Acids Research 8: 1521–1534

Bernards R, Kooter J M, Flavell R A 1979 Gene 6: 265–280

Boyer S H, Margolet L, Boyer M L, Huisman T H J, Schroeder W A, Wood W G, Weatherall D J, Clegg J B, Cartner R 1977 American Journal of Human Genetics 29: 256–271

Bunn H F, Forget B G, Ranney H M 1977 Human Hemoglobins, Saunders, Philadelphia p 312

Chang J C, Kan Y W 1979 Proceedings of the National Academy of Sciences of the United States of America 76: 2886–2889

Chang J C, Kan Y W, Trecartin R F, Temple G F 1980 Annals of the New York Academy of Sciences 344: 113–119

Chang J C, Temple G F, Trecartin R F, Kan Y W 1979 Nature 281: 602–603

Clegg J B, Metaxatou-Mavromati A, Kattamis C, Sofroniadou K, Wood W G, Weatherall D J 1979 British Journal of Haematology 43: 521–536

Cline M J, Stang H, Mercola K, Morse L, Ruprecht R, Browne J, Salser W 1980 Nature 284: 422–425

Comi P, Giglioni B, Barbarano L, Ottolenghi S, Williamson R, Novakova M, Masera G 1977 European Journal of Biochemistry 79: 617–622

Comi P, Giglioni B, Ottolenghi S, Gianni A M, Polli E, Barba P, Covelli A, Migliaccio G, Condorelli M, Peschle C 1980 Proceedings of the National Academy of Sciences of the United States of America 77: 362–365

Conconi F, del Senno L 1974 Annals of the New York Academy of Sciences 232: 54–64

Conconi F, Rowley P T, del Senno L, Pontremoli S, Volpato S 1972 Nature New Biology 238: 83–87

Deisseroth A, Nienhuis A, Lawrence J, Riles R, Turner P, Ruddle F 1978 Proceedings of the National Academy of Sciences of the United States of American 75: 1456–1460

Deisseroth A, Nienhuis A, Turner P, Velez R, Anderson W F, Ruddle F, Lawrence J, Creagan R, Kucherlapati R 1977 Cell 12: 205–218

Dozy A M, Forman E N, Abuelo D N, Barsel-Bowers G, Mahoney M J, Forget B G, Kan Y W 1979a Journal of the American Medical Association 24: 1610–1612

Dozy A M, Kan Y W, Embury S H, Mentzer W C, Wang W C, Lubin B, Davis J R, Koenig H M 1979b Nature 280: 605–607

Efremov G D 1978 Hemoglobin 2: 197–233

Embury S H, Lebo R V, Dozy A M, Kan Y W 1979 Journal of Clinical Investigation 63: 1307–1310

Flavell R A, Bernards R, Kooter J H, de Boer E, Little P F R, Annison G, Williamson R 1979 Nucleic Acids Research 6: 2749–2760

Forget B G, Baltimore D, Benz E J, Housman D, Lebowitz P, Marotta C A, McCaffrey R P, Skoultchi A, Swerdlow P S, Vernon I M, Weissman S M 1974 Annals of the New York Academy of Sciences 232: 76–87

Forget B G, Hillman D G, Cohen-Solal M, Prensky W 1976a Blood 48: 998
Forget B G, Hillman D G, Lazarus H, Barell E F, Benz E J, Caskey C T, Huisman T H J, Schroeder W A, Housman D 1976b Cell 7: 323–329
Fritsch E F, Lawn R M, Maniatis T 1979 Nature 279: 598–603
Goossens M, Dozy A M, Embury S H, Zachariades Z, Hadjiminas M G, Stamatoyannopoulos G, Kan Y W 1980 Proceedings of the National Academy of Sciences of the United States of America 77: 518–521
Higgs D R, Hunt D M, Drysdale C H, Clegg J B, Pressley L, Weatherall D J 1980a British Journal of Haematology 46: 387–400
Higgs D R, Old J M, Pressley L, Clegg J B, Weatherall D J 1980b Nature 284: 632–635
Higgs D R, Pressley L, Clegg J B, Weatherall D J, Sergeant G R 1980c Johns Hopkins Medical Journal 146: 300–310
Higgs D R, Pressley L, Clegg J B, Weatherall D J, Serjeant G R, Higgs S, Carey P 1980d British Journal of Haematology 46: 39–46
Higgs D R, Pressley L, Old J M, Hunt D M, Clegg J B, Weatherall D J, Serjeant G R 1979 Lancet ii: 272–276
Housman D, Skoultchi A, Forget B G, Benz E J 1974 Annals of the New York Acdemy of Sciences 241: 280–289
Huehns E R 1981 In: (eds) Hardisty R M and Weatherall D J. Blood and Its Disorders, 2nd Edn Blackwell Scientific Publications, Oxford (in press)
Huisman T H J, Miller A, Cook L, Gordon S, Schroeder W A 1975 (ed) Aksoy M International Istanbul Symposium on Abnormal Hemoglobins and Thalassemia p 95–110
Huisman T H J, Schroeder W A, Efremov G D, Duma H, Mladenovsky B, Hyman C B, Rachmilewitz E A, Bouver N, Miller A, Brodie A, Shelton J R, Shelton J B, Apell G 1974 Annals of the New York Academy of Sciences 232: 107–124
Hunt D M, Higgs D R, Old J M, Clegg J B, Weatherall D J, Marsh G W 1981 British Journal of Haematology 45: 53–64
Jones R W, Old J M, Trent R J, Clegg J B, Weatherall D J 1981 Nature 291, 39–44
Kan Y W, Dozy A M 1978a Proceedings of the National Academy of Sciences of the United States of America 75: 5631–5635
Kan Y W, Dozy A M 1978b Lancet ii: 910
Kan Y W, Dozy A M, Stamatoyannopoulos G, Hadjiminas M G, Zachariades Z, Furbetta M, Cao A 1979 Blood 54: 1434–1438
Kan Y W, Dozy A M, Trecartin R, Todd D 1977 New England Journal of Medicine 297, 1081–1085
Kan Y W, Dozy A M, Varmus H E, Taylor J M, Holland J P, Lie-Injo L E, Ganesan J, Todd D 1975a Nature 255: 255–256
Kan Y W, Holland J P, Dozy A M, Charache S, Kazazian H H 1975b Nature 258: 162–163
Kan Y W, Lee K Y, Furbetta M, Anguis A, Cao A, 1980a New England Journal of Medicine 302: 185–188
Kan Y W, Trecartin R F, Dozy A M 1980b Annals of the New York Academy of Sciences 344: 141–150
Kattamis C, Metaxatou-Mavromati A, Tsiarta E, Metaxatou C, Wasi P, Wood W G, Pressley L, Higgs D R, Clegg J B, Weatherall D J 1980 British Medical Journal ii: 268–270
Kattamis C, Mataxatou-Mavromati A, Wood W G, Nash J R, Weatherall D J 1979 British Journal of Haematology 42: 109–123
Lawn R M, Fritsch E F, Porter R C, Blake G, Maniatis T 1978 Cell 15: 1157–1174
Lauer J, Shen C-K J, Maniatis T 1980 Cell 20: 119–130
Lie-Injo, L E, Dozy A M, Kan Y W, Lopes M, Todd D 1979 Blood 54: 1407–1416
Little P F R, Annison G, Darling S, Williamson R, Camba L, Modell B 1980 Nature 285: 144–147
Maniatis T 1980 (ed) Goldstein L and Prescott D M Cell Biology, A comprehensive treatise. Vol 3 Academic Press, New York p 564
Maniatis T, Hardison R C, Lacy E, Lauer J, O'Connell C, Quon D, Sim G K, Efstratiadis A 1978 Cell 15: 687–701
Maquat L E, Kinniburgh A J, Beach L R, Honig G R, Lazerson J, Ershler W B, Ross J 1980 Proceedings of the National Academy of Sciences of the United States of America 77: 4287–4294
Mears J G, Ramirez F, Leibowitz D, Bank A 1978a Cell 15: 15–23
Mears J G, Ramirez F, Liebowitz D, Nakaura F, Bloom A, Konotey-Ahulu F I D, Bank A 1978b Proceedings of the National Academy of Sciences of the United States of America 75: 1222–1226
Mulligan R C, Berg P 1980 Science 209: 1422–1427
Na-Nakorn S, Wasi P 1970 American Journal of Human Genetics 22: 645–651
Nathans D, Smith H O 1975 Annual Review of Biochemistry 44: 273–293
Nienhuis A W, Stamatoyannopoulos G 1978 Cell 15: 307–315
Nienhuis A W, Turner P, Benz E J 1977 Proceedings of the National Academy of Sciences of the United States of America 74: 3960–3964
Old J, Longley J, Wood W G, Clegg J B, Weatherall D J 1977 Nature 269: 524–525

Old J M, Proudfoot N J, Wood W G, Longley J I, Clegg J B, Weatherall D J 1978 Cell 14: 289–298
Orkin S H, Alter B P, Altay C 1979a Journal of Clinical Investigation 64: 866–869
Orkin S H, Alter B P, Altay C, Mahoney M J, Lazarus H, Hobbins J C, Nathan D G 1978 New England Journal of Medicine 299: 166–172
Orkin S H, Kolodner R, Michelson A, Husson R 1980 Proceedings of the National Academy of Sciences of the United States of America 77: 3358–3562
Orkin S H, Michelson A 1980 Nature 286: 538–540
Orkin S H, Old J, Lazarus H, Altay C, Gurgey A, Weatherall D J, Nathan D G 1979b Cell 17: 33–42
Orkin S H, Old J M, Weatherall D J, Nathan D G 1979c Proceedings of the National Academy of Sciences of the United States of America 76: 2400–2404
Ottolenghi S, Comi P, Giglioni B, Tolstoshev P, Lanyon W G, Mitchell G J, Williamson R, Russo G, Musumeci S, Schiliro G, Tsistrakis G A, Charache S, Wood W G, Clegg J B, Weatherall D J 1976 Cell 9: 71–80
Ottolenghi S, Giglioni B, Comi P, Gianni A M, Polli E, Acquaye C T A, Oldham J H, Masera G 1979 Nature 278: 654–657
Ottolenghi S, Lanyon W G, Williamson R, Weatherall D J, Clegg J B, Pitcher C S 1975 Proceedings of the National Academy of Sciences of the United States of America 72: 2294–2299
Ottolenghi S, Lanyon W G, Paul J, Williamson R, Weatherall D J, Clegg J B, Pritchard J, Pootrakul S, Wong H B 1974 Nature 251: 389–392
Phillips J A, Scott A F, Smith K D, Young K D, Lightbody K L, Jiji R M, Kazazian H H 1979 Blood 54: 1439–1445
Pressley L, Higgs D R, Aldridge B, Metaxatou-Mavromati A, Tsiarta E, Kattamis C, Wood W G, Clegg J B, Weatherall D J 1980a Nucleic Acids Research 8: 4889–4894
Pressley L, Higgs D R, Clegg J B, Weatherall D J 1980b Proceedings of the National Academy of Sciences of the United States of America 77: 3586–3589
Pressley L, Higgs D R, Pembrey M E, Clegg J B, Weatherall D J 1980c New England Journal of Medicine 303: 1383–1388
Proudfoot N J, Shander M H M, Lanley J L, Gefter M L, Maniatis T 1980 Science 209: 1329–1336
Ramirez F, O'Donnell J V, Marks P A, Bank A, Musumeci S, Schiliro G, Pizzorelli G, Russo G, Luppis B, Gambino R 1976 Nature 263: 471–475
Schroeder W A, Huisman T H J, Shelton R, Shelton J B, Kleihauer E F, Dozy A M, Robberson B 1968 Proceedings of the National Academy of Sciences of the United States of America 60: 537–544
Schwartz E 1969 New England Journal of Medicine 281: 1327–1333
Silvestroni E, Bianco I, Graziani B, Carboni C 1978 Acta Haematologica 59: 332–340
Sophocleous T, Higgs D R, Aldridge B, Trent R J, Clegg J B, Weatherall D J 1981 British Journal of Haematology 47: 153–156
Southern E M 1975 Journal of Molecular Biology 98: 503–517
Stamatoyannopoulos G, Rosenblum B B, Papayannopoulou T, Brice M, Nakamoto B, Shepard T H 1979 Blood 54: 440–450
Taylor J M, Dozy A, Kan Y W, Varmus H E, Lie-Injo L E, Ganeson J, Todd D 1974 Nature 251: 392–393
Temin H M, Mizutani S 1970 Nature 266: 1211
Tolstoshev P, Mitchell J, Lanyon G, Williamson R, Ottolenghi S, Comi P, Giglioni B, Masera G, Modell B, Weatherall D J, Clegg J B 1976 Nature 260: 95–98
Tuan D, Murnanr M J, de Riel J K, Forget B G 1980 Nature 285: 335–337
van der Ploeg L H T, Konings A, Oort M, Roos D, Bernini L, Flavell R A 1980 Nature 283: 637–642
Weatherall D J, Cartner R, Clegg J B, Wood W G, Macrae I. A, MacKenzie A 1975 British Journal of Haematology 29: 205–220
Weatherall D J, Clegg J B 1975 Philosophical Transactions of the Royal Society 271: 411–455
Weatherall D J, Clegg J B 1979 Cell 16: 467–479
Weatherall D J, Clegg J B 1981 The Thalassaemia Syndromes 3rd Edn Blackwells Scientific Publications, Oxford
Weatherall D J, Clegg J B, Wood W G, Old J M, Higgs D R, Pressley L, Darbre P D 1980 Annals of the New York Academy of Sciences 344: 83–100
Weatherall D J, Old J, Longley J, Wood W G, Clegg J B, Pollock A, Lewis M J 1978 British Journal of Haematology 38: 305–322
White J M 1976 British Medical Bulletin 32: 219–222
White J C, Ellis M, Coleman P N, Beaven G H, Gratzer W B, Shooter E M, Skinner E R 1960 British Journal of Haematology 6: 171–177
Wood W G, Clegg J B, Weatherall D J 1979 British Journal of Haematology 43: 509–520
Wood W G, Jones R W 1980 (ed) Stamatoyannopoulos G, Nienhuis A W Proceedings of the 2nd Conference on Hemoglobin Switching, Arlie House, Virginia
Wood W G, Old J M, Roberts A V S, Clegg J B, Weatherall D J, Quattrin N 1978 Cell 15: 437–446

4. The red cell membrane and its abnormalities

Stanley L Schrier

INTRODUCTION

The adult human red blood cell picks up and delivers oxygen to the tissues, transports CO_2, and may participate in certain aspects of haemostasis (Turrito & Weiss, 1980). In order to carry out these functions this $7-8\,\mu$ diameter cell must deform and pass through $3\,\mu$ diameter capillaries, resist shearing forces across the aortic valve, and survive passage through the spleen and other reticuloendothelial (RE) organs where the flow is slow, metabolic depletion occurs, pH falls, and the red cells must pass through narrow sinusoidal slits where they are subjected to intense scrutiny by macrophages. Therefore the red cell must have the capacity to deform, recoil and slide across other red cells without either aggregating, fragmenting, or fusing. Blood flow is modified by the total number of erythrocytes, expressed as the PCV, and the type and amount of plasma proteins, particularly fibrinogen and the immunoglobulins. However, the characteristics of the erythrocyte per se play a critical role in blood flow, especially in the microcirculation.

Normally, the ability of red cells to withstand the stresses of the circulation fails after about 115 days. Red cell changes that would attract the attention of the RE system to remove or remodel the cell include alterations of shape or deformability such that the cells could not traverse the sinusoidal barrier and would therefore be subjected to stasis, acidosis, and metabolic depletion leading to eventual removal. Alteration of the negative charge or some other surface feature could also result in binding to macrophages or endothelial cells.

Shape, deformability, and surface features of the erythrocyte are determined by three interacting compartments: the membrane, haemoglobin, and the non-haemoglobin components, i.e. salts, water, and the substrates, cofactors and enzymes, mainly of glycolysis. Membrane function is affected by the kind and amount of haemoglobin present, by cell water and cation content, and by the energy level of the cell.

The intact erythrocyte has a diameter of 7 to $8\,\mu$, a volume of 85 to 90 fl, and surface area of $140\,\mu^2$. A sphere of volume 90 fl would have a diameter of approximately $5.5\,\mu$ and a surface area of $95\,\mu^2$. The excess surface area allows the red cell to assume a discocytic shape. The red cell differs from other cells in having only a plasma membrane and no intracellular or organelle membranes. The red cell membrane encloses haemoglobin in a manner seemingly designed to optimize its function. It makes good sense to have haemoglobin packaged with the concentrations of hydrogen ion and 2,3-DPG that modulate its function and with the enzymes and cofactors that have the reducing power necessary to protect haemoglobin from oxidative degradation. The membrane barrier allows red cells to control their own internal environment of anions, cations, and water, while the negatively charged outer face may provide the necessary electrostatic repulsive forces that prevent the red cell from aggregating and from adhering to the endothelium.

RED BLOOD CELL MEMBRANE BIOLOGY

General

The quantity of membrane surface area relative to red cell volume (SA/V) is of great importance because this ratio determines the ability of the red cell to preserve its discocytic shape. The qualitative characteristics of the membrane are determined by the assembly of its several components. Several reviews of red cell membranes have recently appeared (Seminars in Hematology 16, No. 1 & 2, January and April 1979; and Normal and Abnormal Red Cell Membranes, 1979, S E Lux, V T Marchesi, C F Fox (eds), Alan R Liss, Inc, New York).

Methods of analysis. The membrane outer surface can be studied in carefully washed red cells, but for studies of the remainder of the membrane, a 'ghost' preparation is usually made by lysing the erythrocytes. However, there is abundant data indicating that ghost membranes are not the same as red cell membranes; therefore results obtained using ghosts should always be interpreted with great caution. There is 'sidedness' in the red blood cell membrane with defined constituents on the external surface and a different set of components on the internal or cytosol surface.

The red cell membrane is composed of lipids, carbohydrates, and proteins. But because the carbohydrates are present mainly in the form of glycolipids and glycoproteins, they will be considered under these two major categories.

Lipids

All of the erythrocytic lipid is in the membrane of which it constitutes about 50 per cent. There are roughly equimolar amounts of phospholipids and non-esterified or free cholesterol and there is no esterified cholesterol.

Phospholipids

The phospholipids of the red cell membrane have a three carbon background (Fig. 4.1), glycerol for the glycerophospholipids and sphingosine in the case of sphingo-myelin. These phospholipids have been described as having a tuning fork appearance because they have one or two non-polar fatty acid side chains on one side of the molecule and polar groups attached to the phosphate on the other (Chapman, 1975). Lecithin or phosphatidyl choline (PC) accounts for 28 per cent of total phospholipids, and sphingomyelin (SM) 25 per cent. The amino phospholipids are phosphatidyl serine (PS, 13 per cent) and phosphatidyl ethanolamine (PE, 26 per cent). There are small amounts of phosphatidyl inositol, phosphatidic acid and lysophospholipids. The latter have only a single fatty acid chain. The phospholipids are arranged in the bilayer with their non-polar fatty acid side chains towards the centre while the polar groups are arranged at the rim. Some of the phospholipid must approach the outer surface of the erythrocyte since externally added non-penetrating phospholipases can attack and degrade them (Allan et al, 1975).

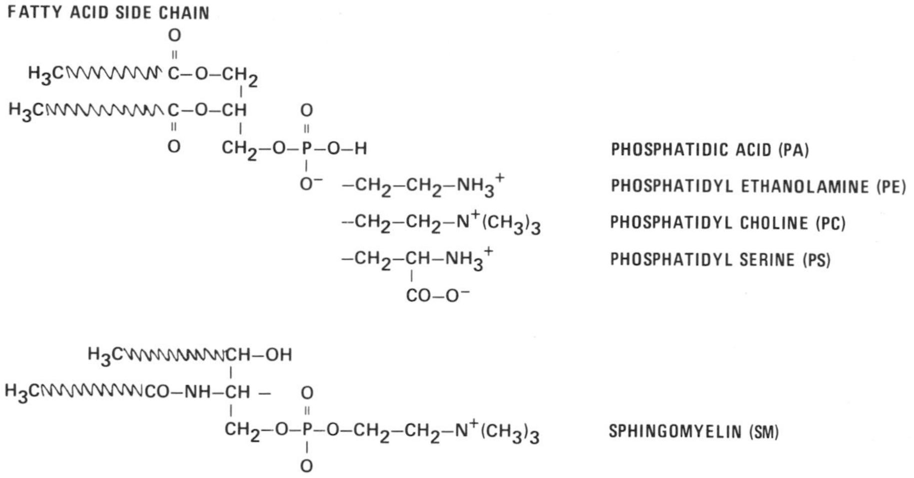

FATTY ACID SIDE CHAIN

$$H_3C\text{\Wwwww}\overset{\overset{O}{\|}}{C}-O-CH_2$$
$$H_3C\text{\Wwwww}\overset{\|}{\underset{O}{C}}-O-CH$$

$CH_2-O-\overset{O}{\underset{O^-}{\overset{\|}{P}}}-O-H$	PHOSPHATIDIC ACID (PA)
$-CH_2-CH_2-NH_3^+$	PHOSPHATIDYL ETHANOLAMINE (PE)
$-CH_2-CH_2-N^+(CH_3)_3$	PHOSPHATIDYL CHOLINE (PC)
$-CH_2-\underset{\underset{CO-O^-}{\|}}{CH}-NH_3^+$	PHOSPHATIDYL SERINE (PS)

$$H_3C\text{\Wwwwww}CH-OH$$
$$H_3C\text{\Wwwwww}CO-NH-\underset{\underset{CH_2-O-\overset{O}{\underset{O}{\overset{\|}{P}}}-O-CH_2-CH_2-N^+(CH_3)_3}{|}}{CH}-$$

SPHINGOMYELIN (SM)

Fig. 4.1 Major phospholipids of the red blood cell membrane. The phosphoglycerides are PS, PE, and PC.

Glycolipids

These are predominantly located in the outer half of the lipid bilayer. Their structure consists of a sphingosine, as the lipid portion, with a series of sugars extending from the carbon-1 of the backbone. Specific enzymes control the addition of sugars and these glycolipids react in turn with glycoproteins to determine the specific blood group antigens of the ABO (H), Lewis, and P systems (Mehta, 1980).

Cholesterol

Cholesterol is probably located towards the core of the bilayer where it may be intercalated between the phospholipid fatty acid side chains (Blau & Bittman, 1978).

Lipid Organization

The phospholipids are arranged asymmetrically with the PC and SM choline phospholipids localized (70 to 80 per cent) to the outer half of the bilayer, whereas the amino phospholipids, PE and PS, are located (80 to 100 per cent) at the inner half (Bretscher, 1972; Marinetti & Crain, 1978; Verkleij et al, 1973). The functional significance of this asymmetry is not known. However, PS may interact with some of the peripheral membrane proteins at the cytosol surface (Mombers et al, 1979). PS is also required for full activation of the pump related Na^+, K^+-ATPase.

Phospholipids move laterally on their side of the bilayer with astonishing rapidity and this lateral diffusion seems to be dampened by the presence of membrane cholesterol. The ability of phospholipids to flip-flop from one side of the bilayer to the other is much slower. Cholesterol apparently is able to cross the bilayer with greater facility than phospholipids and exchange totally with plasma cholesterol (Lange et al, 1977). Therefore circumstances that produce an increase in non-esterified plasma cholesterol will lead to an increase in membrane cholesterol on both sides of the bilayer. This produces an expansion of the red cell membrane surface, a decrease in membrane fluidity and perhaps minor changes in passive Na^+ and K^+ movements (Cooper, 1977, 1978).

Presumably the purpose of this elegant lipid organization is to provide structure to the membrane as well as to enhance the activity of several important membrane enzymes. Nevertheless, the full import of the lipid organization remains to be determined.

Proteins

General

Proteins comprise 50 per cent of the weight of the membrane. Membranes can be dissolved in boiling sodium dodecyl sulfate (SDS) and then characterized by electrophoresis on polyacrylamide gels — SDS-PAGE (Fairbanks et al, 1971) which separate the proteins on the basis of their molecular weight. When the gels are stained with Coomassie blue usually eight banding areas are identified. The nomenclature initially proposed by Fairbanks et al (1971) has generally been accepted. The sialoglycopeptides stain poorly with Coomassie blue but nicely with PAS which usually shows three bands and an additional fourth band is seen when the gels are heavily loaded (fig. 4.2). Two classes of membrane proteins are identified. Easily extracted relatively polar, water-soluble membrane proteins are found at the cytosol face or internal surface and are called peripheral proteins (Steck & Yu, 1973). (The sidedness or asymmetry of the membrane proteins is established by the use of non-penetrable fluorescent or radioisotopic labels.) Integral membrane proteins require more stringent techniques for extraction presumably because of their close association with the membrane lipids. They are relatively non-polar and include all of the membrane glycoproteins and many of the proteins of the outer cell surface.

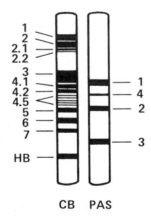

CB   PAS

Fig. 4.2 SDS polyacrylamide gel electrophoresis (PAGE) of red blood cell membrane proteins stained with either Coomassie blue (CB) or periodic-acid-Schiff (PAS) (see text). The Coomassie blue staining bands are labelled according to the system of Fairbanks (Fairbanks et al, 1971) and the PAS according to Marchesi (Marchesi, 1979a).

Early membrane models showed a core of lipid bilayer with proteins stretched out along both external and cytosol surfaces. However, the evidence of lipid bilayer asymmetry, along with the existence of cytosol surface peripheral proteins and transmembrane integral proteins accords better with the fluid mosaic model proposed by Singer & Nicolson (1972). In this model integral membrane proteins, suspended like icebergs, are free to move laterally in a lipid sea while the peripheral proteins are organized on the cytosolic surface and their freedom to move is not detailed in the model. There may be relatively fixed domains or segments consisting of defined associations of proteins, lipids, and enzymes within the membrane (Marchesi, 1978, 1979a; Schrier & Junga, 1980). Therefore the working model used in this review is a fluid mosaic, overlaid with a fixed matrix.

Peripheral or extrinsic membrane proteins
These consist primarily of spectrin bands 1 and 2, actin, band 5, glyceraldehyde phosphate dehydrogenase (G3PD), band 6, ankyrin band 2.1, and bands 4.1 and 4.2. Minor bands 7 and 8 are probably peripheral membrane proteins (Steck & Yu, 1973) (Fig. 4.2).

SPECTRIN
Spectrin is the major peripheral protein (Marchesi, 1979b) and is found almost uniquely in red cells and their precursors. It is confined to the cytosol surface. Spectrin produces bands 1 and 2 which have molecular weights of 240 000 and 220 000. There is a high content of polar amino acids. In vivo, most spectrin is probably tetrameric with two heterodimers associated head-to-head. Elegant techniques identify filaments of spectrin dimer (dimensions 1000 Å × 50 Å) with the two chains coiled about each other. The dimers are associated in a head-to-head manner to form tetramers with a filament length of 2000 Å (Shotten et al, 1979). Band 2 of spectrin can be phosphorylated by membrane associated protein kinases but the idea that the extent of spectrin phosphorylation controls red cell shape cannot be confirmed at this time (Marchesi, 1979b). Nevertheless, the presence of specific protein kinases which may or may not be activated by cyclic AMP (Tsukamoto et al, 1980) and the selectivity of the patterns of spectrin phosphorylation are thought by some investigators to be highly suggestive of a physiologic role which has yet to be identified (Lux, 1979a).

ACTIN
Band 5, MW 45 000, accounts for 4 to 5 per cent of erythrocyte membrane protein, and has all of the characteristics of non-muscle actin (Stossel, 1978; Tilney & Detmers, 1975) including the ability to stimulate the Mg^{2+}-ATPase of myosin (the actin-activated ATPase). In vivo actin is found in the F (filamentous) form where it is usually visible as filaments of 35 Å diameter. Only F, and not G (monomeric) actin, can stimulate the myosin ATPase. In non-muscle cells some actin is found associated with the cytosol face of plasma membranes where it attaches to actin binding proteins and may function in cell motility and phagocytosis. In the red cell, all actin is associated with the membrane and it may exist in an oligomeric or proto-filamentous form, smaller than the size detectable by electron microscopy (Brenner & Korn, 1980). Actin may be involved in membrane contractility or recoil via interaction with a myosin-like analogue.

ANKYRIN (SYNDEIN)
This band, 2.1, MW 210 000 accounts for approximately 5 per cent of membrane protein. Related bands 2.2, 2.3, and 3' are probably proteolytic digestion products of

band 2.1. It is apparently widely distributed in tissues other than red cells (Bennett & Stenbuck, 1979). Ankyrin binds to spectrin heterodimers near their head portion and may also bind to band 3. Ankyrin can be phosphorylated by red cell protein kinases but the importance of phophorylation is not known (Tyler et al, 1979).

BANDS 4.1 AND 4.2

These bands (MW 78 000 and 72 000) account for 4 to 5 per cent of membrane protein and are found only at the cytosol face. Band 4.1 binds to the spectrin heterodimer near its tail (Tyler et al, 1979). Actin also appears to be associated with the band 4.1 spectrin binding site (Sheetz, 1979).

BAND 6, 7, AND 8

Band 6 (MW 35 000) represents a monomeric glyceraldehyde 3-phosphate dehydrogenase (G3PD) which exists in both cytosol and membrane as the active tetrameric enzyme. G3PD binds to a specific site on the integral membrane protein band 3 (see below) (Steck, 1978). It is unclear whether G3PD is mainly a cytosolic or membrane associated enzyme in vivo. It is postulated but unproven that this enzyme in situ could play an important role in providing ATP to the membrane proteins that utilize it (Schrier, 1977).

Very little is known about band 7 (MW 29 000) or band 8 (MW 23 000).

HAEMOGLOBIN

Residual haemoglobin usually appears as a band (MW approximately 16 000) representing monomeric alpha and beta chains. Since the only obvious biologic organization in the human red cell is its membrane, the fact that haemoglobin is part of that membrane could result in extension of this organization into the cytosol (Ponder, 1957). Haemoglobin can associate with the membrane at several sites in vitro but the high affinity site is on band 3 (Shaklai et al, 1977).

Integral membrane proteins

BAND 3

Band 3 (glycoprotein of MW 93 000) accounts for 25 per cent of the membrane proteins (Steck, 1978). Band 3 appears to exist as a non-covalent dimer which pursues a sinuous transmembrane course and some five to seven different segments have been described. The cytoplasmic segments can be phosphorylated. Band 3 dimer modulates anion transport and its cytosolic segment has specific binding sites for G3PD, aldolase and haemoglobin. The linkage of band 3 to the cytosol facing peripheral membrane proteins may occur via association with band 2.1 and 4.2 which in turn bind to spectrin. The external portion of band 3 contains some of the carbohydrates that determine the Ii blood group system (Fukuda et al, 1979).

GLYCOPHORIN

The glycophorins A, B and C are sialoglycopeptides (Marchesi, 1978) and account for 2 to 3 per cent of membrane proteins. They are all transmembrane proteins, some existing as dimers, with all of the oligosaccharides at the outer surface of the red cell. Four PAS staining bands are recognized (Fig. 4.2). PAS band 1 is a glycophorin A dimer, PAS band 2 is glycophorin A monomer, and PAS band 3 is probably glycophorin B. Glycophorin A has a hydrophilic segment which extends beyond the outer surface of the red cell to which oligosaccharides like sialic acid are attached, a central segment consisting of hydrophobic amino acids which penetrates and interacts with the lipid bilayer, and another segment of regulatively polar amino acids which penetrates the cytosolic face. Glycophorin A contains the oligosaccharides defining the M and N antigenic system of red cells and glycophorin B contains the Ss antigenic determinants. The oligosaccharides also contain virus receptor sites and other receptor function is deduced but unproven (Furthmayr, 1978a & b). In addition to providing most of the red cell surface negativity, the glycophorins may serve to delineate specific domains in the membrane with different lipid : protein ratios and different patterns of membrane associated enzymes (Schrier & Junga, 1980).

THE ATPASES

Na^+, K^+-ATPase is both the energy transducer and the molecule mediating the actual translocation of Na^+ and K^+. Against concentration gradients, Na^+, K^+-ATPase transports three atoms of Na^+ out, and two atoms of K^+ in with the conversion of one molecule of ATP to ADP. It is activated by intracellular Na^+ (Km = 25 mmol/l) and extracellular K^+ (2.5 mmol/l) and because the internal Na^+ concentration is about 15 mmol/l while the external K^+ is 3–4 mmol/l, the enzyme is preferentially activated by increments in internal Na^+ and not by changes in external K^+. It migrates in the band 3 area on SDS-PAGE (Dunham & Hoffman, 1970).

Mg^{2+}-ATPase also migrates in the band 3 area and its function is unknown.

Ca^{2+}, Mg^{2+}-ATPase requires phospholipid for full activation, and it mediates Ca^{2+} efflux against a 50 to 100 fold concentration gradient converting one molecule of ATP to ADP for each two molecules of Ca^{2+} extruded (Sarkadi et al, 1977). The entry of Ca^{2+} into the red cell causes the activator protein, calmodulin, to move from the cytosol to the membrane. There calmodulin activates Ca^{2+}, Mg^{2+}-ATPase to extrude Ca^{2+} (Gopinath & Vincenzi, 1977). Calmodulin appears to be identical to the activator of cyclic nucleotide phosphodiesterase (Jarrett & Penniston, 1977).

ACETYLCHOLINESTERASE
The active enzymic site of this glycoprotein faces the external membrane surface. Therefore measurement of acetylcholinesterase activity is used as a marker of the external membrane surface. Its function is unknown.

NADH-OXIDOREDUCTASE
The catalytic site of this glycoprotein is oriented toward the cytosolic face. Therefore the enzyme has been used as a cytosol face marker. It has the capacity to transfer electrons from NADH to a variety of receptors and therefore could play a role in providing reducing power to the membrane cytosol face but no proof of such function exists (Wang & Alaupovic, 1978).

BAND 4.5

Band 4.5 (MW 55 000) contains 11 per cent of the membrane protein, and probably contains several components. The major band 4.5 component contains a cytosolic extension and a segment which reaches the external red cell surface where the carbohydrates contribute to the Ii blood group antigen system (Fukuda et al, 1979). Band 4.5 is also the D-glucose transporting protein.

PROTEIN KINASES

The red cell and its membrane have several protein kinases which can phosphorylate spectrin, band 2.1 and band 3 (Avruch & Fairbanks, 1974; Fairbanks & Avruch, 1974). One of these may be enhanced by the presence of cyclic AMP (Tsukamoto et al, 1980).

Less well-characterized membrane proteins include a myosin-like actin-activated ATPase (Schrier & Hardy, 1979).

CHANNELS OR PORES IN THE MEMBRANE

While there is no morphologic evidence, it is thought that channels or pores exist. Monovalent anions, like chloride and bicarbonate, cross the membrane passively, slower than water, but still rapidly, equilibrating in milliseconds. Monovalent and divalent anions probably penetrate the membrane through the band 3 site. In contrast, the monovalent cations Na^+ and K^+ passively cross the membrane very slowly, probably via separate channels equilibrating in hours.

Supramolecular structure

These molecules are organized so that the assembly results in the identifiable properties of the functioning red cell membrane. Several techniques have been used to study membrane assembly: cross linking agents, freeze cleaving and freeze etching, Triton shells, inside-out (I-O) and right-side-out (R-O) vesicles, external surface charge studies and studies of transmembrane signalling, e.g. effect on the external surface of anti-spectrin antibody.

The cytoskeleton is composed primarily of spectrin along with actin and band 4.1 (Ungewickell et al, 1979). Tetrameric spectrin is the basic unit and higher spectrin multimers occur infrequently (Ji et al, 1980). It is proposed that oligomeric F actin binds to the same band 4.1 which binds the tail portion of the spectrin heterodimer and that these proto F actin filaments cross-link spectrin tetramers to produce the mesh or lattice required (Fig. 4.3) (Lux, 1979a). The cytoskeleton must be linked to the transmembrane proteins to account for transmembrane signalling. Spectrin binds weakly to the amino phospholipids (Marchesi, 1979b) but strongly to ankyrin (Bennett & Stenbuck, 1980). Ankyrin in turn may link spectrin to the integral protein band 3, perhaps through a complex involving band 4.2 (Sheetz, 1979; Bennett & Stenbuck, 1979) (Fig. 4.3). The nature of the association of the cytoskeleton with glycophorin remains to be worked out.

The finding that membrane vesicles and vacuoles are depleted of spectrin (Lux et al, 1977; Hardy & Schrier, 1978; Hardy et al, 1979) supports the idea that spectrin provides a structural framework for the membrane. In further support of the role of spectrin is the observation that the lateral mobility of integral proteins is enhanced when spectrin is removed from the membrane (Fowler & Bennett, 1978). Spectrin deficient mouse hereditary spherocytes undergo spontaneous fusion and budding

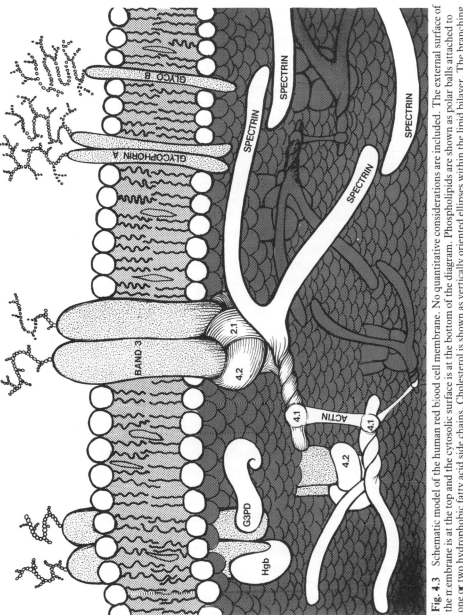

Fig. 4.3 Schematic model of the human red blood cell membrane. No quantitative considerations are included. The external surface of the membrane is at the top and the cytosolic surface is at the bottom of the diagram. Phospholipids are shown as polar balls attached to one or two hydrophobic fatty acid side chains. Cholesterol is shown as vertically oriented ellipses within the lipid bilayer. The branching side chains attached to the integral proteins, band 3 and glycophorin, represent externally oriented carbohydrates carrying blood group antigens and viral receptors. The numbers refer to Commassie blue bands on SDS-PAGE (Fig. 4.2). See text for details of the interactions.

(Shohet, 1979) and the lateral mobility of their integral membrane proteins is vastly increased (Sheetz et al, 1980). The role of other putative cytoskeletal proteins is not so clear.

Red cell shape

Because white ghosts, restored to isotonic conditions, are biconcave discs, it is thought that the disc shape is characteristic of the membrane. The dimple and the annulus of the discocyte are not fixed to specific sites on the membrane surface (Bull & Brailsford, 1973). A tank tread-like motion has been observed in the red cell membrane in which the membrane appears to move as a whole about the cytosol (Fischer et al, 1978). With the discocyte as the norm, several alternative red cell shape changes have been described (Bessis, 1972) in which alteration of the SA/V ratio is a major factor. The SA/V ratio can be reduced by circumstances that either decrease the surface area or increase the cell volume, in which case the discocyte becomes a spherocyte or a stomatocyte. Conversely, if the SA/V ratio is increased, by circumstances that increase the surface area or reduce the cell volume, then the extra surface area will produce a target cell. Membrane surface can be lost either externally or internally. When the discocyte is subjected to ATP depletion, Ca^{2+} accumulation, alkaline pH, phospholipase attack, exposure to lysophosphatidylcholine or amphipathic anions, it sends out sharp external membrane projections and becomes a reversible echinocyte I. If the attack continues, more and more membrane material is trapped in the echinocytic spines and bits of membrane may even be shed (exocytic vacuoles). The resulting decrease in surface area leads to the creation of a spheroechinocyte which eventually becomes irreversible at the spheroechinocyte III stage. Conversely, when the discocyte is exposed to acid pH or amphipathic cations, it becomes a cup-shaped reversible stomatocyte I. If the exposure continues, endocytic vacuoles form along the advancing invaginating stoma, which deprive the membrane of surface area through internal loss, leading eventually to an irreversible spherostomatocyte III. The conversion of discocytes to either echinocytes or stomatocytes is thought to depend on the asymmetry of the lipid bilayer. The amphipathic cations that cause stomatocytosis appear to be attracted to negatively charged PS in the inner half of the bilayer, where, by expanding the inner bilayer, stomatocytosis is produced. Conversely, amphipathic anions repelled by the negatively charged PS seem to be inserted into the outer PC and SM rich half of the bilayer which by expanding would produce echinocytes (Sheetz & Singer, 1974). However, the methods which purported to show insertion of amphipathic materials into membranes may have only shown surface trapping (Conrad & Singer, 1979). Nevertheless, studies with lysophosphatidylcholine (LPC) support the idea that lipid asymmetry is important in red cell shape changes. The insertion of LPC into the outer half of the bilayer causes echinocytosis, and when LPC moves to the inner half of the bilayer, it produces stomatocytosis (Mohandas et al, 1978). The proposal that movement of diacylglycerol could explain red cell shape changes (Allan & Michell, 1975) has been challenged because shape changes can be shown to occur in the absence of parallel diacylglyceride movement (White et al, 1978). Erythrocyte membrane proteins are also asymmetrically distributed and could have a role in shape changes. There was considerable interest in the idea that the extent of spectrin phosphorylation determines shape changes; however, more direct confirmation is required.

Deformability

General

Intrinsic red cell deformability can be considered to be the product of two interacting compartments: the membrane itself and the internal viscosity of the cytosol. Membrane function relates to the quantity of membrane expressed as the SA/V ratio and to the state of the membrane constituents as described above. The internal viscosity of the cytosol relates to its two major components: haemoglobin (30 per cent of the red cell), and water (67 per cent). The kind of haemoglobin present and its physical state have an effect on internal viscosity, the classical example being the gelling of deoxysickle haemoglobin. The relationship between red cell water and haemoglobin is conveniently expressed as the MCHC. Haemoglobin is extraordinarily soluble but at concentrations that exist in the red cell (approximately 30 g/dl) the aqueous solution begins to resemble a gel and when the MCHC increases above 30, the internal viscocity rises hyperbolically (Chien, 1977a). Since there are no circumstances where the amount of haemoglobin synthesized per red cell is increased the MCHC and its related internal viscosity are controlled by circumstances that lead either to decreased amounts of haemoglobin or to variations in red cell water content.

A variety of techniques have been used to obtain quantitative data about red cell deformability (Chien, 1977b) including viscometry (Co-axial cylinder, Cone-Plate, etc.), filters (e.g. polycarbonate sieves), micropipettes, and the ektacytometer which measures the extent of discocytic conversion to ellipsoids upon exposure to fluid shear forces (Bessis & Mohandas, 1975). The results with the ektacytometer show a surprising degree of dependence of deformability on the MCHC and therefore on internal viscosity (Mohandas et al, 1980).

Modulation of membrane function

The function of the erythrocyte and its membrane can be modified over short periods of time by hormones, cyclic nucleotides, Ca^{2+}, and calmodulin.

Hormones

The red cell responds to prostaglandin E_2, epinephrine and acetylcholine by stiffening its membrane and in particular the lipid bilayer (Allen & Rasmussen, 1971; Huestis & McConnell, 1974). Norepinephrine increases the phosphorylation of spectrin (band 2) and band 3 (Nelson et al, 1979) perhaps by mobilizing Ca^{2+} as a messenger (Nelson & Huestis, 1980). However, proof of a physiologic role of such interaction is lacking and the importance of membrane protein phosphorylation remains to be established.

Cyclic nucleotides

Cyclic AMP probably can penetrate the red cell membrane slowly and has specific binding sites on the cytosol face of the membrane. cAMP probably modulates some but not all red cell membrane protein kinases (Tsukamoto et al, 1980; Tao et al, 1980).

Calcium

The red cell membrane regulates Ca^{2+} movement very stringently (Schatzmann & Vincenzi, 1969). With a plasma Ca^{2+} concentration of approximately 2.5 mmol/l, the calcium concentration of the red cell is about 20 μmol/l, much of which is attached to the inner and outer surface of the membrane (Harrison & Long, 1969). Following penetration of calcium into the red cell, calmodulin apparently moves to the membrane where it activates the Ca^{2+}, Mg^{2+}-ATPase to extrude calcium (Cheung, 1980). Depending on its concentration, calcium can cause several membrane-related alterations including: induction of echinocytosis (Bessis, 1972), cross-linking of membrane protein (Lorand et al, 1979), activation of a phosphodiesterase (Allan & Mitchell, 1979), enhancement of endocytosis (Schrier et al, 1978), and reduction in membrane deformability (Palek et al, 1977). The association of spectrin, actin and band 4.1 to form a cytoskeletal gel is sensitive to the concentrations of Ca^{2+} that could exist in the membrane (Fowler & Taylor, 1980). Ca^{2+} entry also causes K^+ and water loss (the Gardos effect) (Gardos, 1959). The Gardos effect is thought to be physiologically important since the erythrocyte controls its intracellular volume and hence internal viscosity by controlling salt and water movement.

Neonatal red cells
Mature adult red cells exposed to concanavalin A do not undergo clustering and endocytosis while neonatal erythrocytes do (Schekman & Singer, 1976). In contrast to adult red cells neonatal erythrocytes undergo spontaneous endocytosis (Holroyde et al, 1969) behaving as though their cytoskeletons are less rigid.

ALTERATIONS IN RED CELL MEMBRANES IN HEALTH AND DISEASE

Age
As the red cell ages in vivo there is a fall in SA/V ratio making the red cell more spheroidal. The MCHC rises as a consequence of water loss thereby increasing the internal viscosity. There is a 10 per cent reduction in sialic acid (Seaman et al, 1977), small amounts of IgG become detectable on the surface of senescent red cells (Kay, 1978), and polymerization of membrane components, particularly spectrin occurs (Jain & Hochstein, 1980). The loss of surface area may represent random loss of membrane from erythrocytes that have been exposed for months to shearing forces, metabolic depletion, and stasis. There may also be a more purposeful membrane remodelling. It is conceivable that weak or damaged segments of the membrane could serve as foci about which endocytic vacuole formation could take place with the spleen then pitting the endocytic vacuoles along with included damaged membrane. In support of this hypothesis is the observation that autophagic vacuoles appear in red cells in splenectomized subjects (Holroyde & Gardner, 1970). The spherocytic shape causes the older red cells to be held up in the RE system where stasis produces further metabolic insult. The reduction in surface negativity could uncover the antigens expressed on senescent red cells to which IgG binds and the combination of decreased deformability and bound IgG could be the signal perceived by macrophages engaged in removing senescent red blood cells.

Storage
Red cell storage results in a fall in ATP which impairs red blood cell survival and a fall in 2,3-DPG which impairs haemoglobin function. There may also be a membrane storage lesion which contributes to the removal of liquid stored red cells. Appearance

of heavy molecular weight complexes on SDS-PAGE and abnormalities in drug-induced endocytosis have been described even after ATP has been restored to normal (Schrier et al, 1979). With prolonged cold liquid storage red cells acquire complement components which may be a factor in their removal (Szymanski & Odgren, 1979).

Disease states

Most haemolytic disorders eventually have some evidence of red cell membrane dysfunction. We propose to consider here only those disorders where the membrane derangement occurs early in the red cell's life span.

Hereditary haemolytic diseases where the membrane is primarily involved

PRESUMED DISORDERS OF MEMBRANE PROTEIN

Hereditary spherocytosis. HS is probably not a single disease but a group of disorders involving subtle but related changes in the red cell membrane. Studies of haemoglobin structure and function and erythrocytic metabolism have shown no consistent abnormalities. A wide variety of membrane abnormalities have been reported in HS, probably reflecting the complicated epiphenomenology of the still elusive primary defect. Normoblasts and reticulocytes in HS are normal. However, as the HS red cell ages, membrane is lost by unknown mechanisms, perhaps by fragmentation. The loss in surface area results in a reduced SA/V ratio, i.e. a spherocyte. These spherocytes, which are more often stomatocytes when viewed by phase microscopy, are damaged so selectively that their infirmity is detected only in the cordal architecture of the spleen. This is in contrast to other forms of spherocytosis such as that seen with autoimmune haemolytic anaemia or microangiopathic haemolysis where other RE organs like the liver can actively participate in the removal of spherocytic cells. Because marrow function is unimpaired, compensation of haemolysis is usually achieved. When the spleen is removed, clinical evidence of haemolysis ceases although labelling with DF^{32}P shows subclinical evidence of continuing haemolysis.

Studies on deformability of HS red cell using micropipettes and the ektacytometer have shown them to be quite rigid (La Celle et al, 1976). However, resealed HS ghosts behave normally in the ektacytometer indicating that the decrease in deformability is due to the reduction in SA/V ratio and not to an intrinsic rigidity in the membrane (Nakashima & Beutler, 1979). HS red cells also have an increased MCHC, which suggests that in addition to losing surface area, they have lost cellular water. The combination of spherocytic shape and increased internal viscosity probably accounts for the selective removal of the affected red cell.

The lipid bilayer is probably normal in HS membranes when analysed quantitatively. Reports of fatty acid abnormalities cannot be confirmed (Zail & Pickering, 1979) There is increased microviscosity at the core of the lipid bilayer in HS (Aloni et al, 1975) but the importance of this observation is unclear since protein is the major contributor to the intrinsic deformability of the red cell and the HS membrane is normally deformable. However, when incubated in vitro under conditions of mild metabolic depletion, HS red cells lose phospholipid and cholesterol where normal cells lose only cholesterol. This well known observation which forms the basis of the diagnostic incubated osmotic fragility test for HS may be the in vitro reflection of the membrane loss which occurs in vivo.

In searching for the cause of the spherocytosis, studies on Na^+, K^+, and H_2O movement in HS red cells were performed. HS red cells are more permeable than normal red cells to passive Na^+ influx, but do not show a parallel increase in passive K^+ efflux. In order to combat the Na^+ influx, the Na^+, K^+-ATPase is activated and extrudes Na^+ at the usual $Na^+:K^+:P$ ratio of 3:2:1. Glycolysis is enhanced as is ATP turnover. Na^+ extrusion is effective because the microspherocyte has a high MCHC, indicating water deficiency, not water loading which would occur with poorly opposed Na^+ entry.

Because it was mistakenly thought that the HS red cell membrane was rigid, Ca^{2+} metabolism was studied because Ca^{2+} can increase membrane rigidity (see above). Reports of increased Ca^{2+} content and decreased activity of the Ca^{2+} pump-related-Ca^{2+},Mg^{2+}-ATPase in HS have not been confirmed.

Spectrin has been studied because mouse spherocytes (Shohet, 1979) are characterized by varying degrees of spectrin deficiency with the extent of deficiency paralleling the degree of haemolysis (Lux et al, 1979). SDS-PAGE of HS membranes has occasionally yielded evidence of minor abnormalities which have not been easily confirmed. However, quantitative analysis of spectrin in HS has yielded repeatedly normal results. The extent of spectrin phosphorylation may be reduced in HS under some (Greenquist & Shohet, 1976) but not all conditions (Wolfe & Lux, 1978; Lux, 1979b) while the kinetics of protein phosphorylation in HS are normal. HS Triton shells are more fragile and easily dispersed in certain batches of aged Triton (Wolfe & Lux, 1978) thereby suggesting the existence of cytoskeletal abnormalities.

Drug induced endocytosis is severely defective in HS and since the membrane is intrinsically normally deformable, it is likely that the defect in endocytosis relates to the function of the membrane components that produce the deep invaginations required (Schrier et al, 1974).

A working hypothesis is that cytoskeletal protein function is affected so that membrane fragmentation or budding occurs early in the life of the HS red cell. The lipid changes observed probably reflect the important association of the lipid bilayer with membrane proteins.

Hereditary elliptocytosis (HE). There are several forms of HE. In one, the gene is linked to the Rh locus, but most cases probably represent the heterozygous state showing morphologically abnormal red cells without evidence of haemolysis. HE, when it causes haemolysis probably represents either the homozygous state, a variant that shows both elliptocytes and microspherocytes and resembles HS, or the rare sporadic haemolysis seen in heterozygous HE (Pearson, 1968). Rarely, infants who appear to develop HE as they grow older may have severe neonatal haemolysis characterized by the appearance of pyknocytes (bizarre variations in red cell shape with fragmentation, buds, ghosts, and iregularly shaped cells) and elliptocytes in the peripheral smear (Carpentieri et al, 1977).

There are no abnormalities of haemoglobin or red cell metabolism in HE. HE ghosts retain the elliptocytic shape as do HE Triton shells, thereby indicating that the disorder involves the membrane and its cytoskeleton. In some, but not all patients with HE, the extracted spectrin seems hypersusceptible to heat denaturation (Lux, 1979b). A new observation is that the spectrin dimer is increased at the expense of tetrameric spectrin in HE and this shift is associated with an increased susceptibility of HE Triton shells to mechanical disruption (Liu & Palek, 1980). It is proposed that the HE defect involves the head area of spectrin heterodimers interefering with their ability to associate into tetramers. While confirmation of this finding is necessary, it seems to support and emphasize the role of tetrameric spectrin in the membrane cytoskeleton (Fig. 4.3). In some cases of HE band 4.1 is deficient.

Hereditary pyropoikilocytosis (HPP). Peripheral blood shows the most extraordinary mixture of erythrocyte buds, ghosts, fragments, and bizarrely shaped cells. Fortunately the extent of haemolysis can be controlled by splenectomy. The term pyropoikilocytosis was initially applied because the red cells fragment in vitro upon only mild heating. Ghosts and Triton shells of HPP red cells retain their bizarre shapes thereby indicating the existence of a membrane disorder (Palek et al, 1979). HPP spectrin becomes virtually inextractable with mild heating, the extent of spectrin phosphorylation is reduced (Walter et al, 1977), and the spectrin appears to be hyperaggregable. Deformability of HPP red cells as measured in the ektacytometer is markedly reduced, in small part because of a slight increase in MCHC. Intact HPP red cells show abnormally high Ca^{2+} influx and studies with HPP ghosts show reduced ^{45}Ca efflux and enhanced membrane retention of ^{45}Ca. It is possible that Ca^{2+} entry via the Gardos effect causes K^+ and H_2O loss with consequent elevation in MCHC. In contrast to the finding in HS, there is a unique enhancement of drug induced endocytosis in intact HPP erythrocytes. The hyperaggregability of HPP spectrin is consistent with the observation of enhanced drug induced endocytosis since the endocytic vacuole probably forms in spectrin depleted zones which would presumably occur more frequently in the presence of hyperaggregable spectrin. It would now be fruitful to study spectrin tethering and spectrin tetramer:dimer ratios in HPP and to pursue its possible relationship to HE.

Rh null. Several families have red cell membranes which express none of the Rh antigens. Rh null red cell are somewhat spherocytic and the patients have compensated haemolysis. The Rh antigen may be a lipoprotein and its absence presumably impairs membrane function. There may be abnormalities in cation flux which have been difficult to confirm (Smith et al, 1973).

Congenital dyserythropoietic anaemia (CDA). These disorders primarily involve the cell nucleus but transmission electron microscopy occasionally shows bundles of microtubules bridging adjacent cells and in some mature red cells double plasma membranes are seen. One form of CDA shows susceptibility to acidified serum lysis (HEMPAS).

ABNORMALITIES OF SALT AND WATER TRANSPORT

Hereditary xerocytosis. Observations made on this rare hereditary haemolytic disorder help to establish several important biologic points regarding separation of passive Na^+ and K^+ channels and the vectorial features of the Na^+,K^+-ATPase. The red cells have a very high MCHC, are rigid, and fragment easily. The basic red cell defect is a passive loss of K^+ in excess of a slight inward leak of Na^+. The pump Na^+,K^+-ATPase is normal and there is no increase in intracellular Ca^{2+}. Since the kinetics of the Na^+-K^+ pump are such that it is activated by increments in internal Na^+ and not external K^+ (see above), the pump is not turned off to allow a compensatory accumulation of Na^+. Consequent on the K^+ loss, there is obligatory water loss and the resulting dehydrated cell is rigid and therefore cannot normally traverse the microcirculation where it may fragment. The fragmentation suggests that there is a membrane defect (in addition to the K^+ leak) which may be a consequence of cellular dehydration (Glader & Sullivan, 1979).

Hereditary stomatocytosis (hereditary hydrocytosis). Acquired stomatocytosis can be seen in alcoholism and pancreatitis. However, in hereditary stomatocytosis considered here, red cells have a decrease in the SA/V ratio because of an increase in red cell volume and not because of a primary loss of surface area. The major defect involves a massively enhanced passive leak in both Na^+ and K^+ with Na^+ influx exceeding K^+ efflux. Despite a supernormally functioning Na^+-K^+ active transport system with concomitant ATP consumption, Na^+ eventually accumulates along with an obligatory water influx producing a swollen, water-loaded cell — the hydrocyte. The MCV is elevated and MCHC decreased. The basic shape of the red cell leads to splenic sequestration and splenectomy improves the clinical picture. There may be membrane defects in addition to the Na^+-K^+ leak. Endocytosis in resealed ghosts is a form of energized endocytosis dependent on Ca^{2+}, Mg^{2+}, and ATP (Schrier et al, 1975) and is grossly decreased in hereditary stomatocytosis. Membrane protein phosphorylation is also decreased. Neither the abnormality in endocytosis nor the abnormality in protein phosphorylation are easily explicable on the basis of abnormal passive cation flux. When hereditary stomatocytic erythrocytes are treated with bifunctional cross-linking agents of a certain size, red ghost endocytosis, monovalent cation leak, and red cell shape all revert to normal (Mentzer et al, 1978). Labelled cross-linking agents interact with PS, PE and membrane proteins but it is not clear how the corrective effect on the disordered physiology of the hereditary stomatocyte is achieved.

Hereditary haemolytic disorders where the membrane is secondarily involved

Sickle cell anaemia (SCA). A single β-chain substitution produces sickle haemoglobin which gels in the deoxy form to produce rigid, elongated erythrocytes. However, the cause of the clinically important vaso-occlusive crises remains poorly understood and therefore, membrane function in SCA has been scrutinized and particularly the role of the irreversibly sickled cell (ISC). The ISC retains its abnormal sickle shape even though its intracellular haemoglobin is restored to the oxy non-sickling form. When homozygous SS red cells are exposed to hypoxia in vitro, the first detectable change, before sickling occurs, is the appearance of a cation leak with K^+ loss exceeding Na^+ gain (Palek, 1977). Then Ca^{2+} enters sickle red cells and because Ca^{2+} affects membrane function, Ca^{2+} metabolism has been extensively studied in SCA with the following results: (a) Ca^{2+} levels are two to three times higher than normal in SS red cells and are even higher in ISC (Eaton et al, 1973); (b) when labelled ^{45}Ca is newly introduced into intact red cells more is sequestered at membrane sites in SCA than in comparable reticulocyte rich controls (Schrier et al, 1980); (c) the Ca^{2+} pump appears to respond abnormally in SCA particularly after sickling has been induced (Bookchin

& Liu, 1980); (d) in sickle ghosts, the Ca^{2+},Mg^{2+}-ATPase with its linked Ca^{2+} efflux pump functions normally but a substantial amount of membrane associated Ca^{2+} is not accessible to this Ca^{2+} pump (Schrier & Bensch, 1976); (e) calmodulin is normally present in sickle erythrocytes but their Ca^{2+} pump is poorly responsive to it (Gopinath & Vincenzi, 1979).

It is not proven that Ca^{2+} accumulation and membrane localization contributes to the pathophysiology of SCA particularly since sickle red cells do not assume the spheroechinocytic shape associated with Ca^{2+} accumulation. Nevertheless, Ca^{2+} may more subtly alter membrane function.

Therefore, membrane proteins have also been studied in SCA with the following results: (a) β^s chains preferentially bind to red cell membranes and sickle red cell membranes generally contain more haemoglobin than normal (Bank et al, 1974); (b) glycoproteins are reduced (Riggs & Ingram, 1977); (c) protein kinase activity is decreased and in consequence there is defective in vitro spectrin phosphorylation (Beutler et al, 1977); (d) Triton shells prepared from ISCs retain the ISC shape indicating that in vitro sickling conditioned and conferred the ISC shape on the proteins of the cytoskeleton (Lux et al, 1976).

Presumably repeated cycles of sickling and unsickling affect the red cell membrane either directly or indirectly possibly via Ca^{2+} accumulation. However, the effect is seen on both cytosol facing proteins and external surface proteins. Probably alterations in membrane proteins lead to the extreme dehydration seen in the ISCs which may have MCHC values of 40 or greater. It is not clear whether there is primary loss of water or primary loss of K^+ with secondary water loss. The result is the very rigid ISC because of increased internal viscosity and cytoskeletal changes. However, ISC become almost normally deformable in the ektacytometer when rehydration is achieved, an observation that conflicts with the evidence of cytoskeletal abnormalities (Clark et al, 1980). In any case, the proportion of ISCs does not correlate with either the frequency or severity of vaso-occlusive crises, only with the extent of haemolysis.

In addition to protein alterations, phospholipid changes have also been described. The aminophospholipids, PS and PE, partly migrate to the outer half of the bilayer where they may serve as foci for coagulation (Chiu et al, 1979).

Monolayers of human endothelial cells bind few normal red cells but many more sickle cells, and the extent of binding seems to correlate with the frequency and severity of the sickle vaso occlusive crises (Hebbel et al, 1980). Conceivably reduced glycoprotein content might facilitate the binding of sickle cells to vascular endothelium where the adherent red cells could become the nidus for propagating aggregates that block the microcirculation.

Therefore, sickle haemoglobin impacts on the red cell membrane causing: salt and water loss with dehydration, Ca^{2+} accumulation, membrane binding of haemoglobin, protein kinase inactivation, phospholipid movement, surface charge reduction, and perhaps adhesion of red cells to vascular endothelium leading in turn to the vaso occlusive crisis.

Haemoglobin CC disease. This has not been as well studied as SCA, but the morphologic picture of target cells can be explained in part. Studies in the ektacytometer indicate that haemoglobin CC erythrocytes have increased internal viscosity presumably due to a water deficit. Therefore, the SA/V ratio is increased.

The mechanism by which haemoglobin CC causes water loss is unknown (Mohandas et al, 1980).

Unstable haemoglobinopathies. Several forms of unstable haemoglobinopathies as well as oxidative haemolysis are characterized by the formation of Heinz bodies. In some cases the Heinz bodies are attached to the membrane either by covalent disulfide bonds or by hydrophobic bonds. Perhaps because of mechanical effects, the attachment of Heinz bodies to membranes interferes with their deformability and they are trapped in the spleen (Rifkind, 1965). Either the oxidative attack or the Heinz bodies leads to a K^+ leak which can produce a dehydrated stiff erythrocyte (Oringer & Parker, 1977).

Thalassaemia. It is thought that α^4 or β^4 tetramers come to lie against the cytosol face of the membrane where they may cause a K^+ leak and membrane rigidity as measured with micropipettes (La Celle, 1975). Lipid analyses of β-thalassaemia major erythrocytes show evidence of peroxidation (Rachmilewitz et al, 1976).

G6PD deficiency. The common forms of G6PD deficiency (A-, Mediterranean, Canton) produce a membrane defect by the formation of Heinz bodies. The 'bite' cell seen in oxidative haemolysis might be the evidence of Heinz body removal. Some of the rarer chronic haemolytic non-spherocytic forms of G6PD deficiency demonstrate clear-cut evidence of membrane damage. In G6PD Long Prairie, SDS-PAGE of red cell membranes shows evidence of high MW complexes which are strikingly similar to those produced in vitro by oxidative attack (Allen et al, 1978). Since the aggregates are dissociable when treated with sulphydryl reducing agents, it is likely that they are cross-linked by intramolecular disulphide bridges. This cross-linking of membrane proteins presumably leads in turn to membrane rigidity and haemolysis.

Wilson's disease. Haemolytic anaemia occurs infrequently at presentation in Wilson's disease (Deiss et al, 1970). The excess copper appears to produce an oxidative attack on erythrocytes, first generating H_2O_2 and then perhaps via interaction with membrane sulphydryls, producing superoxide with further oxidation of the membrane. Documentation of membrane protein oxidation, however, has not yet occurred (Hochstein et al, 1978).

Pyruvate kinase (PK) deficiency. This is a classical example of a metabolic abnormality in which the red cell is unable to maintain its ATP levels, Ca^{2+} enters and K^+ leaks out (the Gardos effect). When water loss follows K^+ loss, the result is a rigid dehydrated red cell (Glader & Sullivan, 1979). Quinine can block K^+ and water flux in energy depleted erythrocytes and when quinine is added in vitro to cyanide treated PK deficient erythrocytes, K^+ and water loss are blocked while ATP depletion and Ca^{2+} entry are unchanged. This observation serves to support the idea that the Gardos effect is capable of producing the highly specific membrane K^+ leak described leading to the production of rigid red cells (Koller et al, 1979).

Acquired haemolytic disorders where membrane dysfunction is prominent and contributes to the haemolysis

IMMUNE ATTACK

In autoimmune haemolytic anaemia the external surface of the membrane is attacked by IgG and complement either alone or in combination. The coated red cells are attacked by macrophages which remove membrane thereby producing spherocytosis with the consequence of reduced deformability and splenic and RE trapping.

PHYSICAL OR CHEMICAL ATTACK

Oxidative drugs or toxins can produce the same membrane damages described above (unstable haemoglobinopathies).

Snake, insect, and bacterial toxins. Clostridia and some snake and insect venoms contain potent phospholipases which can attack the membrane phospholipids so severely that there is loss of surface area, leading to spherocytosis and even intravascular haemolysis. In one study involving Clostridial attack, proteolysis was severe while there was surprisingly no evidence for lipolysis. Therefore both the lipolytic and proteolytic action may be important (Simpkins et al, 1971). Usually there is a loss of surface area leading to microspherocytosis.

Thermal damage. When exposed to temperatures in excess of 45°C the red cell fragments, producing buds and microspherocytes (Ham et al, 1968). The curve of heat denaturation of spectrin is very similar to the red cell heat denaturation curve suggesting that the main effect of high temperatures is directed toward spectrin denaturation (Brandts et al, 1977). Patients with severe burns occasionally have severe haemolysis associated with the fragmented erythrocytes of thermal denaturation.

INFECTIONS

Infection can result in several forms of haemolysis including immune haemolysis and hypersplenism. Some organisms secrete a neuraminidase which could theoretically remove membrane sialic acid thereby reducing the red cell negative charge and its survival (Durocher et al, 1975). There is no proof of this mechanism in humans.

MICROANGIOPATHY

Erythrocytes can be sheared by jets or cleaved on fibrin strands across damaged vessels. There is very little haemoglobin leak when the entire cell is transected perhaps because of the self-sealing properties of the lipid bilayer. The residual fragments have bizarre shapes including sharp corners. Presumably a membrane change of unknown nature occurs that allows the erythrocyte to hold these unusual shapes. The corners of these distorted red cells are further broken off and the remaining fragment, depleted of surface area, becomes a very small rigid microsphere.

ACQUIRED CLONAL DISORDERS

Chronic myeloid leukaemia. In the chronic stable phase, no red cell membrane protein abnormalities occur but as patients enter the stage of metamorphosis and blast crisis, abnormalities of sialic acid content and PAS banding patterns on SDS-PAGE appear, presumably indicating the emergence of more dysplastic erythroid clones (Balduini et al, 1980).

Paroxysmal nocturnal haemoglobinuria (PNH). PNH affects plasma membranes of red cells, neutrophils, and platelets. The red cell membrane acetylcholinesterase activity is low; the cells bind more C3 than normal and for a given amount of bound terminal complexes, there is more lysis of PNH than control cells. The underlying defect that increases the susceptibility of PNH cells to complement action is unknown (Rosse & Adams, 1979).

DISORDERS OF LIPID METABOLISM

Abnormalities of lipid metabolism may be reflected in the circulating red cells because of the ability of cholesterol and the outer bilayer phospholipids to exchange readily with plasma constituents.

Vitamin E deficiency. Premature infants may be deficient in vitamin E which acts as an anti-oxidant protecting against lipid peroxidation. Vitamin E deficiency may be accompanied by haemolysis with irregular shaped red blood cells (Jacob & Lux, 1968).

Liver disease. In several forms of moderately severe liver disease (obstructive jaundice, cirrhosis, hepatitis) there is a symmetrical increase in red cell membrane cholesterol and phospholipid. These molecules intercalate into the membrane, expand its surface area, and by increasing the SA/V ratio produce a target cell. Cholesterol tends to decrease fluidity while the phospholipids, particularly PC, increase fluidity and balance is achieved with the symmetrical increase seen. Haemolysis is not a necessary concomittant perhaps because the lipid fluidity of the membrane is not altered. When normal erythrocytes are transfused into a patient with liver disease and target cells, they develop abnormal shape.

In very severe forms of liver disease, usually alcoholic cirrhosis, the red cell membrane takes up more cholesterol than phospholipid. The relative increase in cholesterol produces an expanded membrane with increased microviscosity and scalloped folded edges presumably due to the intercalation of cholesterol at the core of the lipid bilayer. Perhaps because of this shape or the increased lipid viscosity the cholesterol loaded erythrocyte is detained in the spleen where it is remodelled into the spiny spur cell or acanthocyte which, because of shape and SA/V considerations, is susceptible to subsequent splenic haemolysis (Cooper, 1978).

In severe *protein-calorie malnutrition* and in *anorexia nervosa* acanthocytes and target cells are seen. The complex alterations in lipoproteins may lead to red cell accumulation of both cholesterol and PC in the red cell membrane with a relative increase in cholesterol. The shortened red cell survival occasionally seen is not necessarily related to cholesterol and PC disturbances and may be related instead to lipid peroxidation (Fondu et al, 1980).

Red cell membrane abnormalities where there is no haemolysis

HEREDITARY DISORDERS

The red cell membrane may serve as a surrogate plasma membrane for the study of presumed plasma membrane disorders in diseases where the primarily affected tissue is difficult to sample. Examples of this approach include: (a) Huntington's disease: The red cell membrane, when carrying an electron-spin resonance (ESR) label, responds differently to γ-aminobutyric acid exposure than normal (Butterfield et al, 1978). (b) Duchenne Muscular Dystrophy: ESR probes inserted in red cell membranes indicate that an abnormal environment exists in the non-polar area of the membrane (Sato et al, 1978). (c) Myotonic Muscular Dystrophy: Erythrocytes show membrane permeability to Ca^{2+} (Plishker et al, 1978).

Abnormalities of the red cell surface. (a) The blood group En(a-) phenotype is characterized by the absence of detectable antigens of the MNSs system. SDS-PAGE with PAS staining shows absence of glycophorin A but there is no shortening of red cell survival thereby raising questions about the importance of glycophorin A in maintenance of membrane structure (Tanner & Anstee, 1976).

(b) Duffy negativity {Fy(a-b-)} protects the red cell from attack by the *Plasmodium vivax* parasite of vivax malaria (Miller et al, 1979).

(c) McLeod: Affected red cells lack K_x, a precursor of the Kell antigen system, which is carried on the X chromosome. Male hemizygotes have variable degrees of acanthocytosis and compensated haemolysis (Wimer et al, 1977). While the shape change suggests that there might be a lipid abnormality, it has not been identified.

(d) Acetylcholinesterase: There are two families exhibiting severe hereditary deficiency of red cell membrane acetylcholinesterase without evidence of haemolysis (Shinohara & Tanaka, 1979).

ACQUIRED DISEASES WITH A PROBABLE GENETIC BACKGROUND

Essential hypertension. The diagnosis of primary or essential hypertension has been made in vitro in two laboratories by measuring parameters relating to Na^+ and K^+ transport. The underlying hypothesis is that the red cell may be acting as a surrogate for either renal or vascular plasma membranes. A counter transport system present in normal red cells which can extrude both internal Na^+ and K^+ is functionally deficient in red cells from patients with essential hypertension and some of their relatives (Garay et al, 1980). In addition, a Na^+-Li^+ counter transport system appears to function more rapidly than normal in red cells from patients with essential hypertension (Canessa et al, 1980). The meaning of these observations is not clear but the impact may be substantial, in terms of exploring the pathophysiology of primary hypertension using the red cell membrane.

Diabetes mellitus. Non-enzymatic glycosylation of all red cell membrane protein occurs in the presence of sustained hyperglycaemia and correlates with levels of haemoglobin A_{1c}. This observation confirms the idea that the potential for glycosylation of a variety of proteins exists where there is sustained hyperglycaemia (Miller et al, 1980).

SUMMARY

The pace of the growth of our understanding of red cell membrane biology is much faster than our ability to comprehend disorders of the human erythrocyte membrane. In part this relates to the probable subtlety of red cell membrane disorders because a gross defect interfering with some major function would almost certainly prove lethal in utero. Nevertheless, study of human red cell membranes now offers the opportunity of making diagnoses not only in the case of haemolytic disorders but in situations as diverse as Duchenne muscular dystrophy and essential hypertension. No useful therapeutic intervention has come out of recent studies on human red cell membrane disorders, but the suggestion that bifunctional agents can improve several aspects of impaired function in erythrocytes from patients with hereditary stomatocytosis is intriguing and offers a direction for the future.

REFERENCES

Allan D, Michell R H 1975 Nature 258: 348–349
Allan D, Michell R H 1979 In: S E Lux, V T Marchesi, C F Fox (eds) Normal and abnormal red cell membranes, Alan R Liss, Inc, New York. p 523–529
Allan D, Low M G, Finean J B, Michell R H 1975 Biochimica et Biophysica Acta 413: 309–316
Allan D W, Johnson G J, Cadman S, Kaplan M E 1978 Journal of Laboratory and Clinical Medicine 91: 321–327
Allen J E, Rasmussen H 1971 Science 174: 512–514
Aloni B, Shinitzky M, Moses S, Livne A 1975 British Journal of Haematology 31: 117–123
Avissar N, De Vries A, Ben-Shaul Y, Cohen I 1975 Biochimica et Biophysica Acta 375: 35–43
Avruch J, Fairbanks G 1974 Biochemistry 13: 5507–5514
Balduini C L, Sinigaglia F, Ascari E, Balduini C 1980 British Journal of Haematology 44: 509–510
Bank A, Mears G, Weiss R, O'Donnell J V, Natta C 1974 Journal of Clinical Investigation 54: 805–809
Bennett V, Stenbuck P J 1979 Nature 280: 468–473
Bennett V, Stenbuck P J 1980 Journal of Biological Chemistry 255: 2540–2548
Bessis M 1972 Nouvelle Revue Française d'Hématologie 12: 721–746
Bessis M, Mohandas N 1975 Blood Cells 1: 307–313
Beutler E, Guinto E, Johnson C 1977 Blood Cells 3: 135–152
Blau L, Bittman R 1978 Journal of Biological Chemistry 253: 8366–8368
Bookchin R M, Lew V L 1980 Nature 284: 561–563
Brandts J F, Erickson L, Lysko K, Schwartz A T, Taverna R D 1977 The involvement of spectrin in the A transition. Biochemistry 16: 3450–3454
Brenner S L, Korn E D 1980 Journal of Biological Chemistry 254: 1670–1676
Bretscher M S 1972 Nature (New Biology) 236: 11–12
Bull B S, Brailsford J D 1973 Blood 41: 833–844
Butterfield D A, Braden M L, Markesberry W R 1978 Journal of Supramolecular Structure 9: 125–130
Canessa M, Adragna N, Solomon H S, Connolly T M, Tosteson D C 1980 New England Journal of Medicine 302: 772–776
Carpentieri U, Gustavson L P, Haggard M E 1977 Clinical Pediatrics 16: 76–78
Chapman D 1975 In: G Weissmann, R Claiborne (eds) Cell Membranes, HP Publishing Co, Inc, New York p 13–22
Cheung W Y 1980 Science 207: 19–27
Chien S 1977a Blood Cells 3: 283–303
Chien S 1977b Blood Cells 3: 71–99
Chien S, Cooper G W Jr, Jan K, Miller L H, Howe C, Usami S, Lalezari P 1974 Blood 43: 445–460
Chiu D, Fujimara S, Lubin B 1979 Blood 54: Suppl 1, Abst 8, p 25a
Clark M R, Mohandas N, Shohet S B 1980 Journal of Clinical Investigation 65: 189–196
Conrad M J, Singer S J 1979 Proceedings of the National Academy of Sciences USA 76: 5202–5206
Cooper R A 1977 New England Journal of Medicine 297: 371–377
Cooper R A 1978 Journal of Supramolecular Structure 8: 413–430
Danielli J F 1975 G Weissmann, R Claiborne (eds) Cell Membranes, HP Publishing Co, Inc, New York, p 3–11
Deiss A, Lee G R, Cartwright G E 1970 Annals of Internal Medicine 73: 413–418

Dunham P B, Hoffman J F 1970 Proceedings of the National Academy of Sciences USA 66: 936–943
Durocher J R, Payne R C, Conrad M E 1975 Blood 45: 11–20
Eaton J W, Skelton T D, Swofford H S, Kolpin C E, Jacob H S 1973 Nature 246: 105–106
Elgsaeter A, Branton D 1974 Journal of Cell Biology 63: 1018–1030
Enegren B J, Burness A T H 1977 Nature 268: 536–537
Fairbanks G, Avruch J 1974 Biochemistry 13: 5514–5521
Fairbanks G, Steck T L, Wallach D F H 1971 Biochemistry 10: 2606–2617
Fischer T M, Stöhr-Liessen M, Schmid-Schönbein H 1978 Science 202: 894–896
Fondu P, Mozes N, Neve P, Sohet-Robazza L, Mandelbaum I 1980 British Journal of Haematology 44:
    605–618
Fowler V, Bennett V 1978 Journal of Supramolecular Structure 8: 215–221
Fowler V, Taylor D L 1980 Journal of Cell Biology 85: 361–376
Fukuda M N, Fukuda M, Hakomori S 1979 Journal of Biological Chemistry 254: 5458–5465
Furthmayr H 1978a Journal of Supramolecular Structure 9: 79–95
Furthmayr H 1978b Nature 271: 519–524
Gahmberg C G, Tauren G, Virtanen I, Wartiovaara J 1978 Journal of Supramolecular Structure 8: 337–347
Garay R P, Dagher G, Pernollet M, Devynck M, Meyer P 1980 Nature 284: 281–283
Gardos G 1959 Acta Physiologica Academiae Sci. Hungaricae 15: 121–125
Geiduschek J B, Singer S J 1979 Cell 16: 149–163
Glader B E, Sullivan D W 1979 In: S E Lux, V T Marchesi, C F Fox (eds) Normal and abnormal red cell
    membranes, Alan R Liss, Inc, New York, p 503–513
Gopinath R M, Vincenzi F F 1977 Biochemical and Biophysical Research Communications 77: 1203–1209
Gopinath R M, Vincenzi F F 1979 American Journal of Hematology 7: 303–312
Greenquist A C, Shohet S B 1976 Blood 48: 877–886
Ham T H, Sayre R W, Dunn R F, Murphy J R 1968 Blood 32: 862–871
Hardy B, Schrier S L1978 Biochemical and Biophysical Research Communications 81: 1153–1161
Hardy B, Bensch K G, Schrier S L 1979 Journal of Cell Biology 82: 654–663
Harrison D G, Long C 1968 Journal of Physiology 199: 367–381
Hebbel R P, Boogaerts M A B, Eaton J W, Steinberg M H 1980 New England Journal of Medicine 302:
    992–995
Hochstein P, Kumar K S, Forman S J 1978 In: G J Brewer (ed) The red cell, Alan R Liss, Inc, New York,
    p 669–681
Holroyde C P, Gardner F H 1970 Blood 36: 566–575
Holroyde C P, Oski F A, Gardner F H 1969 New England Journal of Medicine 281: 516–520
Huestis W H, McConnell H M 1974 Biochemical and Biophysical Research Communications 57: 726–732
Jacob H S, Lux S E 1968 Blood 32: 549–568
Jacobson B S, Branton D 1977 Science 195: 302–304
Jain S K, Hochstein P 1980 Biochemical and Biophysical Research Communications 92: 247–254
Jarrett H W, Penniston J T 1977 Biochemical and Biophysical Research Communications 77: 1210–1216
Ji T H, Kiehm D J, Middaugh C R 1980 Journal of Biological Chemistry 255: 2990–2993
Kahlenberg A, Zala C A 1977 Journal of Supramolecular Structure 7: 287–300
Kay M M B 1978 Journal of Supramolecular Structure 9: 555–567
Koller C A, Orringer E P, Parker J C 1979 American Journal of Hematology 7: 193–199
La Celle P L 1975 Blood Cells 1: 269–284
La Celle P L, Weed R I, Santillo P A 1976 In: L Bolis, J F Hoffman, A Leaf (eds) Membranes and disease,
    Raven Press, New York, p 1–17
La Celle P L, Eans E A, Hochmuth R M 1977 Blood Cells 3: 335–350
Lange Y, Cohen C M, Poznansky M J 1977 Proceedings of the National Academy of Sciences USA 74:
    1538–1542
Liu S C, Palek J 1980 Clinical Research (Abst) 28: 318a
Lorand L, Siefring G E Jr, Lowe-Krentz L 1979 Seminars in Hematology 16: 65–74
Lutz H U, Liu S, Palek J 1977 Journal of Cell Biology 73: 548–560
Lux S E 1979a Nature 281: 426–429
Lux S E 1979b Seminars in Hematology 16: 21–51
Lux S E, John K M, Karnovsky M J 1979 Journal of Clinical Investigation 58: 955–963
Lux S E, Pease B, Tomaselli M B, John K M, Bernstein S E 1979 In: S E Lux, V T Marchesi, C F Fox
    (eds) Normal and abnormal red cell membranes, Alan R Liss, Inc, New York, p 463–469
Marchesi V T 1978 Annual Review of Medicine 29: 593–603
Marchesi V T 1979a Seminars in Hematology 16: 3–20
Marchesi V T 1979b Journal of Membrane Biology 51: 101–131
Marinetti G V, Crain R C 1978 Journal of Supramolecular Structure 8: 191–213
Mehta N G 1980 Journal of Membrane Biology 52: 17–24

Mentzer W C, Lam G K H, Lubin B H, Greenquist A, Schrier S L, Lande W 1978 Journal of Supramolecular Structure 9: 275–288
Miller J A, Gravallese E, Bunn H F 1980 Journal of Clinical Investigation 65: 896–901
Miller L H, McAuliffe F M, Johnson J G 1979 In: S E Lux, V T Marchesi, C F Fox (eds) Normal and abnormal red cell membranes, Alan R Liss, Inc, New York, p 497–502
Mohandas N, Greenquist A C, Shohet S B 1978 Journal of Supramolecular Structure 9: 453–458
Mohandas N, Clark M R, Jacobs M, Shohet S B 1980 Journal of Clinical Investigation, in press
Mombers C, Verkleij A J, De Gier J, Van Deenen L L M 1979 Biochimica et Biophysica Acta 551: 271–281
Nakashima K, Beutler E 1979 Blood 53: 481–485
Nelson M J, Huestis W H 1980 Biochimica et Biophysica Acta, in press
Nelson M J, Ferrel J E Jr, Huestis W H 1979 Biochimica et Biophysica Acta 558: 136–140
Nicolson G L, Painter R G 1973 Journal of Cell Biology 59: 395–406
Orringer E P, Parker J C 1977 Blood 50: 1013–1021
Palek J 1977 British Journal of Haematology 35: 1–9
Palek J, Lui S 1979 Seminars in Hematology 16: 75–93
Palek J, Liu A, Liu D, Snyder L M, Fortier N L, Njoko G, Kiernan F, Funk P, Crusbers T 1977 Blood 50: 155–164
Palek J, Liu P Y, Liu S C, Prchal J, Parmley R T, Castleberry R P 1979 Blood 54: Suppl 1, p 31a, Abst 25
Pearson H A 1968 Blood 32: 972–978
Plishker G A, Gitelman H J, Appel S H 1978 Science 200: 323–325
Ponder E 1957 Scientific American 196: 95–102
Rachmilewitz E A, Lubin B H, Shohet S B 1976 Blood 47: 495–505
Rifkind R A, 1965 Blood 26: 433–448
Riggs M G, Ingram V M 1977 Biochemical and Biophysical Research Communications 74: 191–198
Roelofson B, Van Deenen L L M 1973 European Journal of Biochemistry 40: 245–257
Rosse W F, Adams J P 1979 In: S E Lux, V T Marchesi, C F Fox (eds) Normal and abnormal red cell membranes, Alan R Liss, Inc, New York, p 457–461
Rothstein A, Knauf P A, Grinstein S, Shami Y 1979 In: S E Lux, V T Marchesi, C F Fox (eds) Normal and abnormal red cell membranes, Alan R Liss, Inc, New York, p 483–496
Salhany J M, Cordes K A, Gaines E D 1980 Biochemistry 19: 1447–1454
Sarkadi B, Szasz I, Gerloczy A, Gardos G 1977 Biochimica et Biophysica Acta 464: 93–107
Sato B, Nishikida K, Samuels L T, Tyler F H 1978 Journal of Clinical Investigation 61: 251–259
Sauberman N, Fortier N L, Fairbanks G, O'Connor R J, Snyder L M 1979 Biochimica et Biophysica Acta 556: 292–313
Schatzmann H J, Vincenzi F F 1969 Journal of Physiology 201: 369–395
Schekman R, Singer S J 1976 Proceedings of the National Academy of Sciences USA 73: 4075–4079
Schrier S L 1977 Blood 50: 227–237
Schrier S L, Bensch K G 1976 Proceedings of the international conference on biological membranes. In: L Bolis, J F Hoffman, A Leaf (eds) Membranes and disease, Raven Press, New York, p 31–40
Schrier S L, Hardy B 1979 Blood 54: Suppl 1, p 31a, Abst 27
Schrier S L, Junga I 1980 Journal of Supramolecular Structure, in press
Schrier S L, Ben-Bassat I, Bensch K, Seeger M, Junga I 1974 British Journal of Haematology 26: 59–69
Schrier S L, Bensch K G, Johnson M, Junga I 1975 Journal of Clinical Investigation 56: 8–22
Schrier S L, Junga I, Krueger J, Johnson M 1978 Blood Cells 4: 339–353
Schrier S L, Hardy B, Bensch K, Junga I, Krueger J 1979 Transfusion 19: 158–165
Schrier S L, Johnson M, Junga I, Krueger J 1980 Blood, accepted for publication
Seaman G V F, Knox R J, Nordt F J, Regan D H 1977 Blood 50: 1001–1011
Shaklai N, Yguerabide J, Ranney H M 1977 Biochemistry 16: 5593–5597
Sheetz M P 1979 Biochimica et Biophysica Acta 557: 122–134
Sheetz M P, Sawyer D 1978 Journal of Supramolecular Structure 8: 399–412
Sheetz M P, Singer S J 1974 Proceedings of the National Academy of Sciences USA 71: 4457–4461
Sheetz M P, Schindler M, Koppel D E 1980 Nature 285: 510–512
Shinohara K, Tanaka K R 1979 American Journal of Hematology 7: 313–321
Shohet S B 1979 Journal of Clinical Investigation 64: 483–494
Shotten D M, Burke B E, Branton D 1979 Biophysical and electron microscopic studies. Journal of Molecular Biology 131: 303–329
Simpkins H, Kahlenberg A, Rosenberg A, Tay S, Panko E 1971 British Journal of Haematology 21: 173–182
Singer S J, Nicolson G L 1972 Science 175: 720–731
Smith J A, Lucas F V Jr, Martin A P, Senhauser D A, Vorbeck M L 1973 Biochemical and Biophysical Research Communications 54: 1015–1023
Steck T L 1978 Journal of Supramolecular Structure 8: 311–324

Steck T L, Kant J A 1974 Methods in Enzymology 31: 172–180
Steck T L, Yu J 1973 Journal of Supramolecular Structure 1: 220–232
Stossel T P 1978 Annual Review of Medicine 29: 427–457
Szymanski I O, Odgren P R 1979 Vox Sanguinis 36: 213–224
Tanner M J A, Anstee D J 1976 The Biochemical Journal 153: 271–277
Tao M, Conway R, Cheta S 1980 Journal of Biological Chemistry 255: 2563–2568
Tilney L G, Detmers P 1975 Journal of Cell Biology 66: 508–520
Tsukamoto T, Suyama K, Germann P, Sonenberg M 1980 Biochemistry 19: 918–924
Turrito V T, Weiss H J 1980 Science 207: 541–543
Tyler J M, Hargreaves W R, Branton D 1979 Proceedings of the National Academy of Sciences USA 76: 5192–5196
Ungewickell E, Bennett P M, Calvert R, Ohanian V, Gratzer W B 1979 Nature 280: 811–814
Verkleij A J, Zwaal F A, Roelofson B, Comfurius P, Kastelijn D, Van Deenen L L M 1973 Biochimica et Biophysica Acta 323: 178–193
Walter T, Mentzer W, Greenquist A, Schrier S, Mohandas N 1977 Blood 50 (Suppl 1): 98
Wang C S, Alaupovic P 1978 Suppl 2: 220, Abst 556
Weinstein R S, Khodadad J K, Steck T L 1978 Journal of Supramolecular Structure 8: 325–335
White J G, Burris S, Eaton J W 1978 Blood 52 (Suppl 1): 106, Abst 94
Wimer B M, Marsh W L, Taswell H F, Galey W R 1977 British Journal of Haematology 36: 219–224
Wolfe L C, Lux S E 1978 Blood 52 (Suppl 1): 106 Abst 96
Yu J, Fischman D A, Steck T L 1973 Journal of Supramolecular Structure 1: 233–248
Zail S S, Pickering A 1979 British Journal of Haematology 42: 399–402

5. Erythroid colony growth in culture: analysis of erythroid differentiation and studies in human disease states

Jeanette Mladenovic   John W Adamson

Mature erythrocytes arise from a series of differentiation and maturation steps that begin at the level of a pluripotential stem cell which also has the capacity to differentiate into granulocytes, monocytes, and platelets. The study of morphologically recognizable marrow erythroid progenitors has provided much information about the terminal steps of both normal and disordered erythropoiesis. However, early differentiation and maturation events occur in cells which are not morphologically identifiable. Over the last several years, functional in vitro and in vivo assays specific for hematopoietic progenitors have permitted the study of early differentiation steps, providing insight into normal regulatory mechanisms and the complex levels at which they act.

This chapter describes currently available assays for erythroid progenitors in animals and man, and the limitation and application of such assays to the analysis of erythroid differentiation in human disease states.

STUDIES IN EXPERIMENTAL ANIMALS

Colony-forming assays

The original assay for progenitors capable of giving rise to differentiated hematopoietic cells was the spleen colony-forming assay described by Till & McCulloch (1961). When normal mouse marrow cells are injected intravenously into lethally-irradiated syngeneic hosts, macroscopic colonies of hematopoietic cells appear in the spleens of the recipients by 10 to 14 days. Irradiated animals, not rescued by marrow cells, die of hematopoietic failure. Becker et al (1963) formally demonstrated that these complex colonies, which contained all of the usual differentiated myeloid elements found in the blood, arose from a single progenitor termed the spleen colony-forming unit (CFU-S).

In 1965 and 1966 initial reports appeared describing the in vitro growth of colonies of differentiated granulocytes and macrophages in semisolid culture media (Pluznik & Sachs, 1965; Bradley & Metcalf, 1966). These colonies arose from the granulocyte colony-forming unit (CFU-C), and formed in response to a cell-derived growth-promoting material referred to as colony-stimulating activity.

In 1971, Stephenson and Axelrad reported the first successful in vitro growth of erythroid colonies. The development of these colonies required the addition of the hormone erythropoietin to the cultures. In cultures of mouse marrow, colonies of 8 to 64 well-hemoglobinized cells arose from erythroid colony-forming units (CFU-E), reached maximum numbers by 24 to 72 hours, and then disappeared. The number of colonies formed was linearly related to both the number of cells plated and the concentration of erythropoietin added. Subsequently, Axelrad et al (1973) reported the appearance of another type of erythroid colony which grew out over 7 to 10 days in culture. This colony was much more complex and contained up to 10^4 cells. Because the appearance of the clusters of subcolonies in the culture dish was that of a burst, the cell giving rise to a colony was referred to as the burst-forming unit, or BFU-E. Again, the size and number of colonies detected depended on the erythropoietin dose, which was greater than that required for CFU-E growth. More recently, Gregory (1976) described a colony of intermediate size, comprised of 3 to 8 clusters of hemoglobinized cells which are fully mature by day 3 to 4. The cell giving rise to these colonies was termed the day 3 or mature BFU-E. The size, sensitivity to erythropoietin, and time of appearance in culture of these colonies suggest that the day 3 BFU-E is intermediate in its state of maturation between CFU-E and day 8 BFU-E. Various properties of these progenitors are summarized in Table 5.1.

Table 5.1   Characteristics of murine erythroid colony-forming cells

Progenitor	Optimal culture day	Cells/colony	Per cent in DNA synthesis	Sedimentation velocity (mm/hr)	Response to anemia/ hypertransfusion
CFU-E	2	8–64	65–80%	7.0	↑/↓
Day 3 BFU-E	3–4	>100	50%	4.4	↑/↓
Day 8 BFU-E	8–10	>1000	20–40%	3.8	No change

The lineage of differentiation of these progenitors was established by Gregory & Henkelman (1977) using the ingenious analysis of correlation first described by Wu et al (1968). This analysis assumes that the degree of relatedness of progenitors is reflected by the correlation of their numbers in growing clones. Spleen colonies in transplanted, lethally irradiated mice are examples of such clones. In the analysis individual spleen colonies are disaggregated and replated for growth of the various colony-forming cells and the resulting colonies are then enumerated. No correlations between numbers of CFU-E and CFU-S or CFU-C were found, suggesting that CFU-E were separated by several cell divisions from stem cells such that random or regulatory events weakened or abolished possible correlations. In contrast, a close

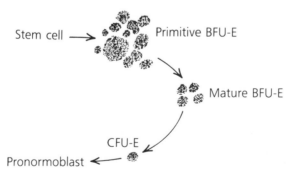

Fig. 5.1   The differentiation sequence of committed erythroid stem cells revealed by in vitro culture techniques. The diagram schematically outlines the in vitro morphology of colonies formed by the various progenitors. Pluripotent stem cells (CFU-S) undergo a restriction or commitment event and become limited in the differentiation program they can express. The earliest detectable erythroid progenitor in culture is the primitive burst forming unit (BFU-E). Further maturation steps result in mature BFU-E and CFU-E. As the colony forming cells mature, they lose proliferative potential and become increasingly sensitive to erythropoietin. Finally, pronormoblasts are seen, the first morphologically identifiable cells of the erythroid marrow. (Reproduced from The Science and Practice of Clinical Medicine, Vol. 6 [Hematology and Oncology], edited by Marshall Lichtman, page 8, 1980, with permission of the publisher.)

correlation was found between CFU-S and primitive BFU-E, and also between BFU-E and CFU-C. This suggested that the primitive BFU-E is the earliest detectable erythroid progenitor (Fig. 5.1). These correlations held, regardless of whether the original spleen colony was predominantly erythroid or myeloid. Thus, it appeared that early restriction or differentiation events occurred either in a random fashion or in a manner independent of later regulatory events.

Physiologic regulation of erythroid colony-forming cells

Normal erythropoiesis is regulated by the glycoprotein hormone, erythropoietin. With anemia or hypoxia, erythropoietin production ordinarily rises, stimulating marrow erythropoiesis in an attempt to correct the deficit in oxygen transport. Conversely, with transfusion-induced polycythemia, erythropoietin levels fall, as does marrow activity. By studying the numbers of the different types of erythroid colony-forming cells under known physiological conditions in an animal model, further insight into factors which influence early and late erythroid differentiation has been obtained.

With phlebotomy- or phenylhydrazine-induced anemia, there is a dramatic increase in the number of CFU-E in the spleen and marrow (Hara & Ogawa, 1976; Adamson et al, 1978). The number of BFU-E in the marrow declines, in concert with an increase in their numbers in circulation and in the spleen. In contrast, hypertransfusion-induced polycythemia results in an 80 per cent decline in the number of CFU-E in marrow and spleen, with little if any change in the number of BFU-E. Injection of erythropoietin restores the number of CFU-E within 1 to 2 days. Thus, the CFU-E population is extremely sensitive to circulating levels of erythropoietin. The fact that hypertransfusion and acute erythropoietic stress have little or no effect on BFU-E implies that this progenitor is insensitive to acute changes in erythropoietin stimulation and is not dependent upon ambient levels of the hormone for maintenance of its numbers.

Further studies reveal that regulatory influences other than erythropoietin significantly affect the number and cell cycle activity of BFU-E (Iscove, 1977). In studies of regenerating marrow, the number and cell cycle activity of BFU-E were compared in anemic and hypertransfused animals. No differences were observed between the two groups. In contrast, recovering CFU-E were markedly reduced in the polycythemic group, confirming the effectiveness of hypertransfusion in the reduction of erythropoietin stimulation. Consequently, under regeneration stress, the response of early BFU-E is independent of erythropoietin stimulation in vivo.

Reports of the response of the intermediate class of BFU-E to physiologic manipulations have differed among investigators (Gregory & Eaves, 1978; Adamson et al, 1978). Since erythropoietic differentiation occurs on a continuum, observed differences in the response of mature BFU-E to changes in erythropoietin levels are likely methodologic.

Cellular and hormonal factors influencing erythroid colony growth

Erythropoietin

The precise mechanism by which erythropoietin initiates erythroid colony growth is unknown, but the hormone is required for hemoglobinization and maturation of the cells of the colony. The time that erythpropoietin acts in culture depends on the progenitor being assayed. CFU-E require erythropoietin throughout most of the period of growth in culture, suggesting that 'triggering', at least in vitro, is not sufficient for full expression of the erythroid program. In contrast, erythropoietin apparently has its predominant action on BFU-E growth later in culture, since it can be added at day 3 or 4 with hemoglobinization of full-sized colonies then appearing on schedule at day 8 to 10 (Iscove, 1978). The early growth of BFU-E, therefore, apparently relies on other factors.

Burst-promoting/enhancing activity

The concept that factors other than erythropoietin influence BFU-E growth was originally suggested by the facts that BFU-E are unaffected by changes in erythro- poietin levels and that their optimal growth in culture depends on carefully selected serum. The demonstration by Aye (1977) that a leukocyte-conditioned medium enhanced erythroid colony growth, and that erythropoietin could be added late in culture with full expression in colony growth also implied the importance of the influence of other factors on early erythroid burst formation.

Wagemaker (1978) has found burst-enhancing activity in mouse serum under experimental conditions designed to promote the release of such factors from populations of marrow cells. An important source of such activity are mitogen- stimulated lymphocytes (Parker & Metcalf, 1974). Under appropriate conditions, mixtures of cells containing lymphocytes release a number of factors capable of promoting the growth of a variety of colony-forming cells. To date, burst-promoting or enhancing activity has not been clearly separated from other factors which promote growth of granulocyte/macrophage or lymphocyte colonies, and the in vivo relevance of such factors in the day-to-day regulation or maintenance of erythropoiesis remains unknown.

Other hormones

A variety of other hormones, including beta-adrenergic agonists, thyroid hormones, growth hormone, and androgenic and non-androgenic steroids, interact with erythro- poietin to enhance the cloning efficiency of CFU-E from a variety of species (Adamson, 1978). Some of these hormones appear to act by different mechanisms in that the populations affected can be separated by physical means. The results of the studies are consistent in that none of the hormones can replace erythropoietin but only augment the effect of erythropoietin on colony growth. It is not certain whether such enhancement represents recruitment of somewhat earlier classes of colony-forming cells, or simply represents enhanced sensitivity of the target tissue to the primary regulatory hormone. This may be brought about through changes in postulated erythropoietin receptor number of avidity or through amplification of other informa- tion/translation steps. These hormonal interactions, defined in vitro, may have in vivo relevance and should be considered as modulating primary regulation events.

STUDIES IN MAN

Colony-forming assays

Colony assays for erythroid progenitors in the mouse have subsequently been applied to studies in man (Tepperman et al, 1974; Gregory & Eaves, 1977). The development of such assays has permitted the identification of three types of erythroid progenitors analogous to those found in the mouse.

In human marrow cell cultures containing erythropoietin, colonies of 8 to 64 hemoglobinized cells arise from CFU-E by 5 to 7 days. At 12 to 14 days, colonies comprised of 3 to 8 well-hemoglobinized subunits appear, those derived from mature BFU-E. Finally, macroscopic bursts containing up to 10^4 cells, originating from primitive BFU-E, are seen in culture after 16 to 21 days. Although the colony-forming cells themselves are not morphologically identifiable, each class of progenitor can be separated by physical and functional properties. As in the mouse, progenitors of increasing maturity are more likely to be in the DNA synthetic phase of the cell cycle, are larger as analyzed by velocity sedimentation (Ogawa et al, 1977a), and show increased sensitivity to erythropoietin.

Erythroid colony-forming cells are also found in human fetal liver (Hassan et al, 1977), umbilical cord blood (Ogawa et al, 1976a), and peripheral blood (Clarke & Housman, 1977; Ogawa et al, 1977b). Under normal circumstances, however, circulating progenitors are limited to BFU-E, while CFU-E are not found. Circulating BFU-E reside in the null-cell fraction of peripheral blood mononuclear cells (Nathan et al, 1978) where they are more easily accessible, more homogenous in terms of many of their properties and more amenable to quantitation than their marrow counterparts. The relationship of these progenitors to those in the marrow and the mechanism which permits their circulation are unknown.

Cellular interactions in erythroid colony growth

T-lymphocytes

In vivo experimental animal studies suggest a potentially important role for lymphocytes in the regulation of early hematopoiesis. Such examples include the appearance of anemia in neonatally thymectomized mice (Metcalf, 1966), increased proliferation of transplanted parent marrow in irradiated hybrid mice by the simultaneous injection of parent thymus cells (Goodman & Shinpock, 1968), and correction of the genetically-determined anemia in W/W^v mice by normal marrow transplantation and its abrogation by serum directed against T-lymphocytes (Wiktor-Jedrzejczak et al, 1977).

This possible 'helper' role of T-lymphocytes has recently been explored in human erythroid cultures. Initial work reported the absolute requirement of T-lymphocytes or a T-lymphocyte product for the optimal expression of size and number of BFU-E colonies from the null cell fraction of peripheral blood (Nathan et al, 1978). This helper function was related to the number of lymphocytes added and was radiosensitive, but was not affected by removal of adherent cells. Both isogeneic and allogeneic cells could function as helpers and a soluble product of tetanus toxoid-stimulated T-lymphocytes could substitute for intact cells. Although other laboratories have not been able to demonstrate the absolute requirement of T-cells for optimal BFU-E growth (Nomdedeu et al, 1978), most data favor the fact that removal and then readdition of T-cells to depleted marrow or peripheral blood mononuclear cells results in the stimulation of burst numbers.

The effect of T-cells on CFU-E and BFU-E growth from human marrow has been less well studied. Zanjani & Kaplan (1979) have suggested stimulation of marrow

CFU-E by unrelated, unfractionated peripheral blood lymphocytes. Although an apparent effect of T-cells on erythroid growth in culture can be demonstrated, further definition of such effects is hampered by lack of adequate techniques to completely remove other interacting cell populations such as monocytes or macrophages, and to reliably and easily separate T-cell populations into those with suppressor and helper activities. These functions may coexist in the same population, masking important but opposing effects (Torok-Storb et al, 1979c).

Monocytes/macrophages
Monocytes and macrophages, which comprise less than 1 per cent of the bone marrow population, are at least one source of colony stimulating factor. They may be crudely removed by adherence to nylon fibers or plastic. Aye (1977) reported that removal of such adherent populations decreased the number of erythroid colonies observed. More importantly, adherent cell removal allowed the detection of more primitive BFU-E when medium conditioned by peripheral blood leukocytes was added back to the culture (Eaves & Eaves, 1978). Such an effect suggested that adherent cells supplied a soluble factor directly or indirectly through interactions with other cells.

However, the issue of monocyte/macrophage effects has been clouded by recent studies showing that peripheral blood BFU-E growth is inversely related to the number of monocytes in culture, with complete inhibition seen with 20 per cent or more monocyte contamination (Rinehart et al, 1978). This effect has not been seen by other laboratories where monocyte contamination of routine cultures may be as high as 20 per cent (Lipton et al, 1980). The reasons for these discrepancies are unknown as is the relevance of such observations to the regulation of erythropoiesis in vivo.

Limitations of human erythroid colony growth
The technology of human erythroid culture has provided a useful tool for the analysis of hematopoiesis. However, the complexities of the technique and the possible divergence from in vivo situations must be recognized. Present culture results are derived from a system in which the stimulators are impure and the culture constituents, of necessity, are not well defined. The serum requirement for normal BFU-E growth is one example of such undefined culture requirements. In addition, even under optimal conditions, colonies may reveal severe morphological abnormalities in the non-nucleated cell progeny, such as hypochromia, microcytosis, and Heinz bodies (Ogawa et al, 1976).

Other limitations are also apparent. In mouse studies, absolute numbers of colony-forming cells may be obtained for a given organ such as the femur or spleen. In studies of man, however, absolute quantitation of precursor cells is not possible due to the marrow sampling error and the uncontrolled peripheral blood contamination. One approach to quantitating alterations in the number of progenitors is to analyze the ratios of various precursors to one another. This may be done for early and late progenitors (CFU-E versus BFU-E) and for early progenitors of different lineages (CFU-C versus BFU-E). In addition, the numbers of such cell types in circulation may be determined in man and expressed as colony-forming cells/ml of blood.

Although erythroid culture techniques possess inherent limitations, the application to studies in man has proved useful. The following sections present studies using erythroid culture techniques in the analysis of human disease states.

Studies in disease states

POLYCYTHEMIA VERA

Polycythemia vera, characterized by increased numbers of circulating erythrocytes, granulocytes, and platelets, is a clonal neoplasm arising from a pluripotent stem cell (Adamson et al, 1976). Erythrocytosis exists despite reduced levels of serum or urine erythropoietin, in contrast to secondary forms of polycythemia.

When bone marrow or peripheral blood cells from patients with polycythemia vera are cultured without added erythropoietin, a variable number of erythroid colonies form (Zanjani et al, 1977; Prchal et al, 1974; Papayannopoulou et al, 1979). The growth of these so-called 'endogenous' colonies is in contrast to cultures of normal bone marrow or of patients with secondary forms of polycythemia in which erythroid colony formation depends upon the addition of erythropoietin to the medium (Mladenovic & Adamson, 1979). Initially thought to be a unique characteristic of polycythemia vera cells, endogenous erythroid colonies have since been reported from cultures of patients with agnogenic myeloid metaplasia, essential thrombocytosis, erythroleukemia and, recently, from patients with familial or congenital erythrocytosis (Greenberg & Golde, 1977; Dainiak et al, 1979). Although some investigators have reported endogenous erythroid colony growth with normal marrow, this is not usually the case. The finding of such endogenous colonies may, therefore, aid in the differential diagnosis of erythrocytosis. To date, the number of endogenous colonies has not correlated with therapy, duration, or severity of disease (Zanjani et al, 1980).

Endogenous erythroid colony formation may be one manifestation of increased sensitivity to erythropoietin of polycythemia vera cells in culture. Curves relating the growth of marrow CFU-E and BFU-E and peripheral blood BFU-E are complex, indicating that at least some population of cells reaches a plateau in response to lower levels of erythropoietin than normal cells (Eaves & Eaves, 1978). Such dose-response curves suggest an abnormal population of progenitors with three possible explanations. One possibility is that the endogenous population might reflect cells with extreme sensitivity to small amounts of erythropoietin present in the culture. Consistent with this is the marked inhibition of endogenous colonies seen upon addition of anti-erythropoietin antibody to the culture (Zanjani et al, 1977). Alternatively, endogenous colony formation may result from 'triggering' in vivo by ambient amounts of erythropoietin. This hypothesis seems unlikely since endogenous erythroid colony-forming cells from peripheral blood do not appear to be in cell cycle, as measured by tritiated thymidine suicide experiments. Finally, these abnormal progenitors may be independent of hormonal regulation. Direct proof of the degree of hormone independence for in vitro growth awaits the development of a completely serum-free culture system.

Cell-marker studies employing heterozygotes for glucose-6-phosphate dehydrogenase (G6PD) have provided new insights into polycythemia vera and other myeloproliferative disorders. Due to X-chromosome inactivation, somatic tissues of females heterozygous at the X-linked G6PD locus for the wild type B gene, and a variant such as A, are a mixture of cells, some synthesizing isoenzyme type B, and the others, type A. In general, all mesodermally derived tissues reflect similar ratios of isoenzyme types in appropriate heterozygotes. While the peripheral blood of hematologically normal G6PD heterozygotes is a mixture of cells with different isoenzyme types, all circulating erythrocytes, granulocytes, and platelets show a single isoenzyme type (Adamson et al, 1976) in polycythemia vera and chronic myelogenous leukemia. This is true whether the disease is clinically active or in remission, and demonstrates that with routine myelosuppressive therapy, cells of the abnormal clone are not replaced by the products of normal progenitors.

Detailed studies of erythroid colony growth in two G6PD heterozygotes with polycythemia vera were undertaken to determine whether colony-forming cells which were not of the neoplastic clone could be detected. This type of study took advantage of the cell proliferation required for colony formation to amplify the constitutive properties of the progenitor — in this case, the G6PD isoenzyme type. When this analysis was carried out, all of the endogenous colonies were found to have the isoenzyme characteristic of the abnormal clone (Prchal et al, 1978). With increasing amounts of erythropoietin, however, colonies were detected which did not contain the isoenzyme of the dominant clone and thus presumably arose from normal progenitors. When the frequency of normal progenitors was calculated, it was clear that had these given rise to mature cells, they should have been detected in circulation. The fact that they were not indicates that somehow the expression of normal progenitors is arrested or blocked in this disorder.

Most recently, such erythroid culture analyses have monitored the frequency of normal colony-forming cells over a period of several years in these patients. The results demonstrated a decline in the number of normal colony-forming cells, suggesting that disease progression is accompanied by a loss of normal progenitors (Adamson et al, 1980). Whether such a mechanism could actually result in the extinction of normal stem cells is uncertain.

Finally, analysis of the response to erythropoietin in culture, combined with the determination of G6PD isoenzyme types, has demonstrated that while endogenous colonies all arise from the neoplastic clone, both neoplastic and presumably normal progenitors participate in the subsequent response to increasing erythropoietin. Consequently, endogenous colony forming cells mark the clone but do not define its extent.

Studies in other hematologic neoplasms
The combination of colony growth and analysis of G6PD in suitable patients has also been applied to the study of chronic myelogenous leukemia and acute non-lymphocytic leukemia. When one patient with chronic myelogenous leukemia was treated aggressively with chemotherapy, the loss of the Philadelphia chromosome in marrow metaphases was accompanied by the re-emergence of normal colony-forming cells (Singer et al, 1980).

The application of these techniques to acute leukemia has shown that some cases involve a stem cell pluripotent for granulocytes, platelets, and red cells; however, in other cases, expression of the neoplastic stem cell is confined to the leukemic blast population (Fialkow et al, 1979). Continued studies of this kind will provide useful information not only about cell of origin but progression of hematologic neoplasms, as well.

Marrow failure states

1. APLASTIC ANEMIA

Severe aplastic anemia is a nearly uniformly fatal illness, not easily treated, and diverse in origin. At present, the treatment of choice is bone marrow transplantation in those individuals fortunate enough to have histocompatible family members as donors. On several occasions, however, preconditioning and subsequent transplantation resulted not in engraftment and growth of donor cells, but reversal of the disease with growth of host cells. This suggested that immunosuppression by the conditioning regimen may have resulted in marrow recovery.

Direct studies in vitro suggesting an immune-mediated etiology for aplastic anemia were presented by Hoffman et al (1977). The addition of varying concentrations of lymphocytes from patients with aplastic anemia to cultures of normal marrow cells led to a marked reduction of CFU-E growth in six of seven instances. Lymphocytes from control patients who had been multiply transfused failed to exert such an inhibitory effect.

Subsequent studies, however, employing granulocyte/macrophage colony growth, failed to implicate an immunologic etiology in the vast majory of patients with this disease (Singer et al, 1979). In addition, culture studies in experimental animals indicated that deliberate transfusion sensitization was capable of promoting the appearance of populations of inhibitor lymphocytes (Torok-Storb et al, 1979a). These results suggested that meaningful in vitro studies could be carried out in aplastic anemia only in the setting of histocompatibility.

The problem of sensitization was circumvented by Torok-Storb and colleagues (1980a) by working in an entirely autologous setting. They demonstrated that the removal of T-lymphocytes by sheep red cell rosetting re-established erythroid burst growth from the peripheral blood cells of 8/32 patients with aplastic anemia. When T-cells were added back to culture, growth was abrogated in 6 out of 8 of these patients. In addition, in vitro studies predicted those patients in whom failure of engraftment might be expected (Torok-Storb et al, 1979b).

A major contribution of this investigation is the recognition that sensitization to non-HLA- and to HLA-associated antigens is important in the interpretation of culture growth patterns. In this context, it is hoped that in vitro growth would predict the response of some patients to immunotherapy. Prospective studies of patients who do not have matched bone marrow donors and their responses to antithymocyte globulin have been undertaken. Such studies are of importance both theoretically and clinically, with hope of providing a less debilitating and more rational form of treatment for some patients with aplastic anemia.

2. ACQUIRED PURE RED CELL APLASIA (PRCA)

Acquired PRCA is a disease characterized by the cessation of red cell production with generally maintained granulopoiesis and megakaryopoiesis. The frequent association of the secondary form of this disease with thymoma has suggested the possibility of an underlying immune mechanism. To date, both humoral and cellular immune mechanisms have been proposed in certain patients with the disease. Krantz & Kao (1967) provided the initial evidence for humorally-mediated inhibition of erythropoiesis. They demonstrated normal erythropoietin responsiveness of bone marrow cells from selected patients with PRCA and inhibition of in vitro hemoglobin synthesis by the addition of the patient's plasma. Such inhibitors were found in the IgG fraction of plasma and were cytotoxic to mature erythroblasts in the presence of complement. The response of the disease to immunosuppressive therapy provided important supporting evidence for the relevance of the in vitro studies.

Humorally-mediated immune suppression has also been demonstrated by erythroid colony assays. When sera from patients with PRCA were substituted for normal sera, marked inhibition of homologous (Hoffman et al, 1976) and autologous (Freedman et al, 1976) CFU-E growth was observed, even in the absence of added complement. Although a humoral factor inhibited colony growth, it was not clear whether the factor was an immunoglobulin, or whether it was directed against a progenitor cell or erythropoietin, itself. However, the factor differed from the complement-dependent cytotoxic inhibitor described previously by Krantz.

Cell-mediated inhibition has also been implicated in some patients with acquired PRCA. When peripheral blood mononuclear cells of two patients with thymoma and immunodeficiency were co-cultured with normal unrelated marrow, decreased CFU-E growth was seen (Litwin & Zanjani, 1977). These results suggested immunologically mediated disease; however, the interpretation was necessarily limited because only one patient had PRCA associated with the illness and inhibition of autologous marrow cell growth was not demonstrated.

In another report of PRCA with transfusion-induced hepatitis, 70 per cent inhibition of CFU-E-derived colony formation was observed when the patient's lymphocytes were co-cultured with homologous marrow. However, only 38 per cent inhibition of autologous marrow growth was found during an active phase of the disease (Wilson et al, 1980). It is uncertain whether such suppression was related to the pathogenesis of the disease, but the difference in results between autologous and random donor marrow cell culture may be related to sensitization arising from prior transfusion therapy.

3. BLACKFAN-DIAMOND SYNDROME OR CONGENITAL HYPOPLASTIC ANEMIA (CHA)

This disease appears in children prior to 18 months of age and is manifested by selective erythroid failure. The disease usually responds to steroid therapy. In contrast to acquired PRCA, a serum inhibitor of erythropoiesis has not been demonstrated, although cell-mediated suppression has been suggested by some observers. In the initial report of six patients, peripheral blood mononuclear cells, co-cultured with homologous normal bone marrow, inhibited CFU-E growth by greater than 90 per cent (Hoffman et al, 1976). Colony growth by normal marrow in the presence of lymphocytes from normal subjects, multiply transfused patients, or patients with acquired PRCA, was not impaired. In another study, two adults with CHA in remission and not receiving therapy demonstrated markedly decreased peripheral blood BFU-E colony numbers which increased when autologous serum was substituted for fetal calf serum in the culture (Steinberg et al, 1979). T-lymphocytes from these patients inhibited BFU-E growth when mixed in culture with random donor mononuclear cells.

In contradictory studies, no inhibition of normal CFU-E growth by CHA peripheral blood lymphocytes was observed, although the studies were not performed with autologous CHA marrow cells (Freedman et al, 1978; Nathan et al, 1978).

Early erythroid culture studies demonstrated the presence of normal CFU-E numbers in four children with this diagnosis (Freedman et al, 1976), but subsequent studies have suggested decreased numbers of CFU-E and BFU-E from bone marrow and a marked decrease or absence of circulating BFU-E (Steinberg et al, 1978; Nathan et al, 1978). Nathan has reported a markedly decreased sensitivity to erythropoietin of circulating BFU-E which subsequently improved toward normal in steroid-responsive patients. The underlying defect was postulated to be a quantitative and/or qualitative decrease in erythroid progenitor numbers. It appears that the underlying pathogenetic mechanism in CHA is uncertain and may be heterogeneous. Interpretation of results has been made difficult by the lack of studies in autologous systems and the inability to quantitate human erythroid progenitors.

PERSPECTIVE

Over the last 10 years, the development of colony forming techniques has provided a valuable tool for the analysis of in vitro erythropoiesis. Studies utilizing this technique have confirmed the importance of erythropoietin as a humoral regulator. In addition, the dependence of early regulation upon cellular interactions and the release of growth stimulators and inhibitors has become apparent. How many such factors exist, the cells they affect, and their physiological significance remain unknown. The serum factor, described as burst promoting activity, is one example of this difficulty. This activity may represent a 'super-molecule' which influences a variety of hematopoietic progenitors; or, it may be one of several closely related 'pathway-specific' molecules, each with a highly selected target cell. Current work is aimed at the definition of such factors and their roles in erythroid growth and differentiation. Resolution of these questions ultimately requires purification of these molecules. Defining the effect of humoral regulators on their target cells at the molecular level requires, in addition, a pure cell population. The definition of cellular interactions in culture also relies upon the ability to separate functional cells. Newer cell sorting methods are becoming available to solve this technical problem.

In hopes of investigating earlier differentiation and commitment events in culture, other colony assays are being developed. For example, the manipulation of culture conditions has permitted the identification of colonies consisting of erythroid/ megakaryocytic, or erythroid/megakaryocytic/granulocytic elements. These mixed colonies are thought to represent the expression of bipotent or multipotent progenitors. Another culture system which maintains progenitor cells for weeks to months has also been described. Such a long term system will further understanding of the hematopoietic micro-environment necessary for growth and differentiation.

Although rapid advances have been made in the understanding of erythropoiesis through in vitro studies, these results must be correlated with the in vivo physiology of marrow regulation. The more detailed our knowledge of the sites and mechanisms of hematopoietic regulation and differentiation, the greater the potential for understanding the pathophysiology of human disease and for devising rational approaches for therapeutic intervention.

REFERENCES

Adamson J W 1978 Clinics in Haematology 7: 555–569
Adamson J W, Torok-Storb B, Lin N 1978 Blood Cells 4: 89–103
Adamson J W, Fialkow P J, Murphy S, Prchal J F, Steinmann L 1976 New England Journal of Medicine 295: 913–916
Adamson J W, Singer J W, Catalano P, Murphy S, Lin N, Steinmann L, Ernst C, Fialkow P J 1980 Journal of Clinical Investigation 66: 1363–1368
Axelrad A A, McLeod D L, Shreeve M M, Heath D S 1973 In: Robinson W A (ed) Hemopoiesis in Culture. Second International Workshop. DHEW Publication 74-205, Washington DC, p 226–234
Aye M T 1977 Journal of Cellular Physiology 91: 69–77
Becker A J, McCulloch E A, Till J E 1963 Nature 197: 452–454
Bradley T R, Metcalf D 1966 Australian Journal of Experimental Biology and Medical Science 44: 287–299
Clarke B J, Housman D 1977 Proceedings of the National Academy of Sciences USA 74: 1105–1109
Dainiak N, Hoffman R, Lebowitz A, Solomon L, Maffei L, Ritchey K 1979 Blood 53: 1076–1084
Eaves C J, Eaves A C 1978 Blood 52: 1196–1210
Fialkow P J, Singer J W, Adamson J W, Berkow R L, Friedman J M, Jacobson R J, Moohr J W 1979 New England Journal of Medicine 301: 1–5
Freedman M H, Saunders E F 1979 Blood 51: 1125–1128
Freedman M H, Amato D, Saunders E F 1976 Journal of Clinical Investigation 57: 673–677
Goodman J W, Shinpock S G 1968 Proceedings of the Society for Experimental Biology and Medicine 129: 417–422
Greenberg B R, Golde D W 1977 New England Journal of Medicine 296: 1080–1084
Gregory C J 1976 Journal of Cellular Physiology 89: 289–302
Gregory C J, Eaves A C 1977 Blood 49: 855–864
Gregory C J, Eaves A C 1978 Blood 51: 527–537
Gregory C J, Henkelman R M 1977 In: Baum S J, Ledney G D (eds) Experimental Hematology Today, Springer-Verlag, New York. Ch 11, p 93–101
Hara H, Ogawa M 1976 American Journal of Hematology 1: 453–458
Hassan M W, Lutton J D, Levere R D, Reider R F 1977 Blood 50 (Suppl 1): 162A
Hoffman R, Zanjani E D, Lutton J D, Zalusky R, Wasserman L R 1977 New England Journal of Medicine 296: 10–13
Hoffman R, Zanjani E D, Vila J, Zalusky R, Lutton J D, Wasserman L R 1976 Science 193: 899–900
Iscove N N 1977 Cell and Tissue Kinetics 10: 323–334
Iscove N N 1978 In: Golde D W, Cline M J, Metcalf D, Fox C F (eds.) Hematopoietic Cell Differentiation, ICN-UCLA Symposia on Molecular and Cellular Biology, Vol X, Academic Press, New York p 37–52
Krantz S B, Kao V 1967 Proceedings of the National Academy of Sciences USA 58: 493–500
Litwin S D, Zanjani E D 1977 Nature 266: 57–58
Lipton J M, Link N A, Breard J, Jackson P L, Clarke B J, Nathan D G 1980 Journal of Clinical Investigation 65: 219–223
Metcalf D 1966 Recent Results in Cancer Research, Springer, New York, 5: 30
Mladenovic J, Adamson J W 1979 Blood 54 (Suppl 1): 143A
Nathan D G, Clarke B J, Hillman D G, Alter B P, Housman D E 1978 Journal of Clinical Investigation 61: 489–498
Nathan D G, Chess L, Hillman D G, Clarke B, Breard J, Merler E, Housman D E 1978 Journal of Experimental Medicine 147: 324–339
Nomdedeu B, Gormus B J, Rinehart J J, Kaplan M E, Zanjani E D 1978 Blood 52 (Suppl 1): 213
Ogawa M, MacEachern M D, Avila L 1977a American Journal of Hematology 3: 29–39
Ogawa M, Gruish O C, O'Dell R F, Hara H, MacEachern M D 1977b Blood 50: 1081–1092
Ogawa M, MacEachern M D, Wilson J M, Fitch M S 1976 Blood 48: 980
Ogawa M, Parmley R T, Bank H L, Spicer S S 1976 Blood 48: 407–417
Papayannopoulou T, Buckley J, Nakamoto B, Kurachi S, Nute P E, Stamatoyannopoulos G 1979 Blood 53: 446–454
Parker J W, Metcalf D 1974 Journal of Immunology 112: 502–510
Pluznik D H, Sachs L 1966 Experimental Cell Research 43: 553–563
Prchal J F, Axelrad A A 1974 New England Journal of Medicine 290: 1382
Prchal J F, Adamson J W, Murphy S, Steinmann L, Fialkow P J 1978 Journal of Clinical Investigation 61: 1044–1047
Rinehart J J, Zanjani E D, Nomdedeu B, Gormus B J, Kaplan M E 1978 Journal of Clinical Investigation 62: 979–986
Singer J W, Brown J E, James M C, Doney K, Warren R P, Storb R, Thomas E D 1978 Blood 52: 37–46

Singer J W, Arlin Z A, Najfeld V, Adamson J W, Kempin S J, Clarkson B D, Fialkow P J 1980 Blood 56: 356–360

Steinberg M H, Coleman M F, Pennehaker J B 1979 British Journal of Haematology 41: 57–68

Stephenson J R, Axelrad A A, McLeod D C, Shreeve M M 1971 Proceedings of the National Academy of Sciences USA 68: 1542–1546

Tepperman A D, Curtis J E, McCulloch E A 1974 Blood 44: 659–669

Till J E, McCulloch E A 1961 Radiation Research 14: 213–222

Torok-Storb B J, Storb R, Thomas E D 1979 Blood 54 (Suppl 1): 231A

Torok-Storb B J, Sieff C, Storb R, Adamson J W, Thomas E D 1980 Blood 55: 211–215

Torok-Storb B, Deeg H J, Atkinson K, Weiden P L, Adamson J W, Storb R 1979 Blood 54: 955–958

Torok-Storb B J, Storb R, Deeg H J, Graham T C, Wise C, Weiden P L, Adamson J W 1979 Blood 53: 104–108

Wagemaker G 1978 In: Murphy M J (ed) in vitro aspects of erythropoiesis, Springer-Verlag, New York, p 44–57

Wiktor-Jedrzejczak W, Sharkis S, Ahmed A, Sell K W 1977 Science 196: 313–315

Wilson H A, Gordon D M, Dworken H J, Tebbi K 1980 Annals of Internal Medicine 92: 196–198

Wu A M, Siminovitch L, Till J E, McCulloch E A 1968 Proceedings of the National Academy of Sciences USA 59: 1209–1215

Zanjani E D, Kaplan M E 1979 In Brown E B (ed) Progress in Hematology. Grune and Stratton, New York, XI: 173–191

Zanjani E D, Lutton J D, Hoffman R, Wasserman L R 1977 Journal of Clinical Investigation 59: 841–848

Zanjani E D, Kaplan M E, Ascensao J L, Banisadre M, Roodman G D, Wasserman L R 1980 Clinical Research 28: 327A

6. Bone marrow culture: leucopoiesis and stem cells

Malcolm A S Moore

INTRODUCTION

The use of in vitro clonal assay systems for quantitation of hematopoietic stem cells and progenitors was pioneered in the mouse (for review see Metcalf & Moore, 1971; Metcalf, 1977), and has been progressively adapted to the study of normal and pathological human hematopoiesis. Chronologically, the assay for human granulocyte-macrophage progenitors (GM-CFC, CFU-c) was the first to be developed (Pike & Robinson, 1970), followed by that for human erythroid progenitors (BFU-e, CFU-e, Iscove et al, 1974), and more recently for megakaryocyte progenitors (CFU-Mk, Vainchenker et al, 1979a, b) and pluripotent progenitors (CFU-GEMM, CFU-MIX, Fauser & Messner, 1978, 1979). Agreement on a uniform nomenclature in the field of hematopoietic research has not yet been reached although a considerable degree of concensus has been reported (Lajtha, 1979) and agreement reached on standardization of culture systems and scoring criteria (Moore et al, 1977). In order to define the unit counted, colonies (C) are defined as aggregates containing greater than 40 cells in semi-solid agar and greater than 20 cells in methylcellulose. Since growth rates may vary depending on the cell type and culture conditions, it is also of value to specify the age of culture. Clusters (C_L or C_1) are defined as containing less than 40 cells in agar culture. Quantitation of clusters in methylcellulose is difficult and dispersion of small cell aggregates in this type of system makes cluster scoring of leukemia cultures unreliable if not impossible. In defining the biological entity and the assay system used, the abbreviations colony former (forming) cell (FC) or unit (FU) are used in conjunction with an abbreviation such as C for in vitro culture or D for diffusion chamber. The use of the unqualified terminology (CFU-c or CFC-c) should be restricted to situations where no information is available on the differentiation potential of the progenitor cell. Advances in our understanding of the functional heterogeneity of hematopoietic progenitor cells detected by in vitro colony assays require additional abbreviations to define the nature of the cell produced. For example, GM is used to define an undefined granulocyte/macrophage colony (i.e. GM-CFC or CFU-GM); whereas, the prefix N (for neutrophil) or Eo (for eosinophil) can be used if more specific information is available concerning differentiation potential. Additional abbreviations include E (erythroid), Mg or Mk (megakaryocyte), M (macrophage), Mo (monocyte), BL and TL (B or T lymphocyte), MIX or GEMM (mixed morphology), and F (fibroblast).

CHARACTERISTICS OF MYELOID PROGENITOR CELLS (GM-CFC)

The results of the GM-CFC assay are dependent on the definition of colony size and the day on which the colonies are scored. The number of human colonies may be maximal at day 10 and colonies scored on day 7 and 14 are not necessarily generated from the same population of precursor cells. When colonies are scored for morphology of the component cells, neutrophil-monocyte colonies account for 97 per cent of all colonies at day 7 but only 75 per cent at day 14, with the remaining colonies being composed of eosinophils. While recognizing the differences in culture techniques and scoring criteria, there is general agreement that the incidence of GM-CFC in normal human marrow is in the range of 30 to $50/10^5$ nucleated cells. Although the frequency may range from 20 to 120 $GM-CFC/10^5$ in any particular subject, the mean frequencies all fall within the narrow range just given. Despite the low incidence of GM-CFC in normal marrow, considerable enrichment of the population has proved possible using density and sedimentation separation. The relative homogeneity and light density of GM-CFC in monkey bone marrow allowed extensive enrichment using a two-step density separation procedure, and in this study morphological identification of GM-CFC as transitional mononuclear cells was possible (Moore et al, 1972). GM-CFC have also been enriched from human bone marrow using a fucose-binding lectin and cell sorting (Morstyn et al, 1980). The most enriched fraction obtained was composed of 23 per cent colony- and cluster-forming cells and blast cells, promyelocytes and myelocytes made up 95 per cent of the cells present.

Direct evidence for the biopotentiality of GM-CFC was reported by Moore et al (1972) who micromanipulated single cells from separated marrow fractions and found that they could form colonies containing both granulocytes and macrophages. This question has been readdressed using a naturally occurring system of cellular mosaicism, the X-linked glucose-6-phosphate dehydrogenase (G6PD) isoenzyme locus as a marker (Singer et al, 1980). In this study of marrow cultures from a number of G6PD heterozygous females, more than 95 per cent of granulocyte-macrophage colonies had either type A or type B G6PD but not both when colony density was less than 20 per dish. At colony densities greater than 30 per dish, between 15 per cent and 75 per cent colonies had both enzyme types and therefore arose from more than one cell. These results are consistent with a unicellular origin for the colonies only when they are cultured at low densities. With increasing colony density, there was a greater frequency of colonies with both type A and type B activity, suggesting that accurate enumeration of committed stem cells can only be performed at low colony concentrations.

In the majority of species, CFC-c are heterogeneous by biophysical and functional criteria. Sedimentation velocity separation of human marrow has shown that the CFC predominantly responsible for colony formation at day 7 with a peak sedimentation rate of 7.1 mm/hr and a high proportion of cells in DNA synthesis can be separated from a population of smaller, more slowly cycling CFC, predominantly forming colonies by day 14. Comparison of these two populations with cells forming granulocytic colonies in diffusion chambers implanted in irradiated mice (CFU-D) has revealed significant differences (Jacobsen et al, 1978, 1979, 1980). CFU-D with a peak sedimentation rate of 5.2 to 5.4 mm per hr could be largely separated from GM-CFC. Additional differences were found in the cycle status of the CFU, since only 8 per cent of CFU-D were in DNA synthesis in contrast to 35 to 45 per cent of GM-CFC. Culturing marrow cell fractions enriched for CFU-D either in suspension culture or diffusion chambers, resulted in generation of greatly increased numbers of GM-CFC, suggesting that the CFU-D is a pre-CFC-c but not a pluripotent stem cell.

Isolation, enrichment and characterization of human hematopoietic progenitor or stem cells would be greatly assisted if specific differentiation antigen markers were available. The Ia antigen has been considered as a differentiation marker since it is expressed at certain stages of human hematopoietic maturation (Winchester et al, 1977, 1978). Ia antigens are recognized by alloantisera, or heteroantisera or mono-clonal antibody directed against purified Ia antigen. The latter biomolecular complex may be isolated from human B-cell line membranes and is the product of genes mapping in the major histocompatibility complex. Biologically and chemically, the human Ia-like antigens are homologous to the murine I region antigen system. In man, Ia antigens are expressed on B-cells, subsets of T-cells, monocytes, normal or leukemic myeloblasts, promyelocytes, pronormoblasts, basophilic normoblasts and megakaryocytes. Early progenitors of myeloid and erythroid lineages also appear to be Ia-positive, since complement-mediated inhibition of GM-CFC (Winchester et al, 1977), BFU-e and CFU-e (Winchester et al, 1978) is seen with titrations of heteroantisera up to 1 to 40 000. An extreme sensitivity to anti-Ia serum is also seen in the pre-CFU-C assay (Moore et al, 1980) and in the diffusion chamber CFU-D assay (Jacobsen et al, 1980).

THE ROLE OF COLONY STIMULATING FACTORS IN NORMAL AND LEUKEMIC MYELOPOIESIS

Granulocyte-macrophage colony stimulating factor (GM-CSF) is the operational name given to the specific factor stimulating the proliferation in semi-solid culture of granulocyte and macrophage progenitors. Alternative names for this factor are colony stimulating activity (CSA) if the material used is impure, or macrophage-granulocyte-inducer (MGI). Awareness of the existence of this factor arose from studies demonstrating that the growth of mouse granulocyte and macrophage colonies depended on the inclusion of underlayers of various cells or the addition of serum, urine or medium conditioned by various cells. Analysis of murine material with colony stimulating activity showed that the activity was wholly ascribable to a carbohydrate-containing polypeptide. Subsequent work with hematopoietic clonal assay systems supporting the growth of erythroid, eosinophil, megakaryocyte and mixed colonies revealed the role of specific stimulating factors comparable to GM-CSF and it is now necessary to identify colony stimulating factors by a prefix indicating the line specificity of the factors (for review see Metcalf, 1977; Burgess & Metcalf, 1980; Moore, 1979a).

GM-CSF for human marrow is elaborated by a variety of normal human cell types including monocytes, macrophages, T lymphocytes and endothelial cells. Other cellular sources of CSF include human placenta, human urine and a variety of human cell lines developed from a pancreatic tumour, a sarcoma, a T lymphoma and a monocyte-like tumor. In contrast to murine CSF species, no human source of CSF has been unequivocally purified to homogeneity. The most studied sources of human-active CSF are human leukocyte conditioned medium and human placental conditioned medium. Both contain CSF's which stimulate cells of both the GM and eosinophil series but other hematopoietic activities, yet to be defined, are also present (Nicola et al, 1979, Burgess & Metcalf, 1980). Placental conditioned medium contains at least two forms of GM-CSF, one of which can be separated from eosinophil CSF and which favors neutrophil production even at low concentrations (Nicola et al, 1979). There is a matching heterogeneity of target cells with subsets of progenitor cells responding selectively to one or other type of CSF. Human active CSF's in media conditioned by placenta, lung, mitogen stimulated leukocytes and various cell lines have apparent molecular weights of 30 000 to 40 000 (Nicola et al, 1979; Wu, 1979; Di Persio et al, 1980; Fojo et al, 1978). In contrast to most murine CSF species, CSF's from human placenta and blood leukocytes do not bind to concanavalin A-sepharose and there is no evidence as yet to indicate that there is carbohydrate associated with these species. Sources of human-active GM-CSF also appear to contain molecules active on murine GM-CFC. Purification of murine-active CSF from human urine (Stanley et al, 1975) and human lung (Fojo et al, 1978) has yielded homogeneous CSF's of molecular weights between 40 000 and 50 000 and distinct from the CSF's derived from murine sources.

Leukemic cells from patients with acute myeloblastic leukemia (AML) or chronic myeloid leukemia (CML) are absolutely dependent upon a source of GM-CSF for their proliferation in vitro. In view of the known heterogeneity of GM-CSF molecules, it has always been possible that leukemic cells might respond preferentially to some minor subset of GM-CSF molecules or even to an abnormal type of CSF perhaps of leukemic origin. To date there is no convincing data that unique forms of GM-CSF exist in leukemic patients and while leukemic cells can produce CSF, studies have so far indicated that such CSF's are similar to those derived from normal cells.

Analysis of dose-response curves for leukaemic GM-CFC has suggested that they do not differ markedly from normal in their responsiveness to CSF (Metcalf et al, 1974; Francis et al, 1979). In contrast, an exceptional responsiveness of certain human myeloid leukemia cells to CSF was reported by Brennan et al (1979). Clonal growth of AML cells was stimulated by a CSF of 45 000 daltons obtained from a human cell line (DiPersio et al, 1980), and leukemic cell sensitivity was 10 to 50 fold greater than normal marrow GM-CFC.

The implication of CSF dependence of human myeloid leukemia cells raises the possibility of biological control of leukemia by either restriction of proliferation by suppression of GM-CSF production or action, or enforced differentiation via a differentiation promoting action of GM-CSF. In this latter context it is of interest that defective CSF production has been reported in patients with preleukemia and in leukemic patients with a poor prognosis following chemotherapy (Greenberg & Mara, 1978; Horsten et al, 1977).

INHIBITORY INTERACTIONS IN NORMAL AND LEUKEMIC HEMATO-POIESIS

There is increasing evidence that mature granulocytes and their products participate as one of the regulators of myelopoiesis. Negative feedback control of granulopoiesis has been reported in various systems and the concept of a granulocyte chalone specifically inhibitory to GM-CFC or to more differentiated myeloid cells has received some experimental support. The studies of Broxmeyer (Broxmeyer et al, 1977a, b, 1978, 1980; Broxmeyer & Moore, 1978) have indicated a more indirect mechanism of granulocyte negative feedback which recognizes the implications of the bipotentiality of the granulocyte-monocyte committed stem cell. 'Spontaneous' colony formation in the absence of an exogenous source of CSF is observed in marrow cultures of all species so far investigated when the cells are cultured at a sufficiently high concentration. This spontaneous colony formation is due to endogenous elaboration of CSF by marrow monocytes and macrophages and is considerably enhanced by the removal of mature granulocytes from the cultured cell population. Addition of mature granulocytes, granulocyte extracts or medium conditioned by incubation with granulocytes markedly inhibits spontaneous colony formation (Broxmeyer et al, 1977a). This granulocyte derived colony inhibitory activity acts in a non-species specific manner to suppress CSF production by monocytes and macrophages. It is not inhibitory to monocyte-macrophage proliferation and is clearly distinct from granulo-cyte chalone, since no inhibition of granulocytic colony formation is observed in the presence of an exogenous source of CSF. A marked and reproducible quantitative defect in this inhibiting activity of mature granulocytes has been reported in patients with CML and the CSF-producing cells in such patients were less sensitive to inhibition by normal mature granulocytes (Broxmeyer et al, 1977a; b). These negative feedback abnormalities in vitro may partially explain the granulocytic hyperplasia associated with chronic myeloid leukemia.

The granulocyte-derived inhibitor has recently been identified as a known and well-characterized metal-binding glycoprotein, lactoferrin (Broxmeyer et al, 1978a) which is present in the specific granules of the mature granulocytes. Lactoferrin acts to decrease both granulocyte and macrophage colony formation in vitro by decreasing production of granulocyte-macrophage colony stimulating activity from normal and leukemic human and murine monocytes and macrophages (Broxmeyer & Moore, 1978). Suppression of CSF production correlates with the iron saturation of lacto-ferrin (LF); apo-LF (depleted of iron) was only active at concentrations greater than 10^{-7} M, native LF (8 per cent iron saturated) was active at 10^{-15} M, and fully iron-saturated LF inhibited at 10^{-17} M. Serum transferrin was only minimally active at concentrations greater than 10^{-6} M (Broxmeyer et al, 1978a). Immunoelectron-microscopic analysis of lactoferrin binding to human monocytes demonstrated surface and intracellular localization (Steinmann et al, 1981).

The relationship between expression of Ia-like antigens on human monocytes and the ability of lactoferrin to inhibit the production of colony stimulatory activity for granulocyte and macrophage colony formation has been investigated by Broxmeyer (1979). The results showed that lactoferrin inhibits production of CSF from an Ia-antigen positive subpopulation of human blood monocytes. This suggests that Ia-antigens may act as receptors of LF; or Ia antigens and receptors for lactoferrin are structurally different but are in close spatial proximity, or a ligand induced alteration of Ia antigens may lead to an interaction with the receptors for lactoferrin. These alternatives remain to be investigated but nevertheless point to a role for Ia-lactoferrin interaction in the regulation of granulopoiesis in vivo.

Pharmacological studies have shown that prostaglandins of the E series (PGE) and other agents capable of elevating intracellular levels of cAMP profoundly inhibit myelopoiesis in vitro, just as CSF promotes continued replication of the GM-CFC and its progeny. PGE limits this effect by an opposing action on the responsiveness of myeloid progenitor cells and their proliferative progeny to stimulation by CSF. Kurland et al (1978, 1979) have shown that prostaglandin synthesized by phagocytic mononuclear cells may be of importance in the modulation of hemopoiesis. Measurement of prostaglandin E production by murine macrophages and human monocytes has been performed using a sensitive radio-immunoassay and has shown a linear relation between the number of phagocytic mononuclear cells and the concentration of PGE in the conditioned medium. This observation explains the lack of correlation between the numbers of monocytes and macrophages used to stimulate granulocyte-macrophage colony formation and the incidence of colonies. Titration of varying numbers of adherent macrophages or blood monocytes as a source of stimulus for human or murine marrow GM-CFC has clearly shown that colony formation is stimulated by low numbers of phagocytic mononuclear cells and inhibited if higher concentrations are used. Parallel studies using monocytes or macrophages treated with indomethacin, a potent inhibitor of prostaglandin synthesis, have revealed a linear relationship between the number of colonies stimulated and the number of phagocytic mononuclear cells used as the source of CSF (Kurland et al, 1978, 1979). These observations point to the unique ability of the macrophage to control the proliferation of its own progenitor cell by elaboration of opposing regulatory influences. A still more intimate interaction between CSF and PGE has been shown since increased levels of CSF produced locally by monocyte/macrophage subpopulations, can in turn, activate increased macrophage prostaglandin synthesis, indicating a very direct relationship between CSF levels and induction of an opposing activity (Kurland et al, 1979).

Morphological examination of bone marrow derived myeloid colonies and clusters proliferating in the presence of exogenously added PGE demonstrated that the effect of PGE on total colony formation resulted from a preferential effect on monocyte-macrophage committed colony forming cells and, to a lesser extent on mixed macrophage-neutrophil colony formation, most likely through an effect on the monocytoid component of these colonies (Pelus et al, 1979). Monocyte-macrophage clonal expansion was sensitive to inhibition by as little as 10^{-10} M to 10^{-11} PGE$_1$ concentrations, whereas inhibition of clonal granulocyte growth required concentrations greater than 10^{-7} M.

Analysis of PGE sensitivity of GM-CFC from patients with CML at various stages of the disease demonstrated that monocyte-macrophage and mixed monocytoid-neutrophilic colonies and clusters were insensitive to inhibition even at concentrations of PGE$_1$ which produce a 70 per cent inhibition of monocyte-macrophage and 60 per cent inhibition of mixed monocytoid and neutrophilic colony and cluster formation by normal bone marrow cells (Pelus et al, 1980).

Exogenous addition of CSF can overcome the inhibitory effects of PGE (Kurland et al, 1978). The altered sensitivity of CML GM-CFC to PGE could not result from a counterbalance by endogenous CSF production, since CSF producing cells were removed based upon their adherence properties. Likewise, removal of adherent PG producing cells and the routine inclusion of indomethacin, a specific prostaglandin synthesis inhibitor, into GM-CFC assays eliminated possible alterations in GM-CFC sensitivity to exogenous PGE due to endogenously produced prostaglandin. Therefore, the altered sensitivity to PGE observed in patients with CML appears to be a direct defect in responsiveness of committed GM-CFC to negative feedback regulation.

The absence of normal hemopoiesis in adult leukemia (AL) not in remission and the recovery of apparently normal blood cells during chemotherapy induced remission suggest that suppressive cell interactions may be involved in the pathogenesis of AL. A number of studies have shown inhibition of normal progenitor cell proliferation and differentiation by cells from patients with leukemia but little or no information was provided regarding the actual characterization of the inhibitory cells or the mechanisms of action. Broxmeyer et al (1978b, c; 1979a, b; 1981) have demonstrated the existence of an S-phase specific inhibitory activity (leukemic associated inhibitory activity, LIA) against normal granulocyte-macrophage progenitor cells which was produced by bone marrow, spleen and blood cells from patients with acute and chronic myeloid and lymphoid leukemia and 'preleukemia'. Greater concentrations of LIA were found in the marrows of patients with AL (newly diagnosed and untreated, or on therapy but not in remission) than with chronic leukemia (Broxmeyer et al, 1978b, c). Remission of AL was associated with low levels of LIA (Broxmeyer et al, 1979). In contrast to its action on normal GM-CFC, LIA was not effective in suppressing the growth of GM-CFC from patients with AL who were not in remission and from patients with AL during remission and with CML. It has been postulated that LIA may thus confer a proliferative advantage to abnormally responsive leukemic cells (Broxmeyer et al, 1978b). LIA has been isolated from extracts of leukemic bone marrow (Bognacki et al, 1981; Broxmeyer et al, 1981). LIA had an apparent molecular weight of about 550 000 and a pI of 4.7 and co-purified with acidic isoferritin. Additionally, purified preparations of LIA were composed almost entirely (greater than 90 per cent) of acidic isoferritins, as determined by radioimmunoassay and isoelectric focusing, and the inhibitory activity in the LIA and in ferritin samples was inactivated by a battery of antisera specific for ferritins, including those prepared against acidic isoferritins from normal heart, and spleen tissues from patients with Hodgkin's disease. LIA and the acidic isoferritin-inhibitory activity had similar physiochemical characteristics as treatment with trypsin, chymotrypsin, pronase and periodate and breakdown of the ferritin into subunits by reduction inactivated the inhibitory activity.

The relevance in vivo of acidic isoferritins as regulators of myelopoiesis is still to be determined but the low concentrations needed for activity on the progenitor cells in vitro suggests that they may be of importance as physiological regulators.

MARROW CULTURE STUDIES IN PATIENTS WITH ACUTE MYELOID LEUKEMIA (AML)

The cloning of normal or leukemic human GM-CFC in either agar or methyl cellulose has permitted analysis of both quantitative and qualitative changes in this cell compartment in leukemia and other myeloproliferative disorders. Changes observed include abnormalities in the maturation of leukemic cells in vitro, defective proliferation as measured by colony size or cluster-to-colony ratio, abnormalities in biophysical characteristics of leukemic GM-CFC, the existence of cytogenetic abnormalities in vitro, and regulatory defects in responsiveness to positive and negative feedback control mechanisms, as will be discussed in the context of CSF responsiveness and control of CSF production and secretion (for review see Moore, 1975, 1976, 1977a, 1979a). Detection of this spectrum of abnormalities has proven to be of clinical use in diagnosis of leukemia and pre-leukemic states, in classification of leukemias and myeloproliferative diseases, and in predicting remission in AML. While considerable variation has been reported among different groups investigating the characteristics of human AML cells in culture, these differences reflect, in part, the heterogeneity of the disease as well as variation in the culture criteria, the source and activity of CSF, and the timing of the culture. Standardized culture and scoring criteria were used in a study of 250 cases of untreated AML and its morphological variants (Moore, 1974a, 1977a, 1978). All cultures were stimulated by feeder layers of 1×10^6 normal white blood cells (WBC) and were scored at 7 days for colonies or clusters of 3 to 40 cells. In this survey, classification of leukemia was performed on the basis of the in vitro growth pattern, and the following categories of growth pattern were observed.

1. *Non-growing* — absence of persisting cells in CSF-stimulated cultures with no colony or cluster formation detected.

2. *Microcluster formation* — absence of colonies and presence of varying numbers of clusters of 3 to 20 cells. The majority of these cases exhibit a pattern of small clusters in marrow culture, generally only 3 to 10 cells with dispersion and degeneration. Included in this category are examples of extensive persistence of leukemic cells in CSF-stimulated cultures without evidence of cluster formation at 7 days. Marrow cultures from these latter patients, when scored prior to 7 days generally show cluster formation with premature dispersion and degeneration of clusters. The majority of microcluster-forming leukemias would be considered non-growing if scored later than 7 days.

3. *Macrocluster formation* — absence of colonies and presence of varying numbers of clusters approaching the lower limit of colony size, i.e. up to 40 cells. If the cultures are scored later than 7 days, the majority of cases would show evidence of colony formation and merge with the fourth type of classification.

4. *Small colonies (microcolonies) with an abnormal cluster-to-colony ratio* — maximum colony size in this group is less than in control cultures, and an abnormal excess of aggregates of less than 40 cells is seen (the normal ratio of colonies to clusters is 1:10).

5. *Colony forming with a normal cluster-to-colony ratio* at 7 days of culture — this category can be further subdivided into cases showing a lower than normal colony incidence and cases with a marked elevation in marrow colony formation invariably associated with a pronounced increase in circulating GM-CFC. Both groups share a similar prognosis; however, the former category is mainly comprised of cases where colony growth is nonleukemic and thus is similar to the pattern seen in ALL, whereas the latter category merges with the growth pattern seen in CML.

Classification of these patients on the basis of a retrospective and prospective correlative analysis between in vitro culture characteristics and remission rate has shown a highly significant correlation between certain growth patterns and response to therapy. As shown in Table 6.1, 37 per cent of all untreated AML cases had growth patterns associated with a poor prognosis. The remaining cases, predominantly comprising examples of microcluster-forming acute leukemia, had a far more favorable response rate. While growth pattern is not an absolute predictor of potential responsiveness of patients to therapy, it provides one of the most significant predictive parameters; other factors (such as the labelling index of the blast cell population, age of patient, or previous history of preleukemic phase) provide additional and interacting prognostic factors. Ten patients included in this survey had acute undifferentiated or stem cell leukemia, and classification into myeloblastic or lymphoblastic type was not possible on the basis of morphology, cytochemistry, or surface markers. Three of these cases showed a myeloid cluster-forming growth pattern in marrow culture, whereas the remainder showed a colony-forming pattern with low plating efficiency and normal granulocytic maturation. The indication that colony formation seen in these cases was due to persisting normal GM-CFC co-existing with a non-myeloid AL was supported by cell separation studies.

Spitzer et al (1976) adopted a simplified classification of agar culture patterns in AL which also proved to be of prognostic significance. Three types of growth were recognized: (1) aggregates of greater than 20 cells, (2) aggregates of 1 to 20 cells and (3) no growth (Table 6.1). The latter category grouped cases of colony forming growth patterns with low plating efficiency, normal cluster-to-colony ratio and normal differentiation, presumed to reflect situations where leukemic cells are non-growing and any clonal growth is due to residual normal GM-CFC. The high proportion of patients with 'no-growth' leukemia in the study of Spitzer et al (1976) can be explained by the inclusion in the study of a number of patients with ALL and undifferentiated leukemia. Significant differences in remission probability were found, and when the value of agar culture results was compared to the value of other known prognostic factors which significantly affect remission by linear logistic regression analysis, in vitro growth pattern was the best predictor of response and made the largest contribution to assessing the probability of response in any individual patient. The MD Anderson Hospital study had the advantage that all patients received identical remission induction therapy (vincristine, prednisone, adriamycin and cytosine arabinoside), although inclusion of patients without consideration of morphological type of AL makes difficult direct comparison with other studies. Vincent et al (1977) developed a still further simplification of marrow culture patterns in acute non-lymphoblastic leukemia (ANLL), recognizing failure of marrow growth in 53 per cent of patients with a 70 per cent complete remission rate and a pattern of abnormal growth with small numbers of diffuse colonies and excessive numbers of cell clusters in the remaining cases with a significantly lower complete remission rate (30 per cent). It should be noted that marrow growth parameters were recorded at 14 days rather than 7 days which significantly alters the distribution of no-growth, cluster forming and colony forming variants.

We have recently completed a study of marrow culture parameter in 202 adult patients with acute leukemia, including 98 consecutive patients with ANLL studied at diagnosis at Memorial Sloan-Kettering Cancer Center (Mertelsmann et al, 1981). A simplified system for classification of GM-CFC incidence and growth pattern was developed to evaluate the feasibility of employing the standard GM-CFC assay as a routine clinical diagnostic procedure of sufficient reproducibility to be performed by technical personnel without the constant need for highly skilled professionals for scoring and interpretation. Aggregate incidence and growth pattern at day 7 of culture were classified as 'no growth' in the absence of significant aggregate formation and as 'normal' when less than 50 colonies and less than 1000 clusters were counted with a less than 30-fold excess of clusters (Table 6.1). The most frequent growth pattern

Table 6.1 Prognostic value of agar culture in acute leukemia

| Growth | 250 Cases ANLL, Moore et al '74, '76 | | 76 Cases AL, Spitzer et al '76 | | 96 Cases ANLL, Mertelsmann et al 1981 | |
	% of cases	% Remission Growth	% of cases	% Remission Growth	% of cases	% Remission
1. Non-growing (blank plate)	2					
2. Macroclusters	22					
3. Microcolony	13					
4a. Single cell	54					
4b. Microcluster						
5. Colony forming (low plating)	4	74				
6. Colony forming (normal-high plating)	5					
P = 0.001						

% Remission Growth — 76 Cases AL, Spitzer et al '76:

Growth	% of cases	% Remission Growth
2. Macrocluster	25	
3. Microcolony / 6. Colony forming (high plating)	21	
4a. Single cells / 4b. Microclusters	47	75
1. Non-growing (blank plate) / 5. Colony forming (low plating)	28	76
P = 0.001		

% Remission Growth — 96 Cases ANLL, Mertelsmann et al 1981:

Growth	% of cases	% Remission
1. Non-growing (blank plate) / 4a. Single cells	26	40
2. Macroclusters / 4b. Microclusters / 3. Microcolonies	57	73
5. Colony forming (low plating)	17	40
6. Colony forming (normal-high plating)		
P = 0.004		

observed in ANLL was termed 'leukemic' or AML-type and revealed a low or absent colony incidence and a more than 30-fold cluster excess. In three of the 96 ANLL cases studied, a very high colony and cluster incidence, but with a colony to cluster ratio of less than 1:30, was observed (Table 6.1). The AML growth pattern was observed in 52 of 96 patients (54 per cent) with ANLL. Three additional patients (3 per cent) showed the high cloning efficiency AML growth pattern (Table 6.1). Sixteen patients with ANLL (17 per cent) showed a normal growth pattern and the remaining 25 patients (26 per cent) revealed no growth in culture. The highest incidence of 'no growth' and 'normal growth' patterns was observed in acute undifferentiated AML (M1:3/4) and, undifferentiated A monocytic L (M5a:3/4). In contrast, a predominance of the 'AML-type' growth pattern was seen in the partially differentiated AML (M2,3:22/29), partially differentiated acute monocytic (M5b:12/22) and in acute myelomonocytic L (M4:4/7). The remission rate by GM-CFC pattern showed a significant correlation between AML-type growth pattern and high remission incidence (Table 6.1). This was true for patients receiving the L-12 protocol (64 per cent CR) or the more recent L-14 protocol (81 per cent CR) the results suggesting that the addition of the anthracycline drug on the L-14 protocol was of special benefit for the group exhibiting a normal growth pattern in the GM-CFC assay.

In a recent morphological analysis of 263 adult patients with ANLL, a significant relationship was documented between the presence of Auer rods on bone marrow smears and both high CR rates as well as long remissions (Mertelsmann et al, 1980). In an analysis of the relationship between Auer rod distribution, marrow growth pattern and their effect on CR rate, Mertelsmann et al (1981) demonstrated that although the highest incidence of Auer rod positive phenotypes was seen in the AML growth pattern group, the association between highest CR rate with AML growth pattern was true for both Auer rod positive and negative groups. The highest remission rate of 89 per cent was observed in patients exhibiting both Auer rods and AML-type growth pattern.

Analysis of remission *duration* patterns by GM-CFC growth category has failed to reveal significant relationships (Mertelsmann et al, 1981). This is in contrast to the observations of Keating et al (1980) but this disagreement might at least in part be due to the fact that the series analyzed by the latter group also included a relatively large proportion of patients with ALL.

Cultures in remission

Unequivocal complete remission in AML is associated with return of a normal growth pattern in marrow culture, a normal colony incidence and granulocytic maturation, and a normal GM-CFC buoyant density distribution. The correlation between return of normal colony formation in marrow culture and onset of remission has been investigated in a study of 57 patients serially (Moore, 1976, 1977a, 1978) analyzed throughout the induction and consolidation phase of therapy. Patients were selected on the basis of marrow growth characteristics prior to therapy, and only examples of non-colony-forming AML were studied, since appearance of normal colony formation during remission induction would provide a simple parameter for detection of non-leukemic progenitor cells. Of the 30 patients who showed return of colony formation at some point during induction, 29 achieved complete remission on the average of 21 days after first detection of colony formation. No examples were observed of a leukemic growth pattern persisting in complete clinical remission. There was no correlation between numbers of colonies observed and the time to remission; however, preliminary analysis indicates some correlation between initial colony incidence and duration of remission.

The value of marrow culture analysis in predicting the onset of relapse has been investigated in a large group of patients in whom complete remission had been achieved. In this analysis, four patterns of relapse emerged: (1) most frequently observed was a concordance of a clinical diagnosis of relapse with a complete return to a cluster-forming leukemic growth pattern. (2) Loss of colony formation and return to a cluster-forming growth pattern 1 to 4 weeks prior to clinical and hematological evidence of relapse. (3) Co-existence of normal and leukemic colony- or cluster-forming cells for varying periods preceding overt relapse. Discrimination between normal and leukemic cells was possible in these cases on the basis of colony size, cell morphology, and the dispersion or degeneration of the leukemic clusters. Density separation and cytogenetic analysis of individual colonies and clusters have further confirmed the co-existence of normal and leukemic GM-CFC in marrow cultures prior to clinical evidence of relapse. (4) This category comprised patients who showed evidence of early relapse based on hematological criteria, including elevated marrow blast cell incidence (without detectable Auer rods), presence of immature cells in the circulation, and, in the case of patients presenting with acute monocytic or myelomono-cytic leukemia, abnormal monocytoid cells in marrow and blood with qualitatively normal colony and cluster formation. In this category there is a clear discrepancy between the interpretation of marrow morphology and the in vitro culture parameters which showed no evidence of leukemic cell proliferation. This paradox was largely resolved by sequential analysis of GM-CFC in the marrows of patients in prolonged remission. A striking variation in the incidence of marrow GM-CFC was observed in a number of patients, which could not be attributed to technical variation or in any direct sense to the maintenance protocol. Correlated with the periodicity of marrow GM-CFC in many patients was a fluctuation in marrow blast cell incidence. A marked increase in the GM-CFC was frequently associated with or closely followed by an increase in marrow blast count to levels compatible with early relapse. The majority of such cases were treated with intensive reinduction therapy; however, a number were continued on maintenance therapy. In the latter type of cases both blast cell and GM-CFC incidence returned to normal levels in subsequent marrow aspirates, and the patients remained in complete remission. In the former cases, a number of patients went on to full leukemic relapse; however, it appears possible that aggressive therapy coinciding with episodes of reactive or regenerating marrow as determined by GM-CFC analysis can severely compromise the status of the normal stem cell compartment, possibly to the extent of allowing the acute leukemic clone to have a proliferative advantage.

Vincent et al (1977) also noted marked variations in marrow growth parameters in remission, ranging from no growth to striking proliferation. When relapse occurred it was possible to identify episodes of abnormal cluster-forming growth patterns in marrow cultures some 21 to 197 days earlier.

It is concluded from the study of Mertelsmann et al (1981) as well as from observations reported previously, that the GM-CFC assay performed at diagnosis can yield valuable diagnostic and prognostic information. Further analysis is required and currently continuing in order to assess the relative prognostic significance of the GM-CFC assay in comparison to other phenotypic markers and clinical and therapeutic parameters. The monitoring of the remission status, however, remains problematic due to spontaneous and therapy induced variations of culture results.

Drug-sensitivity testing
The availability of in vitro methods capable of determining the sensitivity of leukemic cells to specific chemotherapeutic agents would greatly facilitate selection of remission induction regimens appropriate for individual patients. Progress toward achieving such a goal recently has been reported. In one study (Preisler, 1980) marrow specimens from 23 patients with AML were exposed to cystosine arabinoside and/or daunorubicin in vitro and the effects of these agents on colony formation in vitro was determined. The sensitivity of the GM-CFC to the two chemotherapeutic agents did not correlate with each other, indicating that sensitivity to each was independently determined. The relationship between in vitro sensitivity to daunorubicin and cystosine arabinoside and response to in vivo therapy with these two agents administered to 21 patients indicated a clear-cut relationship between in vitro drug sensitivity and in vivo response. Patients whose leukemic cells were sensitive to both agents entered complete remission, whereas patients whose leukemic cells were insensitive to one or both drugs in vitro failed to enter remission.

Park et al (1980) have modified the leukemic colony forming cell assay by introducing daily refeeding of the cultures with fresh medium and CSA. This has the apparent advantage of increasing the frequency and size of leukemic clones, rendering in vitro chemosensitivity studies more applicable. A sensitivity index of relative in vitro response of normal or leukemic GM-CFC was obtained for six commonly used chemotherapeutic agents and a highly significant correlation was observed between selective in vitro toxicity of an agent against leukemic CFC and achievement of remission. It should be remembered that drug sensitivity is only one factor in determining whether or not a patient will enter remission. Patients with drug sensitive disease may fail to enter remission as a result of death due to intercurrent disease. Therefore the ability to predict the outcome of remission induction therapy must depend on multivariate analysis that will take into account clinical prognostic parameters together with marrow culture growth patterns and drug sensitivity of leukemic cells.

Analysis of GM-CFC as well as erythroid progenitors in marrow samples from patients with leukemia has revealed considerable patient-to-patient variation which does not correlate with marrow or blood blast cell incidence. In contrast, a functional clonal measurement related to the leukemic blast cell population has been described recently (Buick et al, 1977; McCulloch et al, 1979). The technique involves culture of cells from the peripheral blood of patients with leukemia in methylcellulose, in growth medium containing fetal calf serum and 5 to 10 per cent conditioned medium harvested from peripheral leukocytes cultured in the presence of phytohemagglutinin (PHA). Compact colonies of more than 20 cells per colony are visible after 5 to 9 days. The cells in the colonies are predominantly peroxidase-negative, and are negative for markers of lymphopoietic populations (surface immunoglobulin or capacity to form E-rosettes). The frequency of colony formation varies markedly from patient to patient and is strongly correlated with the concentration of blast cells in the peripheral blood

($R_s = 0.90$; results for 18 patients). The efficiency of colony formation varies from 10^{-2} to 10^{-4}; only a small minority of cells in the blast cell population have sufficient proliferative capacity in culture to be detected. PHA-leukocyte conditioned medium is also an eminent stimulator of T-lymphocyte colonies in vitro and Lowenberg et al (1980) have reported that, in the PHA assay, growth of colonies from lymphocytic and leukemic cells were sustained equally well. Removal of E-rosette forming cells before culture renders the assay selective for leukemic progenitors as determined by cytogenetic analysis of colonies to confirm the presence of the acquired karyotypic change characteristic of the leukemic cells of the patient. When leukemic blast cell colonies are harvested, the cells dispersed and replated, secondary colonies are usually obtained with characteristics similar to those of the primaries (Buick et al, 1979). The plating efficiency of suspensions obtained from primary leukemic blast cell colonies (plating second efficiency or PE 2), while variable from sample to sample is usually low, indicating that only a minority of cells within colonies have colony forming capacity. Further studies are required before it can be concluded that this blast progenitor assay is detecting a subpopulation of cells identical to a leukemic stem cell fraction. The assay however permits not only evaluation of the effect of potential anti-neoplastic agents on the limited number of cell divisions leading to colony formation but also upon the self-renewal process that is required for extensive growth. A correlation has been reported between in vitro sensitivity of leukemic blast progenitors to adriamycin and subsequent clinical response but colonies surviving exposure to this agent showed no reduction in their content of new blast progenitors (Buick et al, 1979). In contrast, purified human fibroblast interferon inhibited leukemic blast progenitor and normal marrow GM-CFC colony formation to a comparable degree but in marked contrast to adriamycin, which selectively inhibited only plating efficiency, interferon also inhibited secondary plating efficiency of blast progenitors (self-renewal) (Taetle et al, 1980a). Inhibition of primary granulocyte colony formation by interferon has been reported frequently; however, the findings of Taetle et al (1980a) differ from those of Verma et al (1979), in that marked patient-to-patient variation in the effect of interferon on blast progenitors and CFC proliferation was not seen, nor was decreased granulopoietic maturation found in interferon-treated colonies from marrow CFC.

Differentiation of AML blast cells in culture
Evidence for some degree of differentiating ability of myeloid leukemic blast cells has been obtained using semi-solid cloning and liquid culture systems. Particular progress has been made in this area by the use of several human acute myeloid leukemia cell lines that appear to respond to differentiation stimuli.

The HL-60 cell line, derived from a patient with A promyelocytic L proliferates continuously in suspension culture and consists predominantly of promyelocytes. These cells can be induced to differentiate to morphologically and functionally mature granulocytes by incubation with a wide variety of compounds such as dimethyl sulfoxide, butyrate, retinoic acid, leukocyte conditioned medium and phorbol esters (Breitman et al, 1980; Pegoraro et al, 1980; Elias et al, 1980; Koeffler & Golde, 1980).

An alternative approach that has been tested is the ability of leukemic blast cells to differentiate in diffusion chamber cultures which, in spite of the disadvantage that the humoral factors cannot be identified, nevertheless provides growth conditions which might be favourable, namely the detection of earlier progenitors than GM-CFC, differentiation of cells in all hematopoietic cell lines, and the possibility of longer culture periods. In a study of 18 patients with AML, granulopoiesis in diffusion chamber cultures was nearly absent in 3, moderate in 5, and greatly in excess of normal with terminal differentiation up to mature granulocytes in 10 (Hoelzer et al, 1980). In certain cases functional normality of the granulocytes was demonstrated by a normal capacity to phagocytose *Candida albicans* and to reduce nitroblue tetrazolium (NBT). In a further 12 cases of CML in blast crisis, production of immature and mature granulopoietic cells in diffusion chambers, in all cases exceeded normal values and the granulocytes that developed had normal to reduced capacity for phagocytosis and NBT reduction. An at least partially leukemic origin of these differentiating granulocytes was deduced from their excessive numbers, their early time of appearance and from the presence of cytogenetic markers in diffusion chamber cells. Diffusion chamber studies have also been undertaken with the human ANL cell line KG-1 which allows studies of regulation of leukemic cell proliferation and differentiation which need not consider the problem of accounting for residual normal cells. KG-1 cells maintained in mice treated with cyclophosphamide, glucan or endotoxin did not change their degree of maturation despite enhanced cell proliferation (Niskanen et al, 1980). In view of the known species restriction of murine CSA's one may conclude that there are humoral factors other than CSA which are important in stimulating proliferation or differentiation of human leukemic cell growth in diffusion chambers in mice.

MARROW CULTURE IN CHRONIC MYELOID LEUKEMIA (CML) AND BLASTIC CRISIS

CML provides an unrivalled opportunity for exploring genotypic and phenotypic changes paralleling the development and progression of a malignant hematopoietic stem cell clone. The application of tissue culture methodology has resulted in extensive documentation of phenotypic features of hematopoietic progenitor cells, particularly GM-CFC's in CML.

In untreated CML the colony-forming capacity of marrow is normal to increased and greatly increased numbers of GM-CFC's are present in the circulation (Moore et al, 1973a; Moberg et al, 1974). In a study of 103 patients, the incidence of colony-and-cluster forming cells in the marrow was increased on average 15-fold and circulating GM-CFC's were increased 500 times (Moore, 1977a, b, c). Unlike the situation in AML, colony size is normal and the ratio of clusters to colonies is consistently within the lower range of normal (3:1–10:1). A correlation exists between the leukocyte count and total circulating GM-CFC's; however, the magnitude of the absolute increase in the granulocyte committed stem cell compartment is quite out of proportion to the 5- to 20-fold increase in granulocyte production, suggesting that inappropriate overproduction of committed stem cells rather than their excessive differentiation is the underlying defect in CML.

In contrast to cultures of AML bone marrow, normal maturation of GM-CFC's generally is observed in CML with colonies composed of mature neutrophils, eosinophils, monocytes, and macrophages (Moberg et al, 1974; Moore, 1977a, b, c). The proliferation of CML bone marrow in liquid culture is two to threefold greater than normal, presumably reflecting the increased incidence of committed stem cells (Golde et al, 1974). Cellular maturation in such cultures is normal with granulocytes and actively replicating macrophages which are functionally indistinguishable from normal.

In addition to the quantitative abnormality of marked increase in GM-CFC numbers, other qualitative abnormalities serve to characterize leukemic CFC. Separation of marrow and peripheral blood leukocytes in density gradients has revealed a markedly reproducible light density shift of leukemic GM-CFC. This difference in buoyant density of colony- and cluster-forming cells is observed in both marrow and blood and persists in patients undergoing therapy (Moore et al, 1973a, b; Moore, 1977a, b, c). In untreated CML, density separation produces sufficient enrichment of GM-CFC to permit their morphological characterization as myeloblasts (Moore et al, 1973a).

Analysis of the in vitro growth characteristics of marrow or blood from 42 CML patients at the time of clinical diagnosis of blastic transformation revealed, in every case, defects in proliferation and maturation which served to distinguish this phase from the chronic phase (Moore, 1977b, c). Blastic CML exhibited the same spectrum of proliferative abnormalities as has been reported in untreated AML marrow cultures. The most common pattern was that of absence of normal colony formation with persistence of clusters of up to 40 cells (macrocluster type) or presence of small colonies with an excess of clusters (microcolony type). In both categories in vitro maturation was markedly defective, with blasts, promyelocytes, and macrophages predominating and mature neutrophils generally absent. These variants accounted for 50 per cent of the cases studied. Patients with the macrocluster variant tended to present after a shorter duration of chronic phase disease than did the microcolony variant. They had higher leukocyte counts, higher blast incidence, and lower platelet counts. Minimal response to therapy was shown in both categories, remissions were not observed, and survival in blastic crisis was brief. The next most common variants were cases with absence of colony formation in marrow culture with persistence of clusters of 3 to 10 cells (microcluster variant, 14 per cent of cases) and examples of persisting colony formation with high plating efficiency in marrow and blood culture (19 per cent). This latter category cannot be distinguished from chronic phase disease on the basis of growth pattern alone, but morphological analysis of the colonies revealed maturation arrest at the blast-promyelocyte level. The colony-forming category had a high platelet count and a considerably lower blast count in marrow and blood than did any other category and generally the patients had a more subacute course reflected in their longer survival in blast crisis. A final category comprising 14 per cent of cases generally presented with a low leukocyte count and high blast count in marrow and had a very low incidence of colonies and clusters in marrow and blood with normal colony maturation and normal colony-to-cluster ratio.

Leong et al (1979) have reported data on 60 patients in different stages of CML at variance with the preceding observations. Specifically, a normal to greatly increased incidence of colony formation was found in the accelerated-resistant and blastic stages of the disease and no correlation was noted with white cell count, percentage of immature cells, clinical status, survival or terminal transferase (TdT) positivity. This study is instructive in that it demonstrates the restriction of culture analysis to 14 days rather than 7 days and inability to recognize cell aggregates of less than 40 cells can completely eliminate the diagnostic and prognostic value of the GM-CFC assay; furthermore restricting analysis to peripheral blood cultures almost completely prevents any value of culture studies in predicting onset of blastic crisis since changes in circulating GM-CFC populations coincide with rather than precede clinical and morphological evidence of disease progression.

Moore et al (1981) reviewed an additional group of 35 patients with CML on maintenance therapy and subject to regular marrow GM-CFC assay. All cases were clinically stable with normal total white cell counts and in no instance did myeloblasts and promyelocytes exceed 30 per cent in the marrow. 21/35 patients had a normal incidence of colonies and clusters; however, qualitative defects were seen in cultures from the remaining 14 patients. The proliferative defects ranged from a low incidence of small colonies with an excess of clusters (microcolony type) to absence of colony formation with a variable incidence of clusters only (both micro- and macro-cluster variants). On repeat culture, abnormal patterns of GM-CFC growth persisted in some cases whereas in others, variable durations of return to normal culture growth were observed. Where progression to blastic crisis was observed, the same abnormal growth pattern persisted. While detection of abnormal colony and cluster growth patterns can be predictive of blastic transformation; Moore et al (1981), also observed some patients who progressed to blastic crisis without displaying antecedent or associated qualitative defects in GM-CFC proliferation. These patients generally terminated in a TdT-positive blastic crisis.

Table 6.2 Marrow growth patterns in 11 patients with TdT-positive blastic CML

Marrow culture pattern	Marrow/10^5 cells		Blood/10^5 cells	
	Colonies	Clusters	Colonies	Clusters
'Myeloid'	0	82		
,,	0	224		
,,	17	553		
,,	21	600		
,,	71	466	39	511
,,	430	2760		
,,	26	27		
'Lymphoid'	0.1	0.3		
,,	1.2	4.8	6.5	33
,,	6	13		
,,	2	35		

TdT is positive in 30 per cent of patients with CML and other myeloproliferative or myelodysplastic syndromes in blastic crisis (Mertelsmann et al, 1979a, b). The significance of TdT-positive blastic crisis of CML can be considered in the context of marrow culture studies. Table 6.2 shows the pattern of GM-CFC proliferation in the marrow of 11 patients at the time of the first diagnosis of TdT-positive blastic crisis. Four cases displayed a 'lymphoid' marrow culture pattern, comparable to that observed in typical ALL (Moore, 1977b, c). Of the remaining cases, 2 had a normal incidence and ratio of colonies and clusters and 5 had abnormal growth patterns including microcluster, and microcolony variants consistent with a myeloblastic rather than lymphoblastic transformation. Detection of proliferation and maturation abnormalities of GM-CFC observed in a variable proportion of CML patients in stable chronic phase disease and in all patients with CML in myeloblastic crisis suggests that sequential marrow culture studies may be particularly useful in predicting progression to blastic crisis. While predictive in many instances, certain patients may exhibit normal GM-CFC growth patterns alternating with period of abnormal growth over long periods suggestive of prolonged clonal competition between progressively more abnormal leukemic cell subpopulations. In depth studies of such patients may be particularly valuable in determining the crucial variables involved in leukemia disease progression. Concordance of a marrow culture pattern consistent with a lymphoblastic leukemia (no maturation or proliferation defects in GM-CFC) and TdT^+ was noted in only half the total cases of TdT^+ blastic crisis. In cases with AML growth features, TdT^+ most likely represents examples of coincident progression of two acute phase clones independently evolved from the original leukemic pluripotential stem cell clone.

MARROW CULTURE STUDIES IN 'OLIGOLEUKEMIA', PRELEUKEMIA AND MYELODYSPLASTIC DISORDERS

Spitzer et al (1978) used agar culture to delineate various marrow growth patterns and their prognostic significance in 65 patients with a diagnosis of 'oligoleukemia' (myeloid leukemia with less than 50 per cent marrow leukemic infiltrate). Five in vitro growth patterns were observed: (1) low colony and cluster incidence, normal cluster/colony ratio and normal cellular differentiation in colonies; (2) normal to high numbers of colonies and clusters in a normal ratio with normal differentiation; (3) excessive clusters, low numbers of colonies with normal maturation and a high cluster/colony ratio; (4) excessive numbers of clusters of less than 20 cells, and (5) excessive numbers of clusters of greater than 20 cells with or without colonies consisting predominantly of blast cells. Patients with type (1) growth patterns survived longer (p = less than 0.004) and progressed less rapidly to AL (p = less than 0.03) compared to patients with type (4) and (5) growth patterns: also the rate of leukemic blast cell infiltration was slower. Oligoleukemia is a heterogeneous group of leukemic disorders embracing chronic myelomonocytic leukemia, refractory anemia with excess of blasts and smouldering leukemias; thus it is not surprising to observe heterogeneity in culture parameters. However, these latter parameters are clearly of value in the identification of a group of patients with a relatively aggressive leukemic disorder who may be compromised by delaying effective therapy and also those patients with a chronic indolent course who, on the contrary may be compromised by such therapy.

A similar spectrum of abnormal marrow culture patterns is also observed in patients with 'preleukemia', defined as a primary hematological disorder with anemia, neutropenia, thrombocytopenia occurring together or in varying combinations with normal to hypercellular marrow and the presence of dyshemopoiesis in one or more cell lines with marrow blasts always 5 per cent or less but in some cases with elevated promyelocytes. In a study of 19 such patients, Verma et al (1978) reported that the majority (12/19) had a marrow culture pattern of a low incidence of colonies and clusters in a normal ratio with normal cell differentiation. These patients survived significantly longer than patients presenting with cluster forming marrow growth patterns or with abnormal cluster to colony ratios. The latter progressed to acute leukemia more frequently (7/7) and faster (median 20 weeks) than did patients with a low incidence and normal ratio of clusters to colonies (one of 12 at 40 weeks). In an earlier study of patients with idiopathic acquired sideroblastic anemia and chronic myelomonocytic syndrome, (Moore, 1977a), development of acute leukemia was preceded by development of abnormal growth pattern of cells in culture. In a study of 37 patients with idiopathic acquired sideroblastic anemia (Moore, 1977d) 8 cases had refractory anemia only, whereas the remaining cases also had neutropenia, thrombo-cytopenia or both. Marrow colony and cluster incidence was within the normal range in the 8 cases with refractory anemia only. Of the remaining cases, 17 showed a markedly reduced incidence of colony- and cluster-forming cells with normal in vitro granulocytic maturation and a ratio of clusters to colonies within the normal range. Over a period of 6 months to 3 years only one of these cases has progressed to overt AL and then only after showing qualitative defects in marrow culture consistent with those seen in the remaining 12 patients. These latter exhibited one or more qualitative defects similar to those observed in AML. Six of 12 cases showed no colony formation with a peristing micro- or macro-cluster growth pattern and 3 cases showed a pattern of small colonies with an excess of clusters (microcolony type). Of the remaining 3 cases, low numbers of colonies were present of normal size and maturation, but the cluster-to-colony ratio exceeded the normal range. Sequential studies of these latter patients revealed a progressive loss in colony-forming capacity and increase in cluster incidence, suggesting that at the time of initial observation normal colony-forming cells and leukemic cluster-forming cells were co-existing. Eight of the 12 patients showing an abnormal cluster-to-colony ratio progressed to AL between 3 and 14 months after first detection of this in vitro defect. Two patients died without evidence of leukemia and two remained clinically unchanged over periods of 4 and 11 months. Progression to overt leukemia was generally associated with an increasing incidence of cluster-forming cells in the marrow.

Greenberg et al (1976) have also reported abnormal in vitro marrow growth patterns and abnormally light buoyant density of GM-CFC in preleukemic patients a median of 10 months prior to acute transformation. Acute transformation was not observed in patients with idiopathic ineffective erythropoiesis characterized by a normal incidence and density distribution pattern of marrow GM-CFC and normal urinary CSF output. A further variant of the preleukemic state is the chronic myelomonocytic syndrome. In a study of 14 such cases, Moore (1977d) showed an increased incidence of colonies and clusters in marrow and/or blood culture with, in most instances, a normal colony-to-cluster ratio. Biophysical characterization of the GM-CFC was performed using continuous gradient centrifugation in bovine serum albumin or a modified density 'cut' procedure in albumin of density 1.062 g/cm^3. The GM-CFC were of abnormal light density with 58 ± 3 per cent less dense than 1.062 g/cm^3 in contrast to the 0 to 10 per cent of normal GM-CFC in this density region. A similar light density characterizes GM-CFC in CML. Maturation defects were observed in colonies derived from 3 of 14 patients and an abnormal colony-to-cluster ratio in 4 cases. These additional qualitative defects identified the cases of chronic myelomonocytic syn-drome which subsequently progressed to A monocytic or myelomonocytic L associ-ated with loss of colony formation and appearance of a cluster-forming AML growth pattern in marrow and blood culture.

A recent analysis (Mertelsmann et al, 1979) of marrow culture, TdT and clinical data on 29 patients with myelodysplastic syndromes has confirmed earlier observations. The 29 patients included in the analysis were followed for up to 42 months (mean 8.5, range 1 to 42 months). Eleven patients progressed to AL. Of these patients, 6 showed abnormal cluster to colony ratios 1 to 13 months prior to clinically overt leukemia, while in two patients absent colony formation and a high incidence of clusters were detected at the same time as the rapidly emerging leukemia became evident clinically. Marrow cultures performed 2 to 4 months earlier in these two patients were normal. In 3 cases, marrow culture studies performed at the time of clinical diagnosis of AL revealed no growth of marrow cells in culture. In one of these patients, this defect was first detected 5 months prior to the development of leukemia. Of 18 patients with defective colony formation in marrow cultures, 11 progressed to AL after 0–13 (mean 3.3) months. Seven of these 18 patients continue to be in the chronic phase of their disease clinically with a return of normal growth pattern in 3 (mean follow up 26 months, range 4 to 42 months). Eleven of the 29 patients showed no significant culture abnormalities apart from a low incidence of normal colonies and clusters. Significant variations in colony and cluster incidence were observed in several of these patients. However, the cluster-to-colony ratio never exceeded 10 at any time.

Thus, although a normal marrow growth pattern appears to be associated with a favourable prognosis, it has to be kept in mind that AL can develop rapidly. Furthermore, although sequential marrow culture studies in patients with myelodysplastic syndromes allow the identification of a subgroup of patients at high risk of developing AL, not all of these patients will progress to AL, and some will revert spontaneously to a normal growth pattern and continue in chronic form.

MARROW CULTURE STUDIES IN NEUTROPENIC DISORDERS

The neutropenic disorders provide a clinical setting for evaluating abnormalities of granulopoietic regulation and numerous studies have been carried out to determine GM-CFC incidence in such disease states. Greenberg & Schrier (1973) utilized the thymidine suicide technique to determine the proportion of granulocytic progenitor cells in S phase in order to correlate in vitro proliferative activity of neutrophil precursors with peripheral demand in various neutropenic states. When peripheral blood neutrophil counts were at their peak level both GM-CFC and the percentage of these cells in S phase were comparable to controls, whereas at the neutrophil nadir both of these values were strikingly increased. Measurement of CSF production and serum CSF levels in cyclic neutropenia has also revealed a cyclic fluctuation with peak CSF levels coinciding with the neutrophil nadir (Moore et al, 1974b).

In patients with splenomegaly and neutropenia due to acclerated neutrophil removal the incidence of GM-CFC and the percentage in S phase is increased, suggesting the existence of a compensated state characterized by enhanced granulocytic turnover (Greenberg & Schrier, 1973). Decreased production appears to contribute significantly to the neutropenia present in patients with myeloid hypoplasia, Felty's syndrome, and some patients with idiopathic neutropenia and marked decreases in GM-CFC incidence were found.

Chronic idiopathic neutropenia syndrome, characterized by refractory neutropenia despite lack of splenomegaly, history of exposure to toxic drugs or evidence of systemic disease has been explained by a variety of pathophysiologic mechanisms. In a prospective study of 41 patients with this syndrome, Greenberg et al (1980) observed that the marrow GM-CFC incidence was variable but significantly increased and the proportion of CFC in DNA synthesis was normal to increased. Thus a quantitative lack of responsive granulocyte precursors is not the cause of the syndrome. Significantly decreased production of CSF by adherent bone marrow cells was noted and may reflect suboptimal intramedullary levels of this stimulatory factor in the syndrome. The proportion of light density GM-CFC in the marrow of these patients was normal using both the density cut and continuous density gradient procedures. Thus, this biophysical parameter appears to be a useful adjunct to marrow morphology for distinguishing this group of patients who have remained clinically stable from neutropenic patients with preleukemic syndrome or other prodromal myeloproliferative disorders who may otherwise present with clinical similarities.

Children with congenital neutropenia comprise a heterogeneous group of patients for which present classification methods are inadequate. Marrow culture studies have likewise provided substantially heterogeneous findings. Some patients have been described with abnormal maturation of GM-CFC, which mimic the disease (L'Esperance et al, 1973; Tich et al, 1977) and other patients have had paradoxically normal neutrophil colonies (Parmley et al, 1975; Amato et al, 1976; Barak et al, 1971) or defective colony stimulating activity (Nishihara et al, 1977). In a recent report of 6 children with severe congenital neutropenia and repeated life-threatening infections, Parmley et al (1980) observed a normal number of GM-CFC in marrow and blood; CSF production by blood cells and levels in serum was normal or slightly increased. In vitro maturation of the GM-CFC to neutrophils was also uniformly present in colonies. Ultrastructurally dysmorphic neutrophil granulocytes were observed in these patients and Parkley et al (1980) hypothesize that the dysgranulopoiesis in these children results in neutropenia and propose the descriptive name congenital dysgranulopoietic neutropenia for the disorder.

MARROW CULTURE STUDIES IN APLASTIC ANEMIA

Studies of myeloid and erythroid progenitors have revealed a consistent pattern. The incidence of marrow GM-CFC is generally between 1–10 per cent of normal (Table 6.3), and in view of the marked hypocellularity of the marrow aspirates, the absolute reduction in GM-CFC is significantly greater (Moore, 1979b). In the latter study of 39 patients almost all cases showed that the relative proportion of colony forming cells to cluster forming cells was within the normal range and colony maturation was normal. In one of the 39 cases studied marrow culture revealed a growth pattern of excessive

Table 6.3 GM-CFC, CFU-e and BFU-e in aplastic anemia bone marrow

	Number	Marrow/10^5 cells	
		GM CFC	CFC-clusters
Aplastic anemia	38	1.8 ± 0.2	18 ± 2
Aplastic anemia	1	0	3000
Normal	46	31 ± 1.5	270 ± 18
		BFU-e	CFU-e
Aplastic anemia	8	2.8 ± 1.7	7.4 ± 2.9
Normal	32	23.0 ± 5.0	71 ± 8.0

numbers of clusters exhibiting defective maturation, and absence of colony formation (Table 6.3). This growth pattern, typical of the majority of cases of AML, and seen also in a proportion of cases of preleukemia, was not associated with hematological or clinical signs of leukemia. Further observation of the progression of this patient's aplasia was not possible since an HLA matched bone marrow transplant was performed. Erythroid progenitor cell assays were performed on 7 patients and revealed an incidence of BFU-e and CFU-e approximately 10 per cent of normal values (Table 6.3).

While most cases of aplastic anemia have been attributed to congenital or acquired stem cell defects, it seems likely that several diseases of different etiology and pathogenesis exist. The availability of in vitro techniques for detection of myeloid and erythroid progenitor cells has provided an experimental approach for determining the mechanisms leading to aplastic anemia. Using these systems, evidence has been obtained for a reversible immunologically-mediated suppression of hematopoiesis in certain cases of aplastic anemia (Kagan et al, 1976; Ascensao et al, 1976). In these studies, the severe defect in myeloid colony formation in vitro was corrected by removal of small lymphocytes from the patient's marrow by velocity sedimentation or treatment with anti-thymocyte globulin and complement. These candidate suppressor cells were also identified by their ability to inhibit normal GM-CFC when marrow from the patient was co-cultured with marrow from a normal donor in the GM-CFC assay. These preliminary studies on immunologic mechanisms leading to aplasia have been confirmed by others (Haak & Goslink, 1977; Hoffman et al, 1977), and extended to demonstration of suppression of erythroid colony formation by aplastic peripheral blood mononuclear cells. Further evidence for the existence of lymphocyte-mediated suppression of hematopoiesis is provided by the small proportion of aplastic patients who have received either HLA-identical or haploidentical marrow transplants and after rejecting the allograft, spontaneously recovered their autologous marrow function. In a more extensive study of suppressor cell involvement in aplastic anemia, Kagan et al (1979) undertook to co-culture bone marrow from 14 aplastic patients with normal allogeneic bone marrow and showed significant suppression of GM-CFC in 20 per cent of cases with no preincubation and in 54 per cent of cases after a 12-hour preincubation of the cells in suspension culture. In two of these cases complete inhibition of colony formation was observed. The effect on colony formation of anti-thymocyte globulin (ATG) plus complement treatment of the aplastic marrow prior to agar culture was investigated in those cases where suppression was evident in co-culture. In only one case was a significant augmentation of colony formation observed. Considerable criticism has been directed at the in vitro systems used to demonstrate suppressor cell mechanisms in aplastic anemia. In particular, co-culture inhibition has been attributed to transfusion sensitization to major or minor histocompatibility differences in experimental animals and clinical studies (Singer et al, 1978). In the latter report co-culture studies on transfused aplastic patients using HLA-matched, MLC compatible sibling bone marrow target cells produced variable inhibition which correlated with a direct chromium release assay, a known test for sensitization to minor transplantation antigens. Sullivan et al (1980) detected no evidence of cell-mediated inhibition of GM-CFC proliferation in any of 18 patients evaluated by marrow co-culture or anti-thymocyte serum pretreatment. Since most of the patients had received multiple blood transfusions prior to study, the results are at variance with those of Singer et al (1978). This discrepancy could be accounted for by the use of light density peripheral blood mononuclear cells in the Singer co-culture experiments versus the use of marrow cell suspensions by Sullivan et al (1980).

An alternative approach has been used to investigate further the influence of aplastic bone marrow on GM-CFC proliferation (Moore, 1979b). Since suppression due to transfusion-induced sensitization to major or minor histocompatibility antigens is mediated by intact cells and cannot be duplicated by cell extracts or conditioned media, evidence was sought for the possible existence of suppressive mediators contained in, or secreted by marrow cell populations in patients with aplastic anemia. Extracts or conditioned media obtained from control or aplastic marrow were added directly to GM-CFC assays or were preincubated with the target bone marrow and in one of four cases of aplastic anemia, significant and reproducible inhibition of GM-CFC proliferation was observed (Moore, 1979b). This patient received an HLA matched bone marrow graft and no inhibitory activity was detected in the patient's bone marrow following pre-transplant immunosuppression or in the post-engraftment stage. In order to determine the cell population containing the inhibitory activity, aplastic marrow cells were separated by a density cut procedure at $1.070 \, gm/cm^3$ and adherence to plastic. Only extracts from cells present in the non-adherent light density fractions demonstrated significant inhibitory activity. Cell separation procedures using velocity sedimentation and spontaneous sheep red blood cell rosetting were performed to further characterize the inhibitory activity producing cell. Inhibitory activity was detected in a population of slowly sedimenting cells (3.0 to 5.5 mm/hr), which could be separated from the majority of marrow GM-CFC. Dilution of the extract or conditioned media prior to assay demonstrated that the cells sedimenting at 3.0 to 4.0 mm/hr contained more inhibitory activity than more rapidly sedimenting cells. Inhibitory activity was confined to the non-rosetting fraction following separation of marrow with neuraminidase-treated sheep red blood cells.

Evidence for a subgroup of aplastic anemia attributable to an active suppressor mechanism must be reviewed critically in the light of the methodologies employed. It is clear that marrow co-culture studies, even when undertaken with HLA-matched target marrow, may demonstrate GM-CFC inhibition due to transfusion sensitization of the patient to minor histocompatability differences. The duration of co-culture, the source of cells, the cell concentration used and the aplastic to target marrow cell ratio are frequently uncontrolled variables particularly since the cellular composition of aplastic marrow or blood differs so markedly from normal. It is also the case that the human GM-CFC assay is understimulated and is particularly sensitive to enhancement or inhibition both of a specific or non-specific nature.

The available evidence suggests that any suppressor cell activity in aplastic anemia is unlikely to involve classic immunological mechanisms. Abrogation of suppression by treatment of aplastic marrow with anti-thymocyte or anti-lymphocyte globulin plus complement is difficult to interpret since the specificity of such antisera is poorly understood relative to minor subsets of non-T hematopoietic cells with regulatory potential. Similarly, the recovery of normal GM-CFC in the marrow of patients following the onset of pre-transplant immunosuppression does not prove that an immunological suppressor cell mechanism need exist. The existence of an auto-aggressive process in certain patients with aplastic anemia may involve an inappropriately activated hematopoietic regulatory cell or the development of a suppressor cell population not of a classic B or T cell type but possibly related to the natural killer cell population. Finally, it remains unclear whether such suppressor cell populations are acquired as a consequence of the aplastic state or are instrumental in inducing it.

LONG TERM CULTURE OF HUMAN BONE MARROW CELLS

Until recently, quantitation of true pluripotential stem cells with extensive self-renewal capacity has been restricted to an in vivo spleen colony assay (CFU-s) in lethally irradiated rodents. Dexter has reported an in vitro marrow culture system which can sustain for many weeks CFU-s proliferation with differentiation into all hematopoietic progenitor cell pathways (for review see Dexter et al, 1978). In this murine culture system, the environment for stem cell proliferation is provided by an heterogeneous population of adherent bone marrow cells, possibly representative of stromal marrow elements, which develops within 2 to 3 weeks of culture initiation. Upon inoculation with a second population of syngeneic or allogeneic bone marrow, hematopoiesis is sustained for prolonged periods and CFU-s are found intimately associated with the endothelial cells, macrophages and fat-containing cells which comprise the adherent layer.

Adaption of the continuous marrow culture system for use with species other than mouse, particularly human, would have major significance in areas as diverse as transplantation biology and tumor virology, as well as allowing functional charac-terization of pluripotential stem cells in those species in which this is presently not possible. Moore & Sheridan (1979) reported that continuous human bone marrow culture could be established under conditions similar to those used in the murine system (25 per cent horse serum and Fischer's medium) but production of myeloid cells and GM-CFC was limited to only 6 to 8 weeks. Hocking & Golde (1980) also reported GM-CFC and CFU-E maintenance in human marrow culture for 4 to 9 weeks with morphologically recognizable granulopoiesis for 4 to 6 weeks and erythropoiesis for up to 3 weeks. In both studies the adherent marrow population was composed of macrophages, fibroblast cells and flat pavement-like endothelial cells but lacked the giant lipid-laden cells seen in murine long-term marrow cultures. A major limitation in developing an effective long-term human culture system appeared to be an inability to successfully duplicate the components and structural interactions observed in the murine in vitro adherent environment. In an attempt to define a species that would exhibit the efficiency of the murine system in sustaining in vitro hematopoiesis, but would be more closely related to man, hematologically, virologi-cally and immunologically, studies were undertaken with *Tupaia glis* (the tree shrew), a member of the family *Tupaiidae*, regarded as one of the most primitive living Prosimians (Moore & Sheridan, 1979; Moore et al, 1979). The proliferative capacity of a single inoculation of approximately 10^7 *Tupaia* bone marrow cells is illustrated in Figure 6.1. GM-CFC production, neutrophil granulopoiesis and mast cell production can be seen to be sustained for 22 months. Indeed continuous normal myelopoiesis is regularly observed for up to $2\frac{1}{2}$ years. This contrasts with the maximum of 18 to 20 weeks of continuous stem cell replication observed in culture of marrow from certain mouse strains and the 20-week duration of myelopoiesis so far reported in human

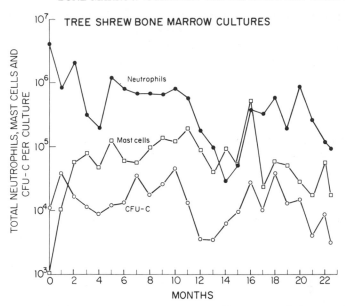

Fig. 6.1   Production of GM-CFC (CFU-c) and mature neutrophils and mast cells in suspension cultures initiated by an inoculum of 10^7. Tree shrew bone marrow cells. Cultures were maintained at 37° C and subjected to weekly demi-depopulation of suspension cells.

marrow culture (Gartner & Kaplan, 1980). The ultimate decline in stem cell replication in the murine system may be attributed to 'aging' of the adherent marrow microenvironment rather than exhaustion of stem cell self-renewal potential. Terminal cultures exhibit detachment of adherent cells, loss of fat-containing cells, and overgrowth by macrophages. A similar process of detachment of the adherent marrow cells is seen at intervals of 1 to 2 months in *Tupaia* cultures. However, in this species, there appears to be a regular cycle of reestablishment of a complex adherent environment from cells present in the suspension. Ultrastructural analysis of the adherent environment reveals large regions dominated by fat cells but in other regions flattened sheets of pavement endothelial cells are seen (Moore et al, 1979). These latter cells are also characteristic of mouse bone marrow cultures and are considered to be derived from the endothelial cells that line the venous sinuses.

Ultrastructural studies on the granulocyte populations in the adherent layer has revealed three main populations; immature progranulocytes, early neutrophils, and relatively mature basophils. The mature basophil cells are characterized by an extremely electrondense cytoplasmic granule population, numerous mitochondria, and condensed peripheral nuclear chromatin. Early cells of the neutrophil series, possibly at the myelocyte stage, show some secondary granule formation and also continued primary granulogenesis of dense-cored small vacuoles in the golgi region, characteristic of neutrophil maturation. Some evidence of early nuclear segmentation is also apparent. The majority of granulocytes in the adherent layer have an overall promyelocyte morphology and differ from the mouse system in that they spread and attach in a characteristic dendritic form. These 'progranulocytes' display a smooth nuclear profile with little peripheral chromatin condensation and prominent nucleoli. The ultrastructural features of the *Tupaia* marrow cultures emphasize the complex interrelationships of sheets of pavement endothelial cells, fat-containing cells, macrophages, and hematopoietic elements previously described in the murine system. The extensive and intimate interactions, including junctional complexes, observed between immature hematopoietic elements and other cellular components of the adherent layer appear not to be dependent on compatibility at major histocompatibility loci both in mouse and *Tupaia* studies. Gartner & Kaplan (1980) have reported a modification of the Dexter system which allows the production of GM-CFC for at least 20 weeks in liquid culture of human bone marrow. Optimal growth conditions consisted of McCoy's medium supplemented with fetal bovine serum, horse serum, and hydrocortisone with incubation at 33°C. Adipocyte-containing confluent stromal layers were readily established and the generation of cells with colony-forming ability appeared to follow two different patterns, designated the 'hyperproliferative' and 'homeostatic' patterns. The hyperproliferative pattern describes cultures in which the number of GM-CFC generated exceeds 100 per 10^5 cells in serial assay over several weeks. In contrast, the homeostatic pattern describes a steady-state situation in which a lower level of GM-CFC, usually between 25 and 75 per 10^5 cells, is continuously present in the cultures. A direct comparison of human marrow from the same donor, cultured in horse serum and Fischers' medium (old system) versus the Gartner & Kaplan (1980) modification ('new' system) shows the advantage of the 'new' at the level of prolonged production of GM-CFC and in all stages of granulocyte differentiation relative to macrophage and lymphocyte proliferation.

The nature of the cell type responsible for sustaining hematopoiesis in long term cultures of human bone marrow has been investigated using antisera directed against Ia-like antigens since numerous studies have identified Ia as an antigen expressed on all classes of immature hematopoietic progenitor cell. The presence of Ia antigen on early hemopoietic progenitors, and its subsequent disappearance with maturation, suggests that it may provide a maturation marker. In order to test this postulate, Moore et al (1980) investigated myelopoiesis, GM-CFC and BFU-e production in human continuous marrow cultures inoculated with marrow cell suspensions depleted of Ia-positive cells.

In the experiment shown in Table 6.4 primary marrow cultures were totally depleted of suspension cells after four weeks, followed by inoculation of fresh autologous marrow treated with 1:100 dilution of anti-Ia serum with complement or with B cell absorbed anti-serum as a control. GM-CFC and BFU-e in the input marrow were reduced to 5 per cent and 3 per cent respectively of control values, recovering to 48 per cent and 72 per cent within one week (Table 6.4). Over a five week period the mean recovery of GM-CFC and BFU-e in four separate experiments was 128 ± 48 per cent and 144 ± 29 per cent of control values. In striking contrast to the extreme sensitivity of the pre-CFU and the various erythroid and myeloid progenitor cells to anti-Ia serum, it appears clear that the predominant cell type, presumably pluripotent, responsible for initiating and sustaining hematopoiesis under conditions of continuous marrow culture is either Ia antigen-negative or extremely resistant to complement-mediated cytotoxicity.

In the mouse, Ia antigens have a major immunoregulatory role and it is probable that the human analogs of Ia antigen expressed on B cells, monocytes and on a subset of circulating T cells may be part of a network through which cell-cell signals are conveyed between subsets on immunocompetent cells. The selective occurrence of the

Table 6.4 Generation of myeloid cells, GM-CFC and BFU-e in continuous marrow culture after treatment of marrow with anti-Ia serum plus complement

Time (days)	Total cells $\times 10^6$		Differential %†			Total GM-CFC per culture		Total BFU-e per culture	
	Control*	Anti-Ia + C'	Myeloid.	Lymphoid.	Mø	Control	Anti-Ia + C'	Control	Anti-Ia + C'
0	15	15				9360 ± 425	480 ± 75	1575 ± 255	45 ± 45
7	7.1	4.4	58(49)	25(24)	17(27)	6095 ± 728	2925 ± 375	570 ± 32	410 ± 45
14	3.1	1.7	48(31)	23(25)	29(44)	5464 ± 376	3949 ± 189	325 ± 13	109 ± 6
21	0.85	0.76	60(60)	12(4)	28(36)	755 ± 133	592 ± 73	84 ± 7	119 ± 11
28	1.4	1.45	22(19)	2(4)	76(77)	75 ± 28	51 ± 29	120 ± 12	413 ± 21
35	0.75	0.65	28(2)	0(0)	72(98)	125 ± 64	16 ± 10	68 ± 8	44 ± 4

*Control = B cell absorbed anti-Ia serum + complement
†Control differential (anti-Ia + C' differential) Mø = monocytes

same Ia glycoproteins on early stages of the granulocytic, erythroid and megakaryocytic series and their subsequent disappearance during differentiation within the bone marrow may represent a phylogenetically earlier role for Ia antigen in hematopoietic regulation. It is clear, for example, that the various lineage-committed hematopoietic progenitor cells require interaction with specific proteins or glycoproteins such as myeloid colony stimulating factors, erythropoietin or thrombopoietin to undergo terminal differentiation. Observations in the continuous marrow culture system further suggests that the interaction of these various 'hemopoietins' with their Ia antigen-bearing progenitor cells occurs locally and involves intimate cell-cell interactions with cellular constituents of the hematopoietic microenvironment. In contrast, the Ia-negative status of candidate human pluripotential stem cells may correlate with their apparent unresponsiveness to lineage-specific 'hemopoietins' and possession of extensive self-renewal capacity.

CHARACTERIZATION OF HUMAN BONE MARROW STROMAL ELEMENTS AND THE PATHOGENESIS OF MYELOFIBROSIS

Myelofibrosis (MF) is defined by pathologists as an accumulation of collagen in bone marrow stroma. Myelofibrosis is the main hematological feature in so-called Primary Myelofibrosis, but it is also associated with many hematological disorders. Since the original description of primary myelofibrosis in 1897, its pathogenesis has remained obscure. Insights into the origin of marrow fibrosis have been obtained by the analysis of cytogenetic markers of hematopoietic cells and marrow fibroblasts from patients with myelofibrosis. Accumulation of collagen in bone marrow appears to be a secondary phenomenon associated with a clonal disease affecting the hematopoietic cells. However, until recently no direct evidence of the reactive origin of fibrosis has been provided. Studies in this direction have been hindered by the lack of in vitro systems for studying (a) the characteristics of collagen-producing cells, and (b) the interaction between hematopoietic cells and marrow stromal cells. Progress in this important area has been reported by Castro-Malaspina et al (1980), who have developed a liquid culture system to clone and to characterize human bone marrow fibroblast

Table 6.5 Bone marrow fibroblast characteristics in normal donors and patients with myeloproliferative disorders

	Normal	MPD, MF⁻*	MPD, MF⁺*
CFU-F			
Adherence, 60 min (%)	9 ± 2	11 ± 3.5	
Cell density, <1.070 g/cm³ BSA	N	N	
Sed. rate in BSA (mm/h)	5.00 ± 0.05	4.95 ± 0.05	
Proliferative status (reduction ³H-TdR)	-2 ± 2	$+1 \pm 1.5$	
PROGENY			
Serum dependence for growth	+	+	+
Contact inhibition of growth	+	+	+
Collagen I, III (IMF)	+	+	+
Fibronectin (IMF)	+	+	+
Plasminogen activator	N	N	N
Karyotype	N	N	N

*MPD: Myeloproliferative Disorders, MF–: Without Myelofibrosis, N – Normal.

colony forming cells (CFC-F). The linear relationship between the number of marrow cells plated and the number of colonies formed suggests that fibroblast colonies originate in a single cell. Bone marrow CFC-F are adherent and non-phagocytic (Table 6.5). The majority (90 per cent + 2 per cent) are less dense than 1.070 g/cu cm. Velocity sedimentation separation demonstrated a heterogeneous CFC-F sedimentation rate, with a modal sedimentation of 4.95 ± 0.15 mm/hr. Analysis of CFC-F proliferative status by the thymidine suicide technique indicated that this cell was non-cycling in individuals with undisturbed bone marrow function. Some of the more distinctive products of fibroblasts, other stromal cells, and hematopoietic colony-forming cells were used as positive and negative markers of CFC-F and the cells derived from them in vitro. Complement-mediated cytotoxicity using anti-Ia and anti-factor VIII antigen antisera did not inhibit fibroblast colony formation, in contrast to the striking reduction of granulocyte-macrophage colony formation seen when bone marrow cells were treated with anti-Ia antiserum. Immunofluorescence staining was used to characterize the cells derived from CFC-F in vitro. No staining was observed after incubation of subconfluent cultures with anti-Ia and anti-factor VIII antisera. A positive immunofluorescent staining was obtained when isolated antibodies against three of the main proteins of bone marrow matrix: type I collagen, type III collagen, and fibronectin were used. Ultrastructural analysis showed that CFC-F progeny, in contrast to endothelial cells, did not contain Weibel-Palade bodies. These data support the fibroblast nature of the colonies described by Castro-Malaspina et al (1980). CFC-F from patients with myeloproliferative disorders such as CML and polycythemia vera exhibited similar density and sedimentation rates as normal CFC-F and their fibroblast progeny had normal functional properties (Table 6.5), (Castro-Malaspina et al, 1981).

The comparison of in vitro growth characteristics demonstrated that fibroblasts from patients with myelofibrosis required anchorage and serum for growth, just as did fibroblasts from normal donors. The growth rate was directly related to the concentration of the source of growth factor(s) (fetal calf serum). Moreover fibroblasts from both sources exhibited contact inhibition of growth. Isolated fibroblasts were also characterized by immunofluoresence staining with specific antibodies for the presence and distribution of fibronectin (FN). Fibronectin was demonstrated with similar staining pattern on the surface and in the cytoplasm of fibroblasts from all groups of donors. Plasminogen activator levels produced by isolated fibroblasts from all sources were also similar. Chromosomal analysis of hematopoietic and collagen producing cells obtained from patients with CML presenting with myelofibrosis showed that only the hematopoietic cells were Ph'+. These studies demonstrate that bone marrow collagen-producing cells derived from patients with myelofibrosis display in vitro the same characteristics as those derived from normal donors and patients with myeloproliferative disease not presenting with myelofibrosis. These findings support the hypothesis that myelofibrosis observed in patients with myeloproliferative disease results from a 'reactive' process rather than from a disorder affecting primarily the marrow collagen producing cells.

Mitogenic activity for marrow fibroblasts has been isolated from cell homogenates of human marrow cell density fractions enriched for megakaryocytes (Castro-Malaspina et al, 1981). The growth promoting activities elicited from homogenates of platelets and marrow fractions enriched for megakaryocytes were similar. The dose-related curves for both were parallel and they were both temperature resistant and trypsin sensitive. These findings implicate megakaryocytes as a source of the growth factor derived from platelets and suggest that megakaryocytes may play a role in the pathogenesis of the marrow fibrosis observed in myeloproliferative disorders by stimulating fibroblast proliferation and collagen secretion. As a result of the preceding in vitro evidence regarding fibrous tissue and its regulation, an hypothesis has been formulated regarding the pathophysiological mechanisms operating in the development of marrow fibrosis associated with myeloproliferative disorders, with particular reference to primary myelofibrosis (Castro-Malaspina & Moore, 1981). Megakaryocytosis of the bone marrow is a predominant feature of primary myelofibrosis, and in many instances megakaryocytes are found in clusters within the marrow parenchyma and marrow sinuses. Quantitative alterations are associated with marked morphological abnormalities which are not seen in other diseases exhibiting megakaryocytosis. Areas of fibroblast proliferation and collagen deposition are often most prominent in areas with large numbers of morphologically abnormal megakaryocytes. Necrotic megakaryocytes are observed in severe forms of myelofibrosis and the progression of myelofibrosis parallels the increase in the proportion of necrotic megakaryocytes. Ultrastructural analysis of fibrotic bone marrow has confirmed that the morphological alterations in megakaryocytes are more prominent in primary myelofibrosis (PMF) than in other myeloproliferative disorders.

Platelet counts in primary myelofibrosis unlike those seen in other myeloproliferative disorders associated with marrow megakaryocytosis are within or below the normal range. High counts are rare, and levels are not comparable to those seen in essential thrombocythemia. Platelet turnover estimations have shown that platelet production is defective in spite of marrow megakaryocytosis and an increased megakaryocyte cytoplasm mass. These observations together with morphological evidence indicate that a high proportion of megakaryocytes in PMF become retarded or arrested in their progress along the megakaryocytopoietic pathway and die within the bone marrow. Imperfect megakaryocyte maturation in primary myelofibrosis results in the intramedullary death of vast numbers of developing megakaryocytes rich in platelet components. As a result megakaryocytic components escape into the marrow intercellular space. We suggest that the process leading to excessive deposition of marrow collagen is initiated by the abnormal presence in marrow intercellular spaces of megakaryocytic derived constituents, particularly megakaryocyte-derived growth factor (MkDGF) and factor 4. High concentrations of MkDGF stimulate fibroblast proliferation and collagen secretion. Increased numbers of

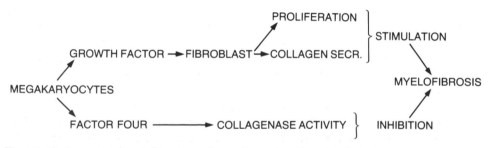

Fig. 6.2 Pathogenesis of myelofibrosis associated with myeloproliferative disorders.

marrow fibroblasts in primary myelofibrosis occurs at a very early stage of the disease and experimental fibrosis studies have shown that one of the earliest stromal reactions morphologically recognizable is fibroblast proliferation, which is followed by collagen deposition. Increased collagen secretion also stimulates the secretion of collagenases and probably of its activator(s). Compensatory breakdown of the excess of collagen by collagenases is inhibited by factor 4 and this imbalance between collagen production and its degradation leads to an excessive accumulation of collagens in marrow stroma.

CLONAL ASSAYS FOR HUMAN PLURIPOTENT PROGENITOR CELLS (CFU-GEMM, CFU-Mix) AND MEGAKARYOCYTE PROGENITORS (CFU-Mk, Mk-CFC)

A clonal assay is now available that facilitates the detection of human pluripotent progenitor cells (Fauser & Messner, 1978, 1979). These pluripotent progenitors give rise to mixed colonies in methylcellulose in the presence of 5 per cent of medium conditioned with leukocytes in the presence of PHA and erythropoietin. The cells of origin sediment at 4.5 mm/hr and are of a density less than 1.077 gm/ml. The cellular composition of mixed colonies may vary greatly and may include neutrophilic and eosinophilic granulocytes, erythroblasts, megakaryocytes and macrophages. In addition, approximately 20 per cent of all mixed colonies contain cells that give rise to different types of secondary hemopoietic colonies when replated as a single cell suspension, indicating the presence of primitive progenitors such as CFU-GEMM, BFU-E and GM-CFC. The clonal nature of the mixed colonies was confirmed by the linear relationship between the number of cells plated and the number of colonies and the absence or presence of Y-chromatin in the mixed colonies in co-culture experiments with male and female cells. Assessment of the proliferative activity of CFU-GEMM by short-term exposure to ^{3}H-thymidine demonstrated that they are quiescent under steady state conditions and actively cycling during phases of bone marrow transplantation. Examination of CFU-GEMM in various stem cell disorders such as polycythemia vera, CML and AML indicated that they are present at a frequency compatible with that observed for normal individuals but a difference was observed when their cycle state was determined. CFU-GEMM in these stem cell disorders were found to proliferate actively. Pluripotent hematopoietic precursors were also shown to be markedly reduced in the marrow of patients with aplastic anemia and indeed were absent in aplastic patients who had repeatedly received transfusions (Hara et al, 1980). This result provides direct evidence that pancytopenia in most patients with aplastic anemia results from a reduced influx into the compartment of maturing hemopoietic cells from the compartment of pluripotent hemopoietic precursors. The availability of this assay provides a powerful tool for detailed analysis of the human stem cell compartment in health and disease and in regenerating situations such as posed by bone marrow transplantation.

Vainchenker et al (1979a, b) reported the growth in plasma clot cultures of megakaryocyte colonies from adult human bone marrow, human blood and fetal liver cells. Megakaryocytes were identified by their morphology and particularly by their polylobulated nucleus when examined by light microscopy. The megakaryocytic nature of large cells was clearly confirmed by the presence of platelet peroxidase, demarcation membranes and α-granules detected by electron microscopy; in addition mature small megakaryocytes were recognized. Megakaryocyte colonies were seen after 9 days of culture and consisted of 2 to 20 cells. The colonies were pure or mixed with the burst erythroblasts. The mixed colonies were numerous in fetal and neonatal cultures, while pure megakaryocyte colonies were seen three times more frequently in those from adult blood and marrow. The total number of colonies was also much lower in adult cultures. In colonies derived from neonatal and fetal cells, megakaryocytes often reached a more complete maturation than in those from adults, proceeding as far as platelet shedding. Megakaryocyte colony formation required a large number of plated cells (greater than 3×10^5/ml) and the presence of erythropoietin-containing preparations. In the absence of erythropoietin, rare spontaneous megakaryocyte colonies could be observed while no erythroid colonies were present. However, erythropoietin induced a fivefold increase in the total number of colonies. These data suggest that erythropoietin is involved in the differentiation of human megakaryocytes, but that it does not act alone, since another factor related to the number of seeded cells appears essential for the formation of human megakaryocyte colonies.

This Mk-CFC assay has yet to be applied to the spectrum of human disorders involving defective megakaryopoiesis and abnormal platelet production. The assay will undoubtedly provide valuable insight into the pathophysiology of such diseases.

REFERENCES

Amato D, Freedman M H, Saunders E F 1976 Blood 47: 531–538
Ascensao J, Pahwa R, Kagan W, Hansen J, Moore MAS, Good RA 1976 Lancet i: 669–671
Barak Y, Paran M, Levin S, Sachs L 1971 Blood 38: 74–80
Bognacki J, Broxmeyer H E, LoBue J 1981 Biochem Biophys Acta (in press)
Breitman T R, Selonick S E, Collins S J 1980 Proc Natl Acad Sci USA 77: 2936–2940
Brennan J K, DiPersio J F, Abboud C N, Lichtman M A 1980 Blood 55: 1230–1239
Broxmeyer H E 1979 J Clin Invest 64: 1717–1720
Broxmeyer H E, Moore M A S 1978 Biochimica et Biophysica Acta 516: 129–166
Broxmeyer H E, Moore M A S, Ralph P 1977a Experimental Hematology 5: 357–373
Broxmeyer H E, Mendelsohn N, Moore M A S 1977b Leukemia Research 1: 3–12
Broxmeyer H E, Smithyman A, Eger R R, Meyers P A, DeSousa M 1978a J Exp Med 148: 1052–1067
Broxmeyer H E, Jacobsen N, Kurland J, Mendelsohn N, Moore M A S, 1978b Journal of the National Cancer Institute 60: 497–512
Broxmeyer H E, Grossbard E, Jacobsen N, Moore M A S 1978c Journal of the National Cancer Institute 60: 513–522
Broxmeyer H E, Grossbard E, Jacobsen N, Moore M A S 1979a New England Journal of Medicine 301: 346–350
Broxmeyer H E, Ralph P, Margolis V B, Nakoinz I, Meyers P, Kapoor N, Moore M A S 1979b Leukemia Research 3: 193–203
Broxmeyer H E, DeSousa M, Smithyman A, Ralph P, Hamilton J, Kurland J, Bognacki J 1980 Blood 55: 324–333
Broxmeyer H E, Bognacki J, Dorner M M, deSousa M, Lu L 1981 In: Modern Trends in Human Leukemia VI. (ed) Neth, R. Springer–Verlag, Berlin (in press)
Buick R N, Till J E, McCulloch E A 1977 Lancet i: 862–863
Buick R N, Messner H A, Till J E, McCulloch E A 1979 J Natl Cancer Inst 62: 249–253
Burgess A W, Metcalf D 1981 Blood 56: 947–958
Castro-Malaspina H, Moore M A S 1981 Submitted
Castro-Malaspina H, Gay R E, Resnick G, Kapoor N, Meyers P, Chiarieri D, McKenzie S, Broxmeyer H E, Moore M A S 1980 Blood 56: 289
Castro-Malaspina H, Rabellino E M, Yen A, Nachman R L, Moore M A S 1981a Blood (in press)
Castro-Malaspina H, Rabellino E M, Yen A, Nachman R L, Moore M A S 1981b In: Evatt B L, Levine R F, Williams N (eds) Megakaryocytes in vitro. North Holland Elsevier (in press)

Dexter T M, Allen T D, Lajtha L G, Krizsa R, Testa N G, Moore M A S 1978 Cold Spring Harbor
    Conference on Differentiation of Normal and Neoplastic Hematopoeitic Cells (eds) Clarkson B, Marks P,
    Till J, p 63–81
DiPersio J F, Brennan J K, Lichtman M A, Abboud C N, Kirkpatrick F H 1980 Blood 56: 717–727
Elias L, Wogenrich F J, Wallace J M, Longmire J 1980 Leukemia Research 4: 301–307
Fauser A A, Messner H A 1978 Blood 52: 1243–1247
Fauser A A, Messner H A 1979 Blood 53: 1023–1027
Fojo S S, Wu M-C, Gross M A, Purcell Y, Yunis A A 1978 Blocken 17: 3109–3116
Francis G E, Berney J J, Chipping P M, Hoffbrand A V 1979 Brit J Haemat 41: 545–554
Gartner S, Kaplan H S 1980 Proc Natl Acad Sci USA 77: 4756–4759
Golde D, Byers L A, Cline M 1974 Cancer Research 34, 419
Greenberg P, Mara B 1978 In: Differentiation of Normal and Neoplastic Hematopoietic Cells. Clarkson B,
    Marks P A, Till J E (eds) Cold Spring Harbor Laboratory, New York p 405–410
Greenberg P L, Schrier S L 1973 Blood 41: 753–761
Greenberg P L, Mara B, Steed S, Boxer L 1980 Blood 55: 915–921
Greenberg P, Mara B, Box I, Brassel R, Schrier S 1976 Am J Med 61: 878–890
Haak H L, Goselink H M 1977 Lancet i: 194
Hara H, Kai S, Fushimi M, Taniwaki S, Okamato I, Ohe Y, Fijita S, Noguchi K, Senba M, Hamano T,
    Kanamaru A, Nagai K 1980 Exp Hematol 8: 1165–1171
Hoelzer D, Harriss E B, Bultman B, Fliedner T M, Heimpel H 1980 In: Cronkite E P, Carsten A L (eds)
    Diffusion Chamber Culture, Springer-Verlag Berlin p 252–250
Hoffman R, Zanjani E, Lutton J D, Zalusky R, Wasserman L R 1977 New Engl J Med 296: 10–13
Horsten P, Granstrom M, Wahren B, Garton G 1977 Acta Med Scand 201: 405–410
Iscove N N, Sieber F, Winterhalter K H 1974 J Cell Physiol 83: 309–312
Jacobsen N, Broxmeyer H E, Grossbard E, Moore M A S 1978 Blood 52: 221–232
Jacobsen N, Broxmeyer H E, Grossbard E, Moore M A S 1979 Cell Tissue Kinet 12: 213–226
Jacobsen N, Broxmeyer H E, Winchester R J, Moore M A S 1980 Scand J Haematol 24: 227–233
Kagan W A, Ascensao J L, Fialk M A, Coleman M, Valera E B, Good R A 1979 Am J Med 66: 444–
    452
Kagan W, Ascensao J, Pahwa R, Hansen J, Goldstein G, Moore M A S, Good R A 1976 Proc Natl Acad Sci
    USA 73: 2809–2894
Keating M J, Smith B S, Gehan E A 1980 Cancer 45: 2017–2029
Koeffler H P, Golde D W 1980 Blood 54: 344–350
Kurland J I, Broxmeyer H E, Pelus L M, Bockman R S, Moore M A S 1978 Blood 52: 388–407
Kurland J I, Pelus L M, Ralph P, Bockman R S, Moore M A S 1979 Proc Natl Acad Sci USA 76,
    2326–2330
Lajtha L G 1979 Blood Cells 5: 447–455
Leong S S, Sokal J E, Gomez G A, Horozewicz J S 1979 Cancer Res 39: 2704–2710
L-Esperance P, Brunning R, Good R A 1973 Proc Natl Acad Sci USA 70: 669–672
Lowenberg B, Swart K, Hagemeijer A 1979 Leukemia Research 4: 243–149
McCulloch E A, Howaston A F, Buick R N, Minden M D, Izaguirre C A 1979 Blood Cells 5: 261–282
Mertelsmann R, Moore M A S, Broxmeyer H E, Cirrincione C, Clarkson B D 1981 Cancer Res (in press)
Mertelsmann R, Moore M A S, Clarkson B D 1979a In: Preleukemia. Schmalzl R, Hellriegel K P (eds)
    Springer Berlin–Heidelberg–New York p 106–111
Mertelsmann R, Koziner B, Filippa D A, Grossbard E, Incefy G, Moore M A S, Clarkson B D 1979b In:
    Modern Trends in Human Leukemia III. Neth R, Gallo R C, Hofschneider P (eds) Springer, Berlin
    p 131–134
Mertelsmann R, Cirrincione C, To L, Gee T S, McKenzie S, Schauer P, Friedman A, Arlin Z, Thaler H T,
    Clarkson B 1980 Blood 56: 773–783
Metcalf D 1977 Springer-Verlag Berlin, New York
Metcalf D, Moore M A S 1971 Haemopoietic Cells, Frontiers of Biology Series, North-Holland Publishing
    Co, Amsterdam
Metcalf D, Moore M A S, Sheridan J W, Spitzer G 1974 Blood 43: 847–853
Moberg C, Oloffson T, Olson I 1974 Scand J Haematol 12: 381–393
Moore M A S 1975 Blood Cells 1: 149–148
Moore M A S 1976 Blood Cells 2: 109–124
Moore M A S 1977a In: Recent Advances in Cancer Research. Gallo R (ed) CRC Press, Cleveland, Ohio
    pp 79–101
Moore M A S 1977b Clinics in Haematology 6: 97–112
Moore M A S 1977c Series Hematology 8: 11–27
Moore M A S 1977d Proceedings, 16th International Congress of Hematology, Kyoto, Japan, September
    1976. Excerpta Medica. International Congress Series No. 415, pp. 99–101

Moore M A S 1978 In: The Year of Hematology Volume II, Gordon A S, Silber R, LobBue J (eds) Plenum Publishing Co, New York pp 33–62
Moore M A S 1979 In: Clinics in Haematology Vol 8: No 2, p 287–309
Moore M A S 1979b In: Aplastic Anemia: Pathophysiology and Approaches to Therapy. Gordon-Smith E C, Heit W, Kubanek B (eds) Springer-Verlag Berlin p 265–271
Moore M A S, Sheridan A P 1979 Blood Cells 5: 297–311
Moore M A S, Mertelsmann R, Pelus L M 1981 Blood Cells (in press)
Moore M A S, Williams N, Metcalf D 1972 J Cell Physiol 79: 283–292
Moore M A S, Williams N, Metcalf D 1973a J Natl Cancer Inst 50: 591–602
Moore M A S, Williams N, Metcalf D 1973b J Natl Cancer Inst 50: 603–611
Moore M A S, Sheridan A P C, Allen T D, Dexter T M 1979 Blood 54: 775–793
Moore M A S, Spitzer G, Metcalf D, Penington D G 1974b Brit J Haemat 27: 47–55
Moore M A S, Spitzer G, Williams N, Metcalf D, Buckley J 1974a Blood 44: 1–11
Moore M A S, Broxmeyer H E, Sheridan A P C, Meyers P A, Jacobsen N, Winchester R J 1980 Blood 55: 682–690
Moore M A S, Burgess A W, Metcalf D, McCulloch E A, Robinson W A, Dick K A, Chevenick P A, Bull J M, Wu A M, Stanley E R, Goldman J, Testa N 1977 British Journal of Cancer 35: 600–508
Morstyn G, Nicola N A, Metcalf D 1980 Blood 56: 798–805
Nicola N A, Metcalf D, Johnson G R, Burgess A W 1974 Blood 54: 614–700
Nishihara H, Nakahata T, Terauchi A, Akabane T 1977 Acta Haematol Jap 40: 52–66
Niskanen E, Koeffler H P, Golde D W, Cline M J 1980 Leukemia Research 4: 203–208
Park C H, Amare M, Savin M A, Goodwin J W, Newcomb M M, Hoogstraten B 1980 Blood 55: 595–601
Parmley R T, Ogawa M, Darby C P, Jr, Spicer 1975 Blood 46: 723–734
Parmley R T, Crist W M, Ragab A H, Boxer L A, Malluh A, Lui V K, Darby C P 1980 Blood 56: 465–475
Pegoraro L, Abrahm J, Cooper R A, Levis A, Lange B, Meo P, Rovera G 1980 Blood 55: 859–862
Pelus L M, Broxmeyer H E, Clarkson B D, Moore M A S 1980 Cancer Research 40: 2523–2525
Pelus L M, Broxmeyer H E, Kurland J I, Moore M A S 1979 J Exp Med 150: 277–292
Pike B L, Robinson W A 1970 J Cell Comp Physiol 76: 77–82
Preisler H D 1980 Blood 56: 361–367
Rich D, Falk P M, Stiehm E R, Feigh S, Golde D W, Cline M J 1977 Pediatrics 59: 396–400
Singer J W, Fialkow P J, Dow L W, Ernest C, Steinmann L 1979 Blood 54: 1395–1399
Spitzer G, Verma D S, Dicke K A, Smith T, McCredie K 1978 Leukemia Research 3: 29–39
Spitzer G, Dicke K A, Gehan E A, Smith T, McCredie K B, Borlogie B, Freireich E J 1976 Blood 48: 794–807
Stanley E R, Hansen G, Woodcock J, Metcalf D 1975 Fed Proc 34: 2272–2278
Steinmann G, Broxmeyer H E, deHarven E, Moore M A S 1981 Brit J Haematol (in press)
Taetle R, Buick R N, McCulloch E A 1980 Blood 56: 549–552
Vainchenker W, Guichard J, Breton-Gorius J 1979a Blood Cells 5: 25–42
Vainchenker W, Bouguet J, Guichard J, Breton-Gorius J 1979b Blood 54: 940–945
Verma D S, Spitzer G, Dickie K A, McCredie K B 1978 Leukemia Research 3: 41–49
Verma D S, Spitzer G, Gutterman J U, Zander A R, McCredie K B, Dicke K A 1979 Blood 54: 1423–1427
Vincent P C, Sutherland R, Bradley M, Lind D, Gunz F W 1977 Blood 49: 903–912
Winchester R J, Meyers P A, Broxmeyer H E, Wang C Y, Moore M A S, Kunkel H G 1978 J Exp Med 148: 613–608
Winchester R J, Ross G D, Jarowski C I, Wang C Y, Halper J, Broxmeyer H E 1977 Proc Natl Acad Sci USA 74: 4012–4017
Wu A M 1979 J Cell Physiol 101: 237–242

7. Bone marrow transplantation

C D Buckner   R A Clift   A Fefer   J D Meyers
K M Sullivan   R Storb   P Weiden   R P Witherspoon
E D Thomas

INTRODUCTION

In a previous volume of Recent Advances in Haematology the subject of marrow transplantation was reviewed (Thomas et al, 1977a). This review will concentrate on the clinical advances that have occurred since 1976 in marrow transplantation for hematologic disease exclusive of the immunodeficiency states.

ADVANCES IN LABORATORY STUDIES

The treatment of acute graft-versus-host disease (GVHD) with steroids or antithymocyte globulin (ATG) is unsatisfactory and new approaches in preventing or treating GVHD must be sought. Recently a new immunosuppressive agent with unique properties, cyclosporin A, has been evaluated. Cyclosporin A suppresses plaque formation in gel, hemagglutinin titers, skin reactivity to oxyzolone and lymphocyte-mediated cytolysis and prevents lymphocyte blastogenesis to various mitogens in different species including man (Thomas et al, 1980). The survival of allografts of hearts in rats and pigs and of kidneys in rabbits, dogs and man can be prolonged with cyclosporin A. Amelioration or prevention of GVHD was observed in histoincompatible mice and rats. The data in rats suggest that the emergence of suppressor cells maintains a stable chimeric state (Tutschka et al, 1979).

We found cyclosporin A to be a very powerful immunosuppressant in the dog, prolonging first and second set skin graft survival and suppressing various in vitro immune functions. However, immunosuppression depended on the continued presence of the drug. Preliminary studies of marrow transplants in mismatched dogs are encouraging, but data showing long-term tolerance is not yet available (Deeg et al, 1980).

Recent interest has also focused on in vitro manipulations of marrow in an attempt to eliminate immune competent cells while retaining viable hematopoietic stem cells. One approach has involved physical separation using albumin gradient techniques (Dicke & van Bekkum, 1971). Another approach was the incubation of marrow with ATG that had been specifically absorbed to remove toxicity to hematopoietic stem cells. Promising results were obtained in murine and canine systems (Korngold & Sprent, 1978; Kolb et al, 1979). The recent availability of monoclonal antibodies that react with subsets of human T cells may provide a way to improve in vitro treatment of marrow.

Interesting results have been obtained in mice and rats with the use of total lymphoid irradiation in a manner analogous to total nodal irradiation for the treatment of Hodgkin's disease (Slavin et al, 1978). Approximately 30 per cent of mice so treated and infused with H2-incompatible hemopoietic cells became long-term chimeras and tolerated skin grafts from marrow donors. The results in dogs are not yet convincing in respect to the establishment of permanent chimerism and tolerance of grafts across a major histocompatibility barrier. Major problems with this approach appear to be rejection of marrow in animals that have received prior transfusions and the length of time for administration of the irradiation.

MARROW TRANSPLANTATION PROCEDURE

Patients with aplastic anemia are given cyclophosphamide (CY) on each of four successive days followed in 36 hours by marrow infusion. Patients with acute leukemia are given CY 60 mg/kg on each of two successive days followed in 3 to 4 days by 1000 rad of total body irradiation (TBI) and immediate marrow infusion. Other regimens have been explored (Santos et al, 1976; Storb et al, 1976; Kim et al, 1977; UCLA Bone-Marrow Transplantation Team, 1977; Oliff et al, 1978; Gluckman et al, 1979; Ramsay et al, 1980).

All patients transplanted in Seattle have large diameter right atrial catheters inserted upon admission and receive prophylactic hyperalimentation (Hickman et al, 1979). Although not proven in a controlled study this approach is thought to decrease significantly the morbidity and mortality of marrow transplantation.

OPPORTUNISTIC INFECTION

Opportunistic infections are a serious and common concomitant of marrow transplantation (Winston et al, 1979). Bacterial infections, including those caused by usually innocuous organisms, are more common in the early granulocytopenic period. Viral and protozoal infections occur later, usually after partial or complete hematopoietic reconstitution. Serious viral infections have occurred as late as 1 to 2 years after transplant. Fungal infections occur both early (up to 50 days after transplant) and late (up to 1 year) and are most common in patients with prolonged granulocytopenia. Finally, patients with active chronic GVHD are very susceptible to bacterial infections (Atkinson et al, 1979; Winston et al, 1979).

Infection prophylaxis

Randomized studies of prophylactic granulocyte transfusions and a protective environment (laminar air flow rooms, sterile food, skin decontamination and oral nonabsorbable antibiotics) have shown that both these modalities effectively decrease the acquisition of serious bacterial infection in the early granulocytopenic period (Clift et al, 1978; Buckner et al, 1978b). The impact of these prophylactic measures on overall survival is more difficult to ascertain as the major causes of death (graft rejection, GVHD, leukemia and interstitial pneumonitis) are not affected by either approach. The prophylactic efficacy of oral or parenteral systemic antibiotics has not been evaluated.

Interstitial pneumonia (IP)

IP due to viruses, protozoa or other unknown ('idiopathic' IP) agents continues to take its toll after allogeneic marrow transplant. The relationship between pretransplant treatment regimens, the immunodeficiency of GVHD and its therapy and IP is not understood.

A review of 525 allogeneic marrow transplant recipients showed a 41 per cent incidence (215 cases) of various forms of nonbacterial pneumonia. Cytomegalovirus (CMV) was the most frequent (85 patients) followed by idiopathic (63 patients) and *Pneumocystis carinii* (34 patients). The incidence of IP was higher in patients with leukemia (48 per cent) than in patients with aplastic anemia (27 per cent).

In our past experience 50 per cent of patients with pure *P. carinii* infection and all patients with mixed infections died despite appropriate treatment. Trimethoprim-sulfamethoxazole is now given as soon as the patient develops 500/mm³ circulating granulocytes and is continued for at least the first 120 days after transplant. Preliminary analysis suggests this may be effective in preventing IP due to *P. carinii*.

CMV infection has been associated with syndromes that include fever, hepatitis, arthritis and leukopenia in addition to fatal dissemination (Meyers & Thomas, 1980). Prophylaxis with adenine arabinoside was unsuccessful as was a therapeutic trial of human leukocyte interferon (Meyers & Thomas, 1980). Prophylactic trials of human leukocyte interferon, of a hyperimmune globulin against CMV and of blood product support exclusively from seronegative donors are presently underway, as is a treatment trial with the combination of human leukocyte interferon and adenine arabinoside for CMV pneumonia.

The etiology and treatment of idiopathic IP remain elusive. Small groups of patients have been examined for evidence of infection with mycoplasma, chlamydia, *P. carinii*, *Legionella pneumophila* and other atypical legionella-like organisms as well as more commonly diagnosed infectious agents, to no avail.

Virus infection

In addition to CMV, infections with herpes simplex virus (HSV) and varicella-zoster virus (VZV) occur in about half of all allogeneic marrow transplant patients. Though most infections are self-limited, 12 patients have died with HSV pneumonia and eight with VZV pneumonia. Infection with VZV is most common within the first year after transplant (median onset 5 months) though cases may occur up to 3 to 4 years after transplant (Atkinson et al, 1980). Most HSV infections occur in the first month after transplant. Our results using adenine arabinoside for the treatment of HSV and VZV infection have been inconsistent, and effective treatment of these infections awaits the development and testing of new antiviral drugs such as acycloguanosine. Preliminary results with this drug in immunosuppressed patients with herpes infections seem promising (Selby et al, 1979).

RESULTS OF MARROW TRANSPLANTATION

Treatment of aplastic anemia

The rationale for treating aplastic anemia by marrow transplantation is the assumption that the disease usually involves hematopoietic stem cell failure. The criteria for severe marrow aplasia warranting treatment by transplantation are a hypoplastic marrow with at least two of the following parameters: granulocyte count less than 500/mm³, platelet count less than 20 000/mm³, and reticulocyte count (corrected) less than 1 per cent in the presence of anemia.

Syngeneic transplants

Aplastic anemia can often be totally corrected by simple marrow infusion from a normal genetically identical twin without any immunosuppressive therapy. A recent review (Appelbaum et al, 1980) of 15 patients with aplastic anemia transplanted with identical twin marrow showed recovery with marrow infusion alone in nine patients and no significant response in three patients. In three patients marrow infusion alone was not successful but recovery occurred after immunosuppression with CY followed by marrow infusion.

Allogeneic grafts from HLA identical siblings

Transplantation of marrow from HLA identical siblings is effective therapy for some patients with severe aplastic anemia (Storb et al, 1976). The Seattle group has carried out 189 allogeneic transplants for aplastic anemia due to a variety of causes. Two of the first four Seattle recipients are now well 9 years after marrow transplantation (Thomas et al, 1972). A prospective cooperative study has shown a significantly better survival for patients undergoing marrow transplantation than for those not transplanted (Camitta et al, 1979). The experience in Seattle before 1975 showed a 46 per cent survival now at 5 to 9 years after transplantation (Storb et al, 1976).

Table 7.1   Identical twin marrow grafts for 34 patients with refractory acute leukemia[a, b]

	No. of patients
Early death	1
Persistent leukemia	9
Complete remission (CR)	24
Relapse	14 (2–16 months; median = 5)
Death in CR	2[c]
Alive in CR	8 (>25, >27, >66, >70, >84, >85, >98, >99 months)

[a] Includes 18 cases of ALL and 16 of ANL.
[b] All received CY, 1000 rad TBI and marrow. Some received additional chemotherapy before CY and/or immunotherapy after transplantation.
[c] Hepatitis at 1 month, interstitial pneumonitis at 4 months.

A problem associated with a high mortality was marrow graft rejection occurring in 25 to 60 per cent of transplant recipients. An analysis of the data from 73 patients showed that positive in vitro tests of cell-mediated immunity against donor cells and a low number of marrow cells infused (less than 3×10^8 cells/kg body weight) were strongly associated with graft rejection (Storb et al, 1977). Most of the 73 patients had been previously transfused, and it was not possible to tell whether the in vitro immune reactivity of recipient against donor was an expression of the underlying disease mechanism or of sensitization to non HLA transplantation antigens induced by blood transfusions. Studies in dogs strongly supported the view that transfusion induced sensitization was the major cause of marrow graft rejection. More than 30 untransfused patients (Storb et al, 1980) have been transplanted with graft failure occurring in only 10 per cent. We conclude that the immunologic mechanisms involved in graft rejection are predominantly induced by blood transfusions and are usually not a manifestation of a pathogenetic mechanism of aplastic anemia.

More intensive immunosuppressive therapy has been given to prevent rejection.

Procarbazine and ATG administered before the standard CY regimen did not alter graft rejection (Storb et al, 1976). TBI, 1000 rad, combined with CY or procarbazine and ATG was successful in preventing rejection but survival was poor because of increased mortality from IP and GVHD related causes.

The transplant group at UCLA has used CY followed by 300 rad TBI (R. P. Gale, personal communication). Although the rejection rate has declined, survival in their patients is projected to be 41 per cent. Gluckman et al (1979) and Santos et al (personal communication) have used CY followed by 800 rad TBI with shielding of the lung to 400 rad in an attempt to reduce IP. Although the rejection rate was low, survival was not apparently improved. The Minneapolis group has explored the use of CY followed by a one day exposure to 750 rad of total nodal irradiation. Nine previously transfused pediatric patients were transplanted (Ramsay et al, 1980). No patient suffered graft rejection and seven of the nine patients are alive.

Another approach to overcome rejection is the infusion of donor peripheral blood mononuclear cells following marrow infusion. The need for more donor cells was suggested by the observation that the larger the dose of marrow cells the less the likelihood of graft rejection (Storb et al, 1977). Peripheral blood mononuclear cells could serve as an added source of pluripotent hemopoietic stem cells and/or lymphoid cells that could enhance engraftment. Pluripotent hemopoietic stem cells have been shown to circulate in the blood of mice, guinea-pigs, dogs and baboons, and, although evidence for pluripotent stem cells in man is missing, studies have shown the presence of circulating committed hematopoietic stem cells. Peripheral blood and thoracic duct lymphoid cells have been shown to enhance allogeneic engraftment in mice and dogs and to increase erythropoiesis in vitro in dogs and man. Initial studies were carried out in patients who, on the basis of in vitro test results of sensitization, were thought to be at high risk for graft rejection. Buffy coat collections were given for 3 to 5 days after marrow infusion. Thirteen of 16 such sensitized patients given only marrow rejected the graft while only three of 23 subsequent patients given marrow plus peripheral blood leukocytes rejected. Survival in the two groups was 25 and 71 per cent respectively. In agreement with previous studies in dogs, the addition of buffy coat did not appear to increase the incidence or severity of GVHD. This approach is currently utilized in all patients who have received blood product transfusions and the overall rejection rate is currently 16 per cent.

In summary, survival among the most recent patients with severe aplastic anemia transplanted in Seattle has increased to 75 per cent compared to 46 per cent before 1975. The reasons for this improvement are the reduction in marrow graft rejection and a decrease in the mortality from acute GVHD.

TREATMENT OF LEUKEMIA

Syngeneic transplants in patients with leukemia

Twin marrow transplantation preceded by CY and TBI has been used to treat endstage leukemia refractory to conventional chemotherapy. The results obtained with a small series of patients were extremely encouraging, with some of the patients remaining in complete unmaintained remission (CR) beyond 5 years (Fefer et al, 1977). The morbidity was tolerable, non-leukemic mortality rare, but the incidence of recurrent leukemia was high. Additional chemotherapy given shortly before CY and

TBI did not decrease the relapse frequency but increased the morbidity and non-leukemic mortality in older patients. An attempt to evaluate immunotherapy after marrow transplantation, in the form of normal twin buffy coat transfusions and injections of killed autologous leukemia cells, was unsuccessful due to the heterogeneity of the patient population. However dramatic differences were not observed between those receiving and not receiving immunotherapy. The results of twin marrow transplantation for refractory acute leukemia are summarized in Table 7.1.

Twin marrow transplantation has also been used to treat chronic granulocytic leukemia (CGL) (Fefer et al, 1979). Remissions can consistently be achieved in patients in blast crisis but relapse usually occurs. Of seven patients transplanted in blast crisis, only one remains in CR at 51 months. Four patients have been transplanted during the chronic phase of CGL with disappearance of all Ph[1]-positive cells (Fefer et al, 1979). One patient relapsed cytogenetically and hematologically and is back into stable CGL 30 months after transplantation, while the others remain cytogenetically, hematologically and clinically well at 37, 40 and 46 months after transplantation. Every patient with CGL who has a normal genetically identical twin should undergo marrow transplantation before blast crisis has occurred.

Since the longest survivor of twin marrow transplantation for hematologic malignancy (more than 116 months) had refractory lymphoma, twin marrow transplantation in lymphomas and other hematologic malignancies should be performed, preferably early before resistance occurs. All patients with a hematological malignancy who have an identical twin should be referred to a transplant center early in their disease course for consideration of transplantation.

Allogeneic transplants for acute leukemia
In a previous issue of Advances in Haematology we reviewed the results of 100 consecutive patients with refractory acute leukemia treated with chemotherapy, TBI and marrow from an HLA identical sibling (Thomas et al, 1977a; 1977b). All patients have now been followed for more than 4 years (Stewart et al, 1979). At the time of the original report four of the 17 surviving patients had relapsed. Three of these four patients have died of their disease and one patient with a solitary testicular relapse remains in CR 62 months after local irradiation without concomitant systemic therapy. One patient died 26 months following transplantation from cardiopulmonary complications following multiple respiratory infections. One patient, who was transplanted despite daunomycin induced cardiomyopathy, died $4\frac{1}{2}$ years after transplantation of congestive heart failure. Of the 12 surviving patients, three suffer from chronic GVHD and nine are living normal lives 51 to 95 months after transplantation.

Analysis of the data from these 100 patients suggested that 70 per cent would have died of leukemia if they had survived transplant complications. We and others have attempted to decrease the relapse rate by developing more intensive treatment regimens. We have added a variety of antileukemic agents to the basic treatment regimen of CY and TBI without decreasing the relapse rate. The UCLA Bone-Marrow Transplantation Team (1977) has reported a decreased relapse rate with a regimen of daunomycin and cytosine arabinoside preceding CY and TBI. However, this regimen is more toxic and ultimate survival is not demonstrably different than with CY and TBI.

Recently we have explored fractionated TBI at doses of 1200 to over 1500 rad given over six or seven days. These regimens have been well tolerated but as yet have made no significant impact on the relapse rate in patients with acute lymphoblastic leukemia (ALL).

Since 1976 we have been conducting a study of transplantation in patients with acute nonlymphoblastic leukemia (ANL) in first remission (Thomas et al, 1979b) and in patients with ALL in second or subsequent remission (Thomas et al, 1979a). Figure 7.1 presents the results of the first 19 patients with ANL transplanted in first remission compared with results in patients transplanted in relapse. The fraction of patients surviving disease free is 65 per cent. The major causes of death are IP and infection related to GVHD. Forty-eight patients have now been entered in this study and relapse of leukemia has occurred in only one patient. These data clearly indicate that the CY + TBI regimen is effective in eradicating leukemia in patients with ANL transplanted in first remission. Efforts are being made to decrease IP and GVHD related deaths without altering the effectiveness of the present antileukemic regimen. The improvement in survival by early transplantation for patients with ANL has now been corroborated (Powles et al, 1980a; Blume et al, 1980).

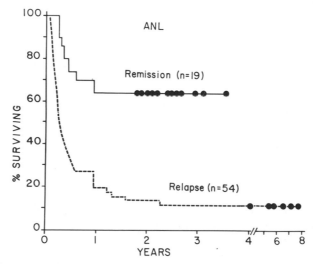

Fig. 7.1 Kaplan-Meier plot of the probability of survival (as of January 1, 1980) of 19 patients with ANL transplanted in first remission and 54 patients transplanted in relapse. The solid circles indicate living patients.

Figure 7.2 shows the survival of patients with ALL transplanted in second or subsequent remission as compared with patients transplanted in relapse. The predominant cause of death in patients transplanted in either remission or relapse is recurrent leukemia and not complications of transplantation. Eleven of 22 patients transplanted in remission and 14 of 26 patients transplanted in relapse developed recurrent leukemia. The relationship of GVHD to leukemia recurrence and survival is discussed below (Weiden et al, 1979b; 1980).

In patients with ALL we are attempting to develop more effective antileukemic regimens. Ongoing studies include an evaluation of increasing doses of fractionated

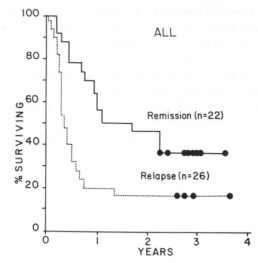

Fig. 7.2   Kaplan-Meier plot of the probability of survival (as of January 1, 1980) of 22 patients with ALL transplanted in second or subsequent remission and 26 patients transplanted in relapse. Solid circles indicate living patients.

TBI, attempts to increase the incidence and severity of GVHD in the hope of manipulating this immunotherapeutic modality, and an evaluation of post-transplant antileukemic therapy beginning with an evaluation of human leukocyte interferon. A study of transplantation in patients with ALL in first remission with poor prognostic features is also being carried out.

Chronic granulocytic leukemia (CGL)
We reported the results of allogeneic marrow transplantation in 14 patients with CGL with blastic transformation or accelerated phase (Doney et al, 1978). Thirteen of these 14 patients died between day 1 and day 194 of transplant complications and one patient achieved a prolonged remission and died on day 492 of recurrent leukemia. Sixteen patients with CGL in various stages of the disease have been transplanted since that report and five are alive and free of disease 4 to 27 months after transplantation.

These data indicate that long-term survival is possible in patients with advanced CGL and the results are probably no worse than for patients transplanted for ANL in relapse (see Fig. 7.1). Whether or not these results can be improved by transplantation in the chronic phase, as has been done with syngeneic transplants, remains to be evaluated.

ALLOGENEIC TRANSPLANTATION AND AGE

The effect of age on post-transplant survival has not been adequately evaluated. There has been a preponderance of children and young adults transplanted and avoidance of transplantation in patients over the age of 50. The median age of all transplant recipients in Seattle is less than 20 years.

We have found that the incidence of GVHD increases with age (Thomas et al,

1980). Camitta et al (1979) found a decreasing survival with increasing age in transplanted patients with aplastic anemia. However the number of patients transplanted in the older age group was very small.

In our transplant series only 11 of 189 patients with aplastic anemia were over the age of 40 and one is a long-term survivor. We have transplanted 20 patients with leukemia over the age of 40 and four are long-term survivors; one of nine with acute leukemia transplanted in relapse, one of six with ANL transplanted in remission and two of five with CGL.

Older patients are probably at greater risk of transplant related complications but more studies are indicated before definitive conclusions about age and survival can be made.

RECOVERY OF IMMUNOLOGICAL FUNCTION

We have reported a study of immune function in 56 long-term survivors after marrow transplantation from HLA identical siblings (Noel et al, 1978). All patients had pronounced impairment of immunologic parameters during the first 4 months. The tempo and pattern of immunologic reconstitution was different in patients with and without GVHD. Quantitative and qualitative antibody responses to neoantigens returned to normal within the first year in patients without GVHD. Patients with chronic GVHD continued to show deficient antibody responses and had an inability to switch from gamma M to gamma G antibody production after repeated challenge. Similarly, patients without GVHD showed return of positive skin test responsiveness while patients with chronic GVHD usually showed absent skin test reactivity. Polyclonal IgG levels in the serum were significantly higher in patients with chronic GVHD than in those without GVHD.

One striking finding was that many parameters of immunity rapidly returned to the normal range. Total lymphocyte counts and the absolute number of T and B cells in the peripheral blood were normal by 3 months. Cells involved in natural killing, antibody dependent killing or lectin dependent killing were generally normal by 1 month. Many patients showed good responsiveness in mixed leukocyte culture testing by 1 to 2 months. These findings suggest that the currently used in vitro tests and lymphocyte markers are not good indicators of immunological status after marrow grafting and demonstrate the necessity of developing new in vitro methodology to study these patients.

Acute and chronic graft-versus-host disease (GVHD)

Current studies indicate that GVHD involves a profound immunodysregulation that may result from an imbalance of regulatory subsets of T lymphocytes (Reinherz et al, 1979; Tsoi et al, 1979). Both an acute and chronic form of GVHD are recognized. Clinical acute GVHD is manifested by abnormalities of the skin, liver and gut. Several prospective studies of the skin (Sale et al, 1977), liver (Sale et al, 1978) and gut (Sale et al, 1979) have helped define the histologic criteria for the diagnosis of GVHD. Such refinements have helped to distinguish GVHD injury from the effects of chemotherapy, irradiation and infection.

Almost every transplant center has employed post-grafting methotrexate (MTX) to prevent or modify acute GVHD (Thomas et al, 1977a). In a recent randomized study the prophylactic administration of horse ATG did not decrease the incidence or severity of GVHD (Weiden et al, 1979a). Powles et al (1980b) have given cyclosporin A to 23 patients and has reported a reduction in GVHD.

Treatment of established acute GVHD remains unsatisfactory. Patients were recently randomized to receive therapy with either corticosteroids or ATG (Weiden et al, 1978). While reduction in disease severity was seen with either therapy, overall results were discouraging as many patients died and one-fourth went on to develop chronic GVHD. Our current approach is to treat acute GVHD with prednisolone and if no response is obtained, therapy is changed to horse ATG for 10 to 20 days. Skin and liver GVHD appear to respond more frequently than gut disease to such therapy. Prolonged periods of gut rest, vigorous parenteral hyperalimentation and close attention to infectious complications are required in the care of such patients.

Over the last decade a curious decrease in the incidence, severity and mortality of acute GVHD has been noted in Seattle. The cause of this is unknown but it may represent earlier transplantation, improvements in supportive care, especially therapeutic and prophylactic parenteral nutrition and a refinement of the diagnostic criteria for GVHD.

In the last 5 years chronic GVHD has been recognized as a major complication of allogeneic marrow transplantation, affecting approximately 25 to 30 per cent of patients surviving 180 days (Lawley et al, 1977; Shulman et al, 1980; Graze & Gale, 1979; Sullivan et al, 1980). Some patients with acute GVHD progress to the chronic phase and some have de novo presentation without evidence of prior acute GVHD (Shulman et al, 1980). Increasing patient age and increasing severity of acute GVHD are associated with a greater likelihood of developing chronic GVHD.

Clinical manifestations of this pleiotropic syndrome resemble the autoimmune diseases. Chronic disease occurs 100 to 300 days after transplant, may persist for years if untreated and affects different target organs than acute GVHD (oral mucosa, lacrimal glands, oesophagus, serosal membranes and muscles). Skin involvement is an almost universal feature. Initial lesions include malar erythema, mottled dyspigmentation, papulosquamous eruptions and desquamation. In untreated patients the disease progresses to dermal induration, ulceration, wasting, scleroderma and joint contracture. Liver function is frequently abnormal and biopsies show a variety of lesions including severe cholestasis with small bile duct proliferation and/or hepatocellular injury with lobular, chronic persistent or chronic aggressive hepatitis (Shulman et al, 1980). Ocular and oral sicca are commonly observed as are oral mucositis, ulceration and striae. Additional clinical features of chronic GVHD include esophagitis with web formation, polymyositis, enteritis and serositis. Antinuclear, antimitochondrial and antismooth muscle antibodies, rheumatoid factor, direct Coombs' reactivity and eosinophilia are detected. Polyclonal hypergammaglobulinemia may be seen but complement levels are normal (Shulman et al, 1980). Direct immunofluorescent studies of skin biopsies reveal deposits of IgM and C'3 along the dermal-epidermal junction (Tsoi et al, 1978).

We found a minority of patients with limited disease that involved only the skin and liver. These patients had a favorable disability-free course without treatment (Shulman et al, 1980). In contrast, extensive chronic GVHD featured multiple organ involvement and without treatment less than 20 per cent of these patients survive without major disabilities. Mortality was often the result of recurrent bacterial infections while morbidity resulted from wasting, sicca and joint contractures. We have used the Karnofsky performance score as the best method of grading the severity and impact of disease.

Attempts to treat chronic GVHD with ATG and/or steroids have been unsuccessful (Sullivan et al, 1980). We have treated patients with a combination of prednisone and either procarbazine, cyclophosphamide or azathioprine. The combination of azathioprine and prednisone was found to be most effective and 76 per cent (16/21) of patients so treated survived more than 2 years after transplant with Karnofsky scores more than 70 per cent (Sullivan et al, 1980). Evidence of GVHD obtained by light microscopy or direct immunofluorescence examination of skin biopsies or findings of keratoconjunctivitis sicca are strongly predictive of subsequent clinical development of chronic GVHD (Sullivan et al, 1980). Early detection of this disorder allows immunosuppressive treatment before clinical deterioration or disability. However, therapy is often prolonged and the long-term hazards of such treatment are currently unknown.

GRAFT-VERSUS-TUMOR EFFECT

A major interest in allogeneic marrow transplantation for treatment of acute leukemia is the possibility that the marrow graft might exert an antileukemic effect. Such an effect might be directed against leukemia associated antigens and be effective in recipients of either syngeneic or allogeneic marrow. Allogeneic marrow transplants, however, might in addition convey an antileukemic effect against histocompatibility antigens found on both leukemic and normal cells.

Evidence for the existence of a graft-versus-leukemia effect in human recipients of allogeneic bone marrow grafts has been difficult to obtain because of the high mortality from non-leukemic causes in patients with severe GVHD (Thomas, 1977b). We have observed progressive leukemia in many patients despite the presence of severe GVHD although dramatic regressions of recurrent leukemia have been reported in two marrow graft recipients with GVHD (Odom, 1978). Recently, the possibility of a graft-versus-leukemia effect was examined by analyzing the results of 242 syngeneic and allogeneic marrow transplants performed in Seattle between 1970 and 1977 (Weiden et al, 1979b). The rate of leukemic relapse in allogeneic marrow recipients with moderate to severe acute or chronic GVHD was 40 per cent of the rate of relapse in allogeneic marrow recipients with minimal GVHD or in recipients of syngeneic marrow. The effect was greater and more significant in patients with ALL than in those with ANL and greater in patients transplanted in relapse compared with patients transplanted in remission. The decreased risk of recurrent leukemia in patients with GVHD transplanted between 1970 and 1977, however, did not result in increased survival, since these patients also had an increased risk of dying from nonleukemic causes (Weiden et al, 1979b).

Patients transplanted during 1977 and 1978 had a lower incidence of GVHD and associated mortality compared with earlier experience (Weiden, 1980). Nevertheless, the antileukemic effect associated with GVHD was unchanged. As a result, the actuarial probability of survival at 2 years after allogeneic marrow transplantation for acute leukemia in 1977–1978 was 0.29 in patients with no or mild GVHD and 0.56 in patients with moderate to severe acute or chronic GVHD (Weiden et al, 1980). This improvement in survival in patients with GVHD appears to be significant for patients with ALL, whether transplanted in remission or relapse, and for patients with ANL transplanted in relapse. Whether or not this immunotherapeutic approach can be manipulated to further decrease the rate of relapse after transplantation remains to be explored.

MISMATCHED DONOR-RECIPIENT PAIRS

The majority of patients do not have HLA genotypically identical siblings and are therefore deprived of important therapeutic options which marrow transplantation would make available. This circumstance has stimulated attempts to identify acceptable alternative donor-recipient combinations. We are studying this problem with a series of transplants in which donors and recipients are HLA genotypically identical for only one haplotype and have some well-defined similarity for the other. With two exceptions these have been sibling or parent-offspring combinations. Preliminary results of this study were published after 21 patients were treated (Clift et al, 1979) and by the end of 1979, 39 patients had been transplanted.

Ten recipients had aplastic anemia and only one of these survives. Four patients died after graft rejection, one died on day 20 from infection and four died as a consequence of GVHD. The survivor is now in good health 3 years after transplantation from her mother with whom she was phenotypically HLA identical at the HLA-A, -B and -D loci. These results are disappointing. Marrow transplantation should be considered in the rare circumstance where a HLA phenotypically identical donor can be identified for an untransfused patient with aplastic anemia. It is probably wise to avoid other donor-recipient combinations in this disease until we have more potent immunosuppressive tools to cope with the additional problems presented by histoincompatibility.

Twenty-nine patients were transplanted as part of the therapy of acute leukemia. The outcome must be considered in the context of the stage and type of leukemia

Table 7.2 'Mismatched' transplants. Patients with acute leukemia transplanted before 1980. Outcome as of April 1, 1980

Diagnosis[a]	Transplants	Survivors (days)	Cause of death[b]
ALL relapse	8	1 (>1056)	IP 3 Leukemia 3 GVHD 1
ANL relapse	7	3 (>125, >250, >328)	Leukemia 1 VOD 1 Rejection 1 Hemorrhage 1
CGL (blast crisis)	2	0	IP 1 Leukemia 1
ALL remission	5	3 (>208, >282, >336)	Glioblastoma 1 Rejection 1
ANL remission	7	5 (>238, >269, >297, >471, >851)	IP 1 GVHD 1

[a] ALL = acute lymphoblastic leukemia; ANL = acute nonlymphoblastic leukemia;
  CGL = chronic granulocytic leukemia.
[b] IP = interstitial pneumonia; VOD = veno-occlusive disease; GVHD = graft-versus-host disease

involved and an analysis is presented in Table 7.2. The results present a pattern indistinguishable from that obtained when donors and recipients are HLA genotypically identical siblings. Thus patients transplanted in remission have a much better prospect of survival than those transplanted in relapse and recurrent leukemia is a major problem in patients with ALL but less so in those with ANL. Nine patients were mismatched with their donors in the HLA-D region. One rejected the transplant and all the others developed sustained engraftment. Five did not develop any GVHD, one had moderate and two had severe GVHD. Six of these patients were transplanted in relapse and all died; three of IP, two of recurrent leukemia and one of graft rejection. Of the three HLA-D mismatched patients transplanted in remission one survives in excellent health at day 851, one has moderate chronic GVHD at day 471 and one died of IP. Seven patients with leukemia were transplanted from donors with whom they were phenotypically but not genotypically identical at all identifiable HLA loci. Six of the donors were parents, one a sibling and one was unrelated to the recipient. All patients achieved sustained engraftment. One developed very mild transient GVHD whereas six, including the patient with an unrelated donor, developed no signs or symptoms suggesting GVHD. Two patients (with parent donors) died, one at day 49 of veno-occlusive disease of the liver and the other on day 200 of recurrent leukemia. Five patients survive between day 188 and day 328.

The number of patients is too small to permit a detailed analysis of the effect of mismatching at any one locus. The overall results in leukemia suggest that appropriate patients may derive benefit from marrow transplantation from donors other than HLA genotypically identical siblings.

AUTOLOGOUS MARROW TRANSPLANTATION

The clinical utilization of cryopreserved autologous marrow has been reviewed (Buckner et al, 1980). Techniques for successful cryopreservation of human marrow have been available for a quarter of a century. Despite this there is little data to support its utility in patients with malignant disease. Lack of progress in this area is due to the difficulties of designing therapy which is truly dose limited by marrow toxicity and is at the same time effective for treatment of a specific malignancy. With the exception of TBI most antitumor agents which have marrow toxicity as the limiting toxicity permit only small additional dose increments before the appearance of other limiting organ toxicity. An additional problem is that the hematological malignancies likely to respond to high dose therapy are diseases in which the marrow may be contaminated with malignant cells. Progress will probably not occur until autologous transplantation is performed early as a form of remission consolidation rather than as a desperate last chance effort in patients with resistant disease.

We have given cryopreserved chronic phase CGL marrow following CY and TBI to seven patients with blastic transformation (Buckner et al, 1978a). In this group of patients, two failed to achieve engraftment and died of infection after 29 and 48 days. Three patients had partial marrow recovery and died on days 55, 58 and 94. Two patients achieved prompt and complete engraftment. One died on day 72 with a fungal pneumonitis and one developed recurrent blastic transformation after 4 months. Goldman et al (1978) have produced remissions, most of which were of short duration, in patients with CGL reconstituted after chemoradiotherapy with stored peripheral blood cells collected in the chronic phase.

We and others have been carrying out studies of the use of cryopreserved marrow in patients with acute leukemia in remission. Marrow is cryopreserved when patients are in remission and stored until relapse at which time CY and TBI are given followed by autologous marrow infusion. We have returned marrow and achieved CR's in two such patients. One relapsed on day 59 and died on day 302 and one relapsed on day 34 and died on day 150. Four patients treated by Gorin et al (1979) all achieved CR and three quickly relapsed with their disease. Similarly, of 24 cases treated by Dicke (1979) 12 achieved CR with a median remission of 4 months (range 2 to 14). Herzig et al (1978) treated 11 patients with hematological malignancies refractory to conventional therapy with high dose CY and TBI followed by autologous remission marrow. Complete remissions lasting 3 to 11 months were obtained in all six patients with acute leukemia. These studies in patients with acute leukemia demonstrate that remission marrow is capable of engraftment after cryopreservation and that remissions, usually of short duration, can be achieved.

Failure to achieve long-lasting remissions may be due to the ineffectiveness of the antileukemic regimen administered to patients in relapse or to the infusion of cryopreserved leukemic cells. Results from transplanting normal syngeneic and allogeneic marrow in patients with resistant leukemia are of paramount importance. As mentioned previously 70 per cent of such patients will relapse following transplantation if they do not die of other causes. In order to distinguish between relapse from residual blasts in the patient and relapse from infused cryopreserved blasts the transplant needs to be done in ANL patients in first remission where the CY + TBI regimen usually eradicates residual blasts (Thomas et al, 1979b, Fig. 7.1). A preliminary report of this approach has been published but follow-up periods are too short to determine the relapse rate (Fay et al, 1979). If autologous transplantation in remission, as consolidation therapy, results in a high relapse rate then efforts to remove tumor cells from the marrow will be of interest. Physical separation (Dicke et al, 1979) and in vitro antibody treatment of human marrow have been attempted (Wells et al, 1979) but are not yet of proven value in man.

PERSPECTIVES

Substantial progress in clinical marrow transplantation has been made since the last review (Thomas et al, 1977a). There has been improved understanding of the basic immunobiology of marrow transplantation (Thomas et al, 1980) although this is not reviewed here in detail. The trend of improvement in clinical results should continue over the next several years. Efforts will be made to decrease the relapse rate in patients with ALL and to decrease the transplant related deaths in patients with ANL transplanted in remission. Undoubtedly, the application of marrow transplantation will be made to diseases other than aplastic anemia and acute leukemia. There should be a major interest in transplanting patients with non-malignant hematologic diseases such as sickle cell anemia and thalassemia which have predictably abbreviated survivals. The lymphoid malignancies with poor risk factors will undoubtedly receive a lot of attention. In all situations transplantation will be most effective when utilized early in the disease course. GVHD will receive major attention in order to decrease transplant related morbidity and mortality and to manipulate its immunotherapeutic effect in patients with leukemia. The renewed interest in autologous marrow transplantation and earlier application in various malignant diseases should allow for significant progress in this area.

This investigation was supported by Grant Numbers CA 18029, CA 18579, CA 15704, CA 18221 and CA 18047, awarded by the National Cancer Institute, DHEW.

Dr Fefer is an American Cancer Society Professor of Clinical Oncology. Dr Meyers is the recipient of Grant BMS 310 from the Graduate School Research Fund, University of Washington and Young Investigator Award AI 15689 from the National Institute of Allergy and Infectious Diseases. Drs Sullivan and Witherspoon are supported in part by Junior Faculty Clinical Fellowships from the American Cancer Society. Dr Thomas is a recipient of a Research Career Award AI 02425 from the National Institute of Allergy and Infectious Diseases.

REFERENCES

Appelbaum F R, Fefer A, Cheever M A, Sanders J E, Singer J W, Adamson J W, Mickelson E M, Hansen J A, Greenberg P D, Thomas E D 1980 Blood 55: 1033–1039

Atkinson K, Storb R, Prentice R L, Weiden P L, Witherspoon R P, Sullivan K, Noel D, Thomas E D 1979 Blood 53: 720–731

Atkinson K, Meyers J D, Storb R, Prentice R L, Thomas E D 1980 Transplantation 29: 47–50

Blume K G, Beutler E, Bross K J, Chillar R K, Ellington O B, Fahey J L, Farbstein M J, Forman S J, Schmidt G M, Scott E P, Spruce W E, Turner M A, Wolf J L 1980 New England Journal of Medicine (in press)

Buckner C D, Stewart P, Clift R A, Fefer A, Neiman P E, Singer J, Storb R, Thomas E D 1978a Experimental Hematology 6: 96–109

Buckner C D, Clift R A, Sanders J E, Meyers J D, Counts G W, Farewell V T, Thomas E D and the Seattle Marrow Transplant Team 1978b Annals of Internal Medicine 89: 893–901

Buckner C D, Appelbaum F R, Thomas E D 1980 In: Karow A M, Pegg D E (eds) Organ preservation for transplantation. Marcel Dekker, Inc, New York (in press)

Camitta B M, Thomas E D, Nathan D G, Gale R P, Kopecky K J, Rappeport J M, Santos G, Gordon-Smith E C, Storb R 1979 Blood 53: 504–514

Clift R A, Sanders J E, Thomas E D, Williams B, Buckner C D 1978 New England Journal of Medicine 298: 1052–1057

Clift R A, Hansen J A, Thomas E D, Buckner C D, Sanders J E, Mickelson E M, Storb R, Johnson F L, Singer J W, Goodell B W 1979 Transplantation 28: 235–242

Deeg H J, Storb R, Weiden P L, Graham T, Thomas E D 1980 In: Gale R P, Fox C F (eds) Biology of bone marrow transplantation. Academic Press, New York, pp 281–284

Dicke K A, van Bekkum D W 1971 Transplantation Proceedings 3: 666–668

Dicke K A, Zander A R, Spitzer G, Verma D S, Peters L J, Vellekoop L, Thomson S, Stewart D, Hester J P, McCredie K B 1979 Experimental Hematology 7 (Suppl 5): 170–187

Doney K, Buckner C D, Sale G E, Ramberg R, Boyd C, Thomas E D 1978 Experimental Hematology 6: 738–747

Fay J W, Silberman H R, Moore J O, Noell K T, Huang A T 1979 Experimental Hematology 7 (Suppl 5): 302–308

Fefer A, Buckner C D, Thomas E D, Cheever M A, Clift R A, Glucksberg H, Neiman P E, Storb R 1977 New England Journal of Medicine 297: 146–148

Fefer A, Cheever M A, Thomas E D, Boyd C, Ramberg R, Glucksberg H, Buckner C D, Storb R 1979 New England Journal of Medicine 300: 333–337

Gluckman E, Devergie A, Bussel A, Bernard J 1979 In: Touraine J L (ed) Bone marrow transplantation in Europe. Excerpta Medica, Amsterdam, pp 42–47

Goldman J M, Catovsky D, Galton D A G 1978 Lancet 1: 437–438

Gorin N C, Najman A, Salmon Ch, Muller J Y, Petit J C, David R, Stachowiak J, Hirsch Marie F, Parlier Y, Duhamel G 1979 European Journal of Cancer 15: 1113–1119

Graze P R, Gale R P 1979 American Journal of Medicine 66: 611–620

Herzig G P, Phillips G L, Mill W, NaPombejara C, Bernard S, Wolff S 1978 Blood 52 (Suppl 1): #536 (abstract)

Hickman R O, Buckner C D, Clift R A, Sanders J E, Stewart P, Thomas E D 1979 Surgery, Gynecology and Obstetrics 148: 871–875

Kim T H, Kersey J, Sewchand W, Nesbit M E, Krivit W, Levitt S H 1977 Radiology 122: 523–525

Kolb H J, Rieder I, Rodt H, Netzel B, Grosse-Wilde H, Scholz S, Schaffer E, Kolb H, Thierfelder S 1979 Transplantation 27: 242–245

Korngold R, Sprent J 1978 Journal of Experimental Medicine 148: 1687–1698

Lawley T J, Peck G L, Moutsopoulos H M, Gratwohl A A, Deisseroth A B 1977 Annals of Internal Medicine 87: 707–709

Meyers J D, Thomas E D 1980 In: Young L S, Rubin R H (eds) Clinical approach to infection in the immunocompromised host. Plenum Press, New York, Chapter 15 (in press)

Noel D R, Witherspoon R P, Storb R, Atkinson K, Doney K, Mickelson E M, Ochs H D, Warren R P, Weiden P L, Thomas E D 1978 Blood 51: 1087–1105

Odom L F, August C S, Githens J H, Humbert J R, Morse H, Peakman D, Sharma B, Rusnak S L, Johnson F B 1978 Lancet 2: 537–540

Oliff A, Ramu N-P, Poplack D 1978 Blood 52: 281–284

Powles R L, Palu G, Raghavan D 1980a In: Roath J (ed) Topical reviews of haematology. John Wright & Sons, London, pp 186–219

Powles R L, Clink H M, Spence D, Morgenstern G, Watson J G, Selby P J, Woods M, Barrett A, Jameson B, Sloane J, Lawler S D, Kay H E M, Lawson D, McElwain T J, Alexander P 1980b Lancet 1: 327–329

Ramsay N K C, Kim T, Nesbit M E, Krivit W, Coccia P F, Levitt S H, Woods W G, Kersey J H 1980 Blood 55: 344–346

Reinherz E L, Parkman R, Rappeport J, Rosen F S, Schlossman S F 1979 New England Journal of Medicine 300: 1061–1068

Sale G E, Lerner K G, Barker E A, Shulman H M, Thomas E D 1977 American Journal of Pathology 89: 621–635

Sale G E, Storb R, Kolb H 1978 Transplantation 26: 103–106

Sale G E, Shulman H M, McDonald G B, Thomas E D 1979 American Journal of Surgical Pathology 3: 291–299

Santos G W, Sensenbrenner L L, Anderson P N, Burke P J, Klein D L, Slavin R E, Schacter B, Borgaonkar D S 1976 Transplantation Proceedings 8: 607–610

Selby P J, Jameson B, Watson J G, Morgenstern A, Powles R L, Kay H E M, Thornton R, Clink H M, McElwain T J, Prentice H G, Ross M, Corringham R, Hoffbrand A V, Brigden D 1979 Lancet ii: 1267

Shulman H M, Sullivan K M, Weiden P L, McDonald G B, Striker G E, Sale G E, Hackman R, Tsoi M S, Storb R, Thomas E D 1980 American Journal of Medicine 69: 204–217

Slavin S, Fuks Z, Kaplan H S, Strober S 1978 Journal of Experimental Medicine 147: 963–972

Stewart P S, Buckner C D, Clift R A, Sanders J E, Storb R, Leonard J M, Thomas E D 1979 Experimental Hematology 7: 509–518

Storb R, Thomas E D, Weiden P L, Buckner C D, Clift R A, Fefer A, Fernando L P, Giblett E R, Goodell B W, Johnson F L, Lerner K G, Neiman P E, Sanders J E 1976 Blood 48: 817–841

Storb R, Prentice R L, Thomas E D 1977 New England Journal of Medicine 296: 61–66

Storb R, Thomas E D, Buckner C D, Clift R A, Deeg H J, Fefer A, Goodell B W, Sale G E, Sanders J E, Singer J, Stewart P, Weiden P L 1980 Annals of Internal Medicine 92: 30–36

Sullivan K M, Shulman H M, Weiden P L, Storb R, Tsoi M S, Thomas E D 1980 In: Gale R P, Fox C F (eds) Biology of bone marrow transplantation. Academic Press, New York, pp 69–73

Thomas E D, Buckner C D, Storb R, Neiman P E, Fefer A, Clift R A, Slichter S J, Funk D D, Bryant J I, Lerner K G 1972 Lancet 1: 284–289

Thomas E D, Buckner C D, Clift R A, Fefer A, Neiman P E, Storb R 1977a In: Hoffbrand A V, Brain M C, Hirsch J (eds) Recent advances in haematology. No 2 Churchill Livingstone, Edinburgh, pp 111–125

Thomas E D, Buckner C D, Banaji M, Clift R A, Fefer A, Flournoy N, Goodell B W, Hickman R O, Lerner K G, Neiman P E, Sale G E, Sanders J E, Singer J, Stevens M, Storb R, Weiden P L 1977b Blood 49: 511–533

Thomas E D, Sanders J E, Flournoy N, Johnson F L, Buckner C D, Clift R A, Fefer A, Goodell B W, Storb R, Weiden P L 1979a Blood 54: 468–476

Thomas E D, Buckner C D, Clift R A, Fefer A, Johnson F L, Neiman P E, Sale G E, Sanders J E, Singer J W, Shulman H, Storb R, Weiden P L 1979b New England Journal of Medicine 301: 597–599

Thomas E D, Fefer A, Storb R 1980 In: Mihich E (ed) Immunological aspects of cancer therapeutics. John Wiley & Sons, Inc, New York (in press)

Tsoi M S, Storb R, Jones E, Weiden P L, Shulman H, Witherspoon R, Atkinson K, Thomas E D 1978 Journal of Immunology 120: 1485–1492

Tsoi M S, Storb R, Dobbs S, Kopecky K J, Santos E, Weiden P L, Thomas E D 1979 Journal of Immunology 123: 1970–1976

Tutschka P J, Beschorner W E, Allison A C, Burns W H, Santos G W 1979 Nature 280: 148–151
UCLA Bone-Marrow Transplantation Team 1977 Lancet 2: 1197–1200
Weiden P L, Doney K, Storb R, Thomas E D 1978 Transplantation Proceedings 10: 213–216
Weiden P L, Doney K, Storb R, Thomas E D 1979a Transplantation 27: 227–230
Weiden P L, Flournoy N, Thomas E D, Prentice R, Fefer A, Buckner C D, Storb R 1979b New England
    Journal of Medicine 300: 1068–1073
Weiden P L and the Seattle Marrow Transplant Team 1980 In: Gale R P, Fox C F (eds) Biology of bone
    marrow transplantation. Academic Press, New York, pp 37–48
Wells J R, Billing R, Herzog P, Feig S A, Gale R P, Terasaki P, Cline M J 1979 Experimental Hematology
    7 (Suppl 5): 164–169
Winston D J, Gale R P, Meyer D V, Young L S and the UCLA Bone Marrow Transplantation Group 1979
    Medicine 58: 1–31

8. Acute leukaemia

H E M Kay

AETIOLOGY OF LEUKAEMIA

It is established that leukaemia can be caused by viruses, by radiation or by chemical agents and it is probable that it is often the interaction of these agents — either necessary or effective causes, according to the circumstances — which initiates in the susceptible individual a clone of cells whose growth leads to acute leukaemia.

Recent research into the aetiology of human leukaemia has been of two main kinds. Firstly epidemiological surveys have sought either to link the incidence of each form of the disease to particular antecedent causes, such as chemicals or radiation, or else to identify non-random irregularities — 'clustering' — in the incidence since that might indicate the existence of any causative agent, including an infective virus. Secondly traces of virus in leukaemic cells have been looked for by antigenic or enzymic analysis or by demonstration of nucleic acid homologies.

Epidemiology

Many 'clusters' of leukaemia cases have been reported from time to time — either as an increased number in a short period of time in a large area or as high frequency in a localised area over a longer period of time. These have been claimed as evidence of a common local cause but the significance has often been difficult to determine.

The theory and analysis of case-clustering has received attention from statisticians in recent years in an effort to discover how to distinguish random from nonrandom clusters. The method of Knox (1964) which determines whether there are more patients developing the disease at about the same time and living in close proximity than would be expected by chance is generally used, but its value depends on there being a relatively short and constant incubation period and on a relatively static population; neither of these assumptions can be relied upon. The topic has recently been reviewed by Smith (1978) who concluded that: 'Clustering of cases of leukaemia in space and time has not been consistently observed and the epidemiologic evidence does not strongly suggest an infectious aetiology for this group of diseases.'

Recent increases of leukaemia observed in Lancashire (Birch et al, 1979), in children in Utah who may have received radiation from nuclear bomb fallout (Lyon et al, 1979) and in nuclear shipyard workers (Najarian & Colton, 1978) are of marginal significance. Those exposed to fall-out from the 'Smoky' atom bomb test may show a significant increase in AML and CML incidence (Caldwell et al, 1980).

Radiation

The fact that radiation can be leukaemogenic is not in doubt but the relationship of quality of radiation, of dose, dose-rate, age and other circumstances to the incidence and type of leukaemia have yet to be fully described. Also the mechanism is uncertain:

in radiation leukaemia in the C57BL mouse an essential step is the conversion of provirus to virus which can then induce leukaemia in cells which need not themselves have been irradiated. It is possible that such a step is involved in human radiation-induced leukaemia although virus has not been observed (but see below).

The question of dose, and dose rate and age are much more complex than might be supposed since the two processes of leukaemia-induction and cell sterilisation have counteracting effects and because susceptibility seems to decline sharply with age Thus it is possible to account for the occurrence of leukaemia due to small doses of prenatal radiation by presuming a high susceptibility before birth, the dose being too low to kill significant numbers of cells, whereas a large dose as given in the radiation-treatment of cervical carcinoma yields no excess of leukaemia, presumably because the cell sterilisation effect overcomes the increase in leukaemia-induction (see Mole, 1975). The reduction of X-ray doses for pre-natal diagnostic examination has more or less eliminated one minor cause of childhood leukaemia (and other childhood neoplasms) and the data from other circumstances of irradiation are limited. The excess of leukaemia seen after treatment of Hodgkin's disease and other neoplasms is more closely related to chemotherapy (see below) and the number of radiation accidents is mercifully too low to yield analysable figures. The Japanese survivors of the 1945 bombs ceased to have a significant increase of acute or chronic myeloid leukaemia after about 20 years (Finch, 1979) but the incidence of solid tumours has increased with the lapse of time; whether any increase of CLL (which is rare in the Japanese) will occur remains to be seen.

Chemical carcinogenesis

Benzene has been known as a leukaemogenic agent for many years and still causes some sporadic cases. Small epidemics may occur as has happened among leather workers in Turkey who used benzene as a glue-solvent (Aksoy, 1978). Identification of the cause and its withdrawal has subsequently brought the epidemic to a close. The role of other solvents remains suspect but unproven.

Iatrogenic leukaemia

In medicine, the increasing use of cytotoxic chemotherapy and the consequent prolonged survival of patients with Hodgkin's disease, other lymphomas, myeloma, carcinoma of breast, lung and ovary, and melanoma has resulted in an increasing tally of leukaemias (Harris, 1979; Auclerc et al, 1979). The characteristic type of leukaemia has been AML, often myelomonocytic, sometimes erythroleukaemia and sometimes subacute or even chronic. On epidemiological and experimental evidence alkylating agents and procarbazine can be assumed to be the main culprits and other anti-leukaemic agents, e.g. methotrexate and mercaptopurine, are more or less exonerated. All immunosuppressives, however, e.g. azathioprine, cyclophosphamide, cyclosporin A, especially when used to support a tissue transplant seem to predispose to the induction of lymphomas, the nature and manifestations of which may be unusual (Kinlen et al, 1979). There is a widespread assumption that the immunosuppression acts by permitting the proliferation of cells — perhaps virus-transformed cells — which are otherwise held in check through immunological surveillance, and the demonstration of EB virus antigen in three such tumours supports this idea (Hanto et al, 1980).

Alternatively, lymphomas may arise because of a homeostatic imbalance in the immune system.

Other drugs which are on the list of suspects are the phenylbutazones, widely used as analgesics and probably responsible for some cases of aplasia but not yet reliably indicated as leukaemogens. One piece of circumstantial evidence relating to chemicals in leukaemogenesis concerns chromosome changes. It has been observed that chromosome changes are more frequent and more diverse where drugs or other chemical agents might have been causative (Mitelman et al, 1978), partial or complete deletion of Numbers 5 and 7 being especially common (Rowley, 1980); but in other series (Lawler et al, 1979) this association has not been confirmed and there is a need for further data.

Viral leukaemogenesis

The part played by some RNA viruses — retroviruses — and some DNA (herpes-type) viruses in leukaemia in many animal species has prompted the search for positive evidence in human leukaemia. One strong piece of circumstantial evidence that can be adduced is the recurrence of leukaemia in the donor cells following bone marrow transplantation. Five, possibly six, cases have now been reported (see Elfenbein et al, 1978) and others, where the origin of the recurrence was not looked for or not identifiable, can be assumed. This pattern of events is reminiscent of the leukaemia induced in C57BL mice by radiation, where the radiation is assumed to change provirus to a virus which can then infect and transform unirradiated cells to a leukaemic condition.

Direct evidence for virus in leukaemic cells can be gained from the occasional demonstration of C-type RNA virus particles, from the presence of virus-type reverse transcriptase in leukaemic cells, from virus-induced antigens common to virus-infected cells to other species and from RNA homologies with viruses found in other primates and in some murine leukaemias (see Thiry, 1979). The situation is immensely complex since the evidence points mostly to defective virus or virus components which may become complemented and thus activated by combination with a helper virus. Many of the proven leukaemogenic viruses in animals seem to be hybrids related to natural non-oncogenic viruses from other species. Furthermore, lack of all traces of virus does not eliminate its possible implication. Thus in feline leukaemia which can be proved conclusively to be caused by a virus (FeLV) the signs of virus are very variable. In epidemics horizontal infection can cause a number of syndromes – marrow hypoplasia, immunodeficiency etc. — which may or may not be followed by leukaemia. Virus can then sometimes be found but mostly in cells other than the leukaemic cells, e.g. the nasal mucosa, and in other cases may be inferred from the presence in leukaemic cells of viral antigen, homologous RNA or transcriptase. On the other hand in epidemics due to FeLV, one-third of the leukaemia cases occur in cats where the only evidence of FeLV is the presence of the FOCMA (feline oncorna-virus associated cell membrane antigen) (Francis et al, 1979). It was concluded that 'If the virus-negative feline tumours can be shown to be caused by FeLV they may provide important clues (as to) whether retroviruses might cause virus-negative tumours in man'.

The other main suspect virus for human neoplasms is the EB virus as related to the Burkitt tumour, to nasopharyngeal carcinoma and to post-transplant lymphomas.

Epidemiological surveys show that the pattern of EB infection in Burkitt prone areas is no different from elsewhere in Africa, leading to the supposition that another circumstance, e.g. early malarial infection, is the effective cause although the EB virus may well remain a necessary cause. Cases of acute leukaemia show no consistent pattern in relation to prior infection by EBV nor do they exhibit biochemical or immunological evidence of virus, except in some instances of the rare B-cell acute leukaemia which can resemble morphologically and chromosomally the Burkitt tumour (see Magrath & Ziegler, 1980).

THE CLASSIFICATION OF ACUTE LEUKAEMIA

The instincts in most post-Linnaean scientists to classify their material have found fulfilment among students of leukaemia throughout the century. Recently this quest has been greatly reinforced and diversified by new methods of cell characterisation. Many of the techniques for the analysis of enzymes, antigens and chromosomes are described in Chapters 10 and 11; with further refinements, for example through the use of monoclonal antibodies, these methods may achieve a precision, consistency and, through follow-up studies, a relevance which would enable them to displace the traditional basis of classification by morphology.

Meanwhile, the FAB (Franco-American-British) (Bennett et al, 1976, 1981) group have tried to construct a more consistent system for distinguishing separate types of both acute lymphoblastic and acute myeloid leukaemia (Table 8.1). In ALL, three subdivisions are recognised, of which L3 is both the rarest and the most distinctive; the basophilic vacuolated cytoplasm is a readily recognised feature and this type is, with a few exceptions, correlated with the presence of B-cell properties, especially surface immunoglobulin. The distinction between the relatively uniform, small celled L1 and the more heterogeneous L2 type is, however, much more subjective and less closely correlated, although L2 seems to be commoner in T-ALL, in null ALL and in adults. There are six aspects of the cells which may vary independently — mean size, variation in size, nuclear shape, nuclear chromatin, quantity of cytoplasm and nucleolar prominence. A scoring system has recently been devised (Bennett et al, 1981) but it is arguable whether the weight given to each characteristic is the most appropriate for predictive purposes and the interpretation remains a subjective one. Thus it is not suprising that there is some disagreement about the prognostic importance of cell type in ALL. In most series, however, there is a definable group with small uniform cells (L1 or microlymphoblastic) which have a favourable prognosis (for refs. see Viana et al, 1980). It may be difficult to agree on where the dividing line should be drawn (e.g. 26 per cent group I microlymphoblastic or 60 to 70 per cent L1 in several series of childhood ALL), and it is probable that the prognostic significance of the typing will vary with the particular regime of chemotherapy. Indeed, little purpose is served by such a subjective and unrefined system of classification unless it be to indicate a preferred treatment. The possibility that the difference between L1 and L2 represents a difference in kinetic behaviour which might in turn indicate desirable differences in the type and scheduling of drug regimes, should encourage the search for such correlations. At present, no conclusions have been drawn as to the appropriateness of different regimes for each subtype of ALL, exceppt that L3 B-ALL with a universally poor outlook might be best

Table 8.1 Classification of acute leukaemia

General term	FAB	Distinctive morphology	Additional tests	Type name	Chromosomes
Acute lymphoblastic	L1	Small, uniform with little cytoplasm	c-ALL antigen, TdT, HUTL Ag, Ia Ag, Ac ph'ase, PAS, CIgM	Common ALL / T-cell ALL / Null ALL	Variable / Some Ph' +
	L2	Pleomorphic, larger with cytoplasm + and nucleoli +			
	L3	Vacuolated, basophilic cytoplasm	SIgM	B-ALL	Some 14q+, 8q−
Acute undifferentiated leukaemia	—	Pleomorphic, no positive criteria	c-ALL neg, HUTLA neg, (TdT+), Ia+	Undifferentiated not readily distinguished from null ALL	?
Acute myeloid leukaemia	M1	Minimum evidence of granulopoietic differentiation	Peroxidase or Sudan Black	Myeloblastic	Variable
	M2	Moderate granulopoietic differentiation (Auer bodies)	Peroxidase or Sudan Black	Myelocytic	
	M3	Hyper- or micro-granular promyelocytes		Promyelocytic	Normal or t(15; 17)
	M4	Granulocytic and monocytic differentiation	Non-specific esterase ++ Lysozyme +, Monocytes in blood +	Myelomonocytic	
	M5	Monoblasts and monocytes	Non-specific esterase +++ Lysozyme ++	Monocytic	Variable
	M6	Erythroid precursors incl. dysplastic forms	(PAS + erythroblasts)	Erythro-leukaemia	
	?M7	Atypical often small megakaryocytes	Specific peroxidase Coarse PAS + granules ? Reticulin increase	Megakaryocytic	?

managed through immediate intensive cytoreduction followed by marrow transplantation.

The FAB proposals are on a surer ground in AML; in particular the distinction of Acute Promyelocytic Leukaemia (M3) from other varieties and its correlation with a special tendency to intravascular coagulation and bleeding, to relatively long remission and in several series, to a unique chromosome anomaly, $t(15q+; 17q-)$ is valuable. But the recent description of a microgranular variant of this disease with only a few of the typical promyelocytes present is a warning that expert microscopy is needed for accurate diagnosis (Golomb et al, 1980). Among the other varieties there is the problem of introducing lines of division into a continuum. The distinctions of myeloblastic leukaemia with (M2) or without (M1) conspicuous myeloid differentiation, and of myelomonocytic (M4) and monocytic (M5) types have a general utilitarian value, but as yet lack a precise pathogenetic basis. It is likely that the degree of monocytic or myelocytic differentiation is often related to the disturbance of homeostatic regulators, especially CSA (see below), and the presence of a large erythropoietic element in the leukaemic clone in M6 disease may indicate the retention of susceptibility to erythropoietin stimulation.

To only a limited extent is the morphological type related to the potentiality of the stem cell in which the disease has arisen. Most cases of AML probably arise from multipotential myeloid stem cells but an origin from a more restricted precursor cell may be surmised where it can be shown that the erythroid precursors in the leukaemic marrow do not share the enzymic characteristics of the leukaemic clone (Fialkow et al, 1979).

Another way of classifying AML is by the ability of the cells aspirated from the marrow to grow in agar culture (see Ch. 6). The patterns of growth — as microclusters, macroclusters or microcolonies with excess clusters — presumably reflects the formation and dependence upon regulatory substances, especially CSA. But it also gives some prognostic guidance since the common microcluster growth pattern is associated with a higher rate of remission than are other forms.

As guides to therapy the systems of classification in AML have a long way to travel. The need for heparin treatment when M3 disease is diagnosed is clear enough, but in other respects progress, slow at best, will probably depend upon the demonstration of particular biochemical characteristics as, for example, the association of a response to corticosteroids with the presence of TdT and also, perhaps, with high levels of steroid receptors (see Koeffler et al, 1980; Marks et al, 1978) (see also Preissler, 1980).

One morphological characteristic, the presence of Auer rods, has now been shown to have prognostic significance since in cases with Auer rods the remission rate, 68 per cent and median survival, 13.5 months, are better than in those without, 40 per cent and 6.2 months respectively (Mertelsmann et al, 1980).

FAILURE OF DIFFERENTIATION IN ACUTE LEUKAEMIA

The ability to grow normal and some leukaemic haemopoietic cells in culture and the discovery of factors which govern haemopoiesis has led to some progress in unravelling the pathogenesis of leukaemia. Short-term growth in agar culture can be accomplished for most cases of AML and for some ALLs (see Ch. 6 and Smith et al, 1978; McCulloch, 1979) but since it is only a short-term culture it may only tell us about the differentiating cells and not the true stem cells of the clone. Long-term liquid culture on the other hand is only rarely achieved and its very rarity may indicate that the cell lines derived are not typical of leukaemia as a whole.

Failure to differentiate is a classical characteristic of the cells of acute leukaemia; such failure may be relatively slight as in M2 AML for example and in all cases of acute leukaemia, a thorough dissection, biochemical and antigenic, will show some signs of lymphoid or myeloid differentiation (see Ch. 10) although this is always incomplete. In some circumstances it seems that the block to differentiation can be partly overcome. Compounds such as dimethyl sulphoxide or sodium butyrate are powerful inducers of erythrocytic or granulocytic differentiation by leukaemic cells in culture (see Gallagher et al, 1979) but some variation in the propensity to differentiate occurs with the more physiological agents, such as corticosteroids (Tsiftsoglou et al, 1979) and the known regulators of haemopoiesis — CSF, lactoferrin etc. (see Ch. 6). The possibility that remission may be the result of induced differentiation of the leukaemetic clone is suggested by rare cases where there is both morphological and cytogenic evidence of such a change (Craddock et al, 1975), but remission in acute leukaemia is generally due to the replacement of the leukaemic clone by a cytogenetically normal clone of cells.

The influence of some of the regulatory factors in some forms of leukaemia has now been partly elucidated (Adamson, 1979; Eaves & Eaves, 1978; Broxmeyer et al, 1979).

Erythropoietin (EPO)
Erythropoietin which is derived mainly from the kidney, affects the late stages of erythropoiesis. In crythroleukaemia the leukaemic cells appear to retain a normal sensitivity to EPO since hypertransfusion can virtually abolish the erythroid differentiation. In polycythaemia vera, by contrast, there appears to be an excessive sensitivity, both of late and early erythropoietic cells, to very small quantities of EPO, as shown by in vitro cultures using EPO-antiserum. Sensitivity of leukaemic cells to the burst promoting activity (BPA) factor which influences predominantly the early stages of erythropoiesis has not yet been worked out.

Colony-stimulating factors (CSF) or activity (CSA)
A factor (or factors) derived from monocytes or other tissues is required for normal granulopoiesis. As might be expected, their formation may be increased in monocytic leukaemias. In some cases of AML, there may be a qualitative difference from normal CSF and in others there is partial failure of the leukaemic cells to respond. The existence of these related factors leads to a highly complex interaction of normal differentiating and leukaemic cells.

Lactoferrin
Saturated lactoferrin formed by granulocytes, inhibits the formation of CSF by monocytes. There appears to be reduced formation in CGL and in some cases of AML; it is probable that leukaemic monocytes fail to respond to this normal inhibitor.

Leukaemic-associated inhibitory activity (LIA)
The presence in AML cells of a substance which inhibits normal haemopoietic cells

appears to supply the mechanism whereby the leukaemia clone is able to supplant normal haemopoietic cells. However, it is present not only in AML bone marrow in relapse, but also in remission, so it is uncertain whether it is a product of the AML cells themselves or whether they are able to proliferate because they (and also normal remission cells) have acquired a resistance to its activity.

Other factors
It is probable that many other factors will be discovered which control the rate of proliferation and differentiation at the various stages of haemopoiesis. The interaction of these factors derived from normal and leukaemic clones (perhaps also from different leukaemic subclones) will lead to a great variety of homeostatic imbalances in acute and chronic leukaemias which will be difficult to unravel. Even in the apparently simple case of polycythaemia vera, where an excessive sensitivity to erythropoietin can explain the major abnormality in the disease, the customary hyperplasia of granulopoiesis and thrombocytopoiesis is not accounted for.

In lymphoblastic leukaemias, the discovery of factors for T-cell and B-cell maturation may eventually be worked into the account of pathogenesis. At present, all that is known is that thymic extracts may induce T-cell properties in the cells of 'null' (i.e. c-ALL) ALL (Pasmino et al, 1977) and that there may be an inhibitor of thymic hormone in the serum in ALL (Twomey et al, 1980).

TREATMENT OF ACUTE LEUKAEMIA

General considerations
In the last decade a substantial improvement in the number of long-term remissions in childhood ALL has been accompanied by small but significant improvements in ALL in adults and in AML at all ages. Although these advances have been well-documented through the clinical trials of the main cooperative groups and large centres, the greater precision of classification of disease which is now possible (see p. 164) means that future trials must be evaluated on a different basis. Small differences, which might have been attributable to random heterogeneity between the groups of cases being compared, may, in future, more reliably be ascribed to differences in the treatment if care has been taken to ensure comparability of the groups.

In ALL, the prognostic factors which have been found to be important are as follows (scoring for adversity) (Miller et al, 1980):

1. *Blood leucocyte count*. The prognosis is inversely related to the initial count (mainly, of course, of blast cells) all the way from 5 to more than 500×10^9 per litre.

2. *CNS disease at onset*. Although rare, the presence of symptoms or signs of CNS leukaemia at first diagnosis, is almost always a fatal sign, although other obscure neurological episodes may be associated with a good final outcome (Kay, 1979).

3. *Cell morphology* (see Viana et al, 1980). The standard morphology of the leukaemic Romanovsky-stained blasts may be related to remission duration. Microlymphoblasts, cells less than 12 μm across, or uniform (L1) blasts, seem to give the best prognosis in

some series, but not in all. Similarly, PAS-positivity has been a good prognostic indicator in some series. This may be because the criteria for classification are somewhat subjective and arbitrary or possibly because some regimes do make a distinction between varieties of disease whereas others do not. In any case, it would be important to determine what is the basis of the morphological distinction; it might be the proportion of cells in cell cycle or the concordance of pleomorphism with biochemical diversity and hence liability to drug resistance.

4. *Cell phenotype* (Greaves et al, 1981). It is not yet clear to what extent the antigenic and enzyme properties affect prognosis independently of other variables. Most T-cell and many null-cell cases have high leucocyte counts; the prognosis in both these groups is certainly worse than for c-ALL and in some series it seems that, even at equivalent leucocyte counts, the outcome is poorer in T-ALL than in c-ALL. The prognosis in B-ALL is universally poor but the pre-B phenotype is not prognostically different from other c-ALL cases.

5. *Sex*. Males tend to do worse than females, partly because there is at all ages a higher proportion of high count cases among males, especially T-ALL, partly because of the chance of testicular relapse, and perhaps for other reasons.

6. *Karyotype*. Insufficient studies have been published to determine the effect of chromosome abnormalities except that the presence of Ph' anomaly (present in 1 to 2 per cent of childhood ALL and in about 30 per cent of adult ALL) is correlated with a high relapse rate. Preliminary observations suggest that hyperdiploidy may be a favourable factor; pseudodiploidy (Secker-Walker et al, 1978) and chromosome translocations (Bloomfield et al, 1981) seem to be adverse factors.

7. *Serum immunoglobulins*. A low serum immunoglobulin at onset is associated with a poor prognosis partly because of a lower remission rate, partly because of early relapse.

Many other variables have been analysed for their relation to outcome and further analytic studies will be needed. Even a simple variable, such as age, may be difficult to evaluate because although the prognosis deteriorates with increasing age, that may be accounted for in some degree by the higher leucocyte count, male predominance and Ph' + proportion. Also each analysis will be valid for the treatment given and not necessarily for other treatments.

Treatment of ALL (Mauer, 1980)

Remission induction

Clinical remissions have been achieved in such a high proportion of cases that only marginal benefits could have been expected from the addition of other agents to the standard combination of vincristine plus prednisolone. In c-ALL the rate of remission with the two agents is nearly 100 per cent, failures being most often due to infection or haemorrhage, especially in adults over the age of 40, but with T-ALL, B-ALL and null types of disease, the rate of remission is lower. The addition of an anthracycline or asparaginase or perhaps other agents increases this rate, but further detailed series are needed to establish optimal regimes for the minority subtypes of ALL.

Perhaps of greater importance is the effect that the induction regime and the subsequent consolidation treatment have on the final rate of sustained remission. Data from ALGB (Jones et al, 1977) suggest that omission of asparaginase decreases the number of long-term remissions and at St Jude, the regime with the poorest long-term remission rate (Total VII) was the only regime without an additional agent (e.g. asparaginase or daunorubicin) or a period of intensification immediately after remission was obtained (Simone, 1976). Similarly, in the MRC UKALL trials, the proportion of long-term remissions — in boys at least — was highest in UKALL I which included a 28-day period of asparaginase in contrast to later 8-day courses (Kay, 1977). Recent regimes of the CCSG include a 3-week course of asparaginase and this may in part account for their good results, while smaller studies showing excellent prolonged remission rates have been reported from Boston (Sallan et al, 1980) and from Berlin. The latter has an exceptionally intensive early treatment and even those with adverse features (high leucocyte counts, etc.) have a more than 50 per cent probability of long-sustained remission (Riehm, 1980).

The number of variables of treatment and classification in all these studies and trials as well as the variable length of follow-up makes it extremely difficult to make valid comparisons and to reach firm conclusions. At present, however, there seem to be no adequate data to deny the need for an intensive early treatment in which high or prolonged dosage with asparaginase and perhaps the inclusion of an anthracycline drug are valuable.

'Intensification' of the early treatment in ALL will undoubtedly lead to a few serious infections and fatalities, but clearly there is now a strong case for the maximum tolerable addition of good remission-induction agents. What these should be and how they should be scheduled has yet to be fully determined. It may be hoped that the same regime which increases the number of long-term remissions in c-ALL will also be of greatest value in treating the other varieties of ALL.

CNS prophylaxis

Since the introduction of cranial irradiation at St Jude, it has been generally agreed that some sort of prophylaxis against the development of overt CNS leukaemia is needed, both in children and adults (Omura et al, 1980). However, it should be noted that the benefit in terms of survival is not as great as might have been expected since where CNS disease has been prevented, marrow relapse becomes more likely and it is probable that energetic treatment of CNS-leukaemia when it is manifest can sometimes be successful.

The best form of CNS prophylaxis is still quite undecided and is not likely to be determined in the near future owing to the number of variables and the length of time needed to assess the results — including the long-term neurotoxicity and perhaps the oncogenicity of irradiation. Variables which are not always considered in evaluation are the effect of steroids and asparaginase which may have profound effects according to their dosage and schedule. Although asparaginase is scarcely detectable in the CSF, the fluid is rendered asparagine-free and this must have a powerful inhibitory effect which might be related to the dose and length of asparaginase treatment. In this situation, moreover, there may be an antagonistic effect between asparaginase and methotrexate.

A widely used regime of 2400 r cranial radiation plus five intrathecal doses of methotrexate forms a useful basis for comparison of other regimes. It is effective as a prophylaxis in over 90 per cent of cases, but carries a perceptible risk of cerebral damage. Price has described two main types of lesion, a demyelinating encephalo-pathy and mineralising angiitis, see Table 8.2 (Price & Jamieson, 1975; Price & Birdwell, 1978). Mild or moderate intellectual defects, notably difficulty with arithmetic, are not uncommon in children who have received maximal prophylaxis, especially if that has included appreciable doses of intrathecal or intramuscular methotrexate after 2400 r cranial irradiation (Eiser, 1979). The impairment of learning is most severe when the prophylaxis has been at the age of one to three. Evidence of cerebral damage can also be seen in CT scans in the form of ventricular dilation and sometimes cortical atrophy (for references see Green et al, 1980), while intracranial calcification is common where much methotrexate has been given parenterally.

The effects on the endocrine system, probably mediated via the hypothalamus and pituitary, include a retardation of growth but these are mild and reversible (Shalet & Beardwell, 1979; Swift et al, 1979).

A lower dose of 1800 r cranial irradiation is now widely used, both in the CCSG and elsewhere. Initial results (Nesbit, 1980) suggest that it is not significantly less effective than 2400 r and may be associated with fewer bone marrow relapses as well as with less neurotoxicity. However, the type of disease is an important variable and more intensive CNS prophylaxis may be needed for high count T-cell cases where CNS involvement is especially frequent and is manifest earlier. To forestall this complica-tion, treatment at the Memorial Hospital includes the insertion of an Ommaya reservoir so that adequate concentrations of methotrexate throughout the CSF can be ensured. An alternative strategy is to give the methotrexate by intravenous infusion (500 mg/m^2) combined with an intrathecal dose by the lumbar route. Neither is entirely successful or free of complications. A recent comparison of radiation versus non-radiation regimes shows that some cranial radiation is needed to prevent CNS leukaemia, but that survival in standard risk disease may in the long run be equally good if methotrexate infusions are given (Green et al, 1980). A totally different strategy is to give 15 fractionated doses of radiation to cranium and spine over a period of three years. This gives an 87 per cent CNS disease-free rate, but three cases out of 76 developed AML which raises the possibility that such a schedule is leukaemogenic (Zuelzer, 1978).

Testicular disease

Another sanctuary site in leukaemia is the testis, perhaps because there is a blood testis barrier (Dym & Fawcett, 1970). Leukaemic infiltration of the testis has been found with increasing frequency in some series, but not in all (MRC, 1978a; Nesbit et al, 1980). Cumulative incidences as high as 25 per cent have been reported (Rosenkrantz et al, 1978; Eden, 1980) and such rates are associated with a higher marrow relapse rate and shorter survival for boys than for girls. It is not entirely clear why this phenomenon has been so capricious. The testis is involved in both T-ALL

Table 8.2 Neurological complications of ALL and its treatment

	Postmeasles encephalitis	Leukaemic infiltration	Leucoencephalopathy	Mineralising angiopathy	Somnolent syndrome
Pathogenesis	Subacute encephalitis: virus inclusions in glial cells and neurones.	Invasion of subarachnoid space from pial vessels.	Demyelination and degeneration of cerebral white matter	Calcific degeneration of cerebral blood vessels. Degeneration of grey matter.	Reversible demyelination of cerebral neurones.
Causation	Measles while on ALL treatment.		Radiation and/or methotrexate.	Methotrexate (? and radiation)	Radiation 6–10 weeks earlier
Manifestations	Convulsions, ataxia, athetosis, coma.	Headache, vomiting, nerve palsies, diabetes insipidus.	Lethargy — coma, convulsions, ataxia, spasticity.	Defects in learning? Convulsions, ataxia, etc.?	Transient somnolence, irritability.
Diagnosis	Measles 2–20 weeks earlier. (Antibodies in CSF or serum)	Leukaemic cells in CSF.	History. Ventricular dilation on CT scan.	Calcification on X-ray	History. (CSF protein +)
Course and treatment	Usually fatal (? Interferon)	Intrathecal MTX (Ara-C) Radiation.	Progressive. No treatment.	? Not progressive. No treatment.	Spontaneous recovery.
Reference	Kay, 1979	Price, 1979	Price, 1979	Price, 1979	Freeman et al, 1973

and c-ALL and in the latter it has been most often diagnosed within nine months of stopping chemotherapy.

However, duration of chemotherapy does not seem to influence the final incidence, nor is there any common factor to those regimes of maintenance therapy where it has been most frequent. On the other hand, regimes with an intensive early phase, especially with prolonged asparaginase, may result in lower rates of testicular disease, implying that maintenance treatment (MP + MTX) does no more than suppress the manifestations.

Treatment of the complication is relatively simple and 2400 r (not a lower dose as was once thought) to both testes is generally recommended. It may be possible to detect the infiltrate by biopsy at the end of the period of systemic therapy but a false negative rate of 10 per cent or more diminishes the value of the procedure. Alternatively prophylactic testicular irradiation at the same time as CNS prophylaxis has been tried and where given in conjunction with radiation of other supposed sanctuary sites in CCSG trial CCG 101, it was effective not only in preventing relapse in the testis but perhaps to some extent also in the bone marrow. A justification for this drastic measure is that males are very seldom fertile after standard anti-ALL treatment and that irradiation does not impair interstitial cell function.

Maintenance treatment in ALL

Convenience and the consistent attainment of reasonably good results have led to the adoption of a standard regime of daily mercaptopurine and weekly methotrexate as the bread-and-butter routine anti-ALL treatment. Exceptions have been the complicated multidrug regimes of the Memorial Hospital (Gee et al, 1976) but for the ordinary case of childhood ALL these appear to have no advantage (see Frei & Sallan, 1978).

The unanswered questions concern the necessary duration of treatment, the extra benefit if any from added vincristine and prednisolone, the route of administration for the methotrexate and the avoidance of the infections which the immunosuppression permits. Comparisons of three and of five years of treatment show no benefit for the longer treatment and indeed two years may be adequate for all, although for boys, at least, a period of 19 months was not as good as three years (MRC, 1977). Extra steroid and vincristine are customarily given but the original demonstration of their value may no longer be valid if otherwise optimal treatment is given. Immunosuppression can probably be attributed to the continuous MP for the most part, but no other regime, for example with interrupted dosage, has been discovered which is maximally antileukaemic and less immunosuppressive. The consequences can be partly avoided by passive immunisation with immunoglobulin to prevent varicella and measles and by the use of cotrimoxazole to counter pneumocystis and other respiratory infections.

Methotrexate

It has been known for some time that methotrexate resistance may be present or acquired by leukaemic cells in various ways. The introduction of rapid and easy assay techniques for measuring plasma methotrexate levels has shown that wide individual variations occur in the rate of absorption, excretion and/or metabolism so that the peak level in the plasma after a standard dose of $12.5 \, mg/m^2$ can vary from as little as 20 ng to over 1000 ng/ml — a 50-fold variation. Moreover, the shape of the curve showing plasma concentration versus time can be either a sharp peak at one hour or a slow increase up to five hours. The correlation of these patterns with the outcome of treatment has yet to be fully explored but in some treatment schedules a low serum level is a warning of probable relapse (Craft et al, 1980).

Treatment of T-ALL
Neoplasms of the T-cell lineage in childhood and early adult life comprise some very variable tumours ranging from 'Stage I' thymic lymphomas which can be relatively benign and curable tumours to T-cell ALL with blood blast counts as high as $10^{12}/l$. This variation and their comparative rarity makes it exceedingly difficult to decide upon the best lines of treatment. New agents which have been used with at least partial effect include deoxycoformycin (Prentice et al, 1980) which is selectively active against T cells on account of their content of adenosine deaminase, antithymocyte globulin (Fisher et al, 1978) and thymidine (Fox et al, 1979; Howell et al, 1980). Alternatively, where a bone marrow transplant is possible, high dose cyclophosphamide and whole body irradiation may succeed even though remission cannot be obtained by other means (Garrett et al, 1980).

ALL in adults (Henderson et al, 1979)
The principles of treatment in adults are not different from those in childhood ALL; prophylaxis is needed to prevent CNS leukaemia but does not prolong survival. Results comparable to those in children can be expected in young adults when adverse factors — high leucocyte count, T or null cell disease, Ph' positivity — are absent but long remissions over the age of 30 are distinctly rare.

Acute myeloid leukaemia (Gale, 1979)
The advances in the treatment of AML have been much less dramatic than in ALL, but it is now appreciated that long-term remissions, presumptive cures, are attainable in a small but significant minority of cases. At present it is only possible to measure the increased incidence of remission which is attributable to better supportive therapy and the use of relatively intensive multidrug regimes, but a few long term trials are now being reported which, if actuarial assumptions are sustained, may give long survival rates among remitters of 20 to 35 per cent (Bloomfield, 1980; Weinstein et al, 1980). These, and results shortly to be published, must be compared with the prospects after bone marrow transplantation (see Ch. 7) and we must hope that the work in the next few years will promote optimum treatment strategies for patients with AML in groups as defined by age, cell type, chromosome analysis, biochemical characteristics, etc.

Supportive treatment
Treatment to mitigate the effects of haemopoietic failure may be needed by patients with many types of malignant disease or with bone marrow aplasia but the commonest single condition has been AML which has thereby become the testing ground for the employment of various regimes.

PREVENTION OF BLEEDING
Platelet transfusion has become a routine measure and requires little comment.

Sensitisation to platelet antigens is seldom a problem in AML since the period when they are required is short: nevertheless, there may be difficulties in preventing fatal haemorrhage especially in the presence of serious infection and/or if there is some degree of disseminated intravascular coagulation.

The problem is epitomised in the management of acute promyelocytic leukaemia where lysis of the leukaemic promyelocytes is presumed to initiate intravascular coagulation. It is generally agreed that anti-leukaemic cytotoxic agents should be withheld until full heparinisation is established. Large numbers of platelets are nearly always needed and they may with advantage be supplemented by fibrinogen and perhaps by fresh frozen plasma. In normal circumstances the phagocytic system exerts a buffering effect on the chemical reactions inherent in thrombosis, coagulation and fibrinolysis so that the addition of transfused granulocytes may also be beneficial. Vigorous treatment, monitored by estimations of fibrinogen and FDP may suppress the vicious circle of coagulation, fibrinolysis and platelet consumption, but even the best equipped and most experienced centres fail to save all their cases of acute promyelocytic leukaemia. Figure 8.1 illustrates a successful remission induction.

INFECTION

The successful management of infection in acute leukaemia is mainly dependent on

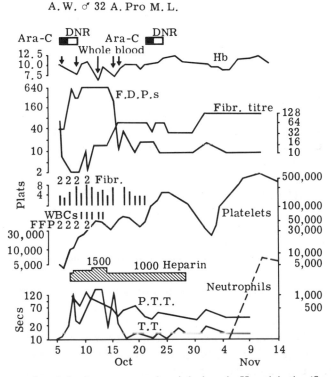

Fig. 8.1 Attainment of remission in acute promyelocytic leukaemia. Heparinisation (figures show units per hour) begun in this case after cytosine arabinoside (Ara-C) and daunorubicin (DNR). Note elevation of fibrin degradation products (FDPs) and lowering of fibrinogen when anti-leukaemic treatment starts. Units of fibrinogen, platelets, leucocytes and fresh frozen plasma (FFP) as shown.

the experience, sufficiency and continuity of the medical and nursing staff, but because it is difficult and politically unwise to measure those variables, studies and trials have been concentrated on the efficacy of antibiotic regimens, protective isolation and granulocyte transfusion. Comparative trials of therapeutic antibiotic regimes have shown the benefit of having a fixed protocol of management and the hazard of combining two nephrotoxic antibiotics, but the precise choice will always have to be determined by circumstances such as the local prevalence of antibiotic resistant strains. The value of alimentary antibiotics remains controversial. There is little to be said for the expensive combination of gentamycin, vancomycin and nystatin (GVN) but neomycin or framycetin with colistin and nystatin (Neocon or Fracon) has trial-proved worth (Storring et al, 1977) and cotrimoxazole (not strictly a gut decontaminant) with nystatin may be equally effective.

Protective isolation has both advocates and detractors. It probably ensures a consistent standard of remission attainment by avoiding epidemics of cross-infection but it is difficult to demonstrate more than a marginal benefit for AML remission induction. For bone marrow transplants, on the other hand, where infection and graft-versus-host reactions may combine to increase morbidity and mortality, the benefit of isolation and some measure of antibiotic decontamination seems more secure.

Granulocyte transfusions are considered in Chapter 15. In acute leukaemias they have been used for local infections or septicaemias not responding to antibiotics with good effect. Their use as prophylaxis in neutropenic patients is said to be helpful but the cost is high.

LEUCOSTASIS

One complication that has recently come to be recognised is leucostasis — a condition where fatal cerebral anoxia is caused by sludging in the cerebral capillaries. This occurs in AML where a high leucocyte count is accompanied by high haemoglobin levels. Occasionally it may be unavoidable but sometimes it is caused by giving red cell transfusion before chemotherapy has lowered the concentration of leucocytes in the blood (Harris, 1978).

Drug regimes in AML

Increasing experience has shown that, for the majority of patients with AML, remission is most readily gained if the initial treatment is intensive. This may be achieved by giving three or more agents — an anthracycline, cytosine arabinoside and thioguanine — but comparable rates are claimed if only two drugs are given for long enough — an anthracycline (three consecutive days) and cytosine arabinoside (seven days or even 10 days) (Holland et al, 1976; Preisler et al, 1979). The success of these intensive and extended courses may be because there is rapid recruitment of non-cycling leukaemic blasts into proliferation after the first three days of treatment so that a maximum differential effect is achieved towards the end of one week of treatment (Vaughan et al, 1980). Whether that be the explanation or no, it is being increasingly appreciated that the treatment must be given with determination and without hesitancy. Furthermore, this applies even in the elderly patients, where caution has hitherto prevailed (Reiffers et al, 1980). It will now be difficult with a standard remission rate of over 70 per cent to determine the value of minor amendments and of additional drugs, but the length of the subsequent remission may be a good measure of total cytoreduction by the induction regime.

Anthracyclines (Jacquillat et al, 1976)
Few valid comparisons have been made of the three anthracyclines — daunorubicin, adriamycin and rubidazone. Their pharmacology is slightly different in that the metabolism to daunorubicinol and other products occurs at different rates and might affect both toxicity and antileukaemic activity. Mole for mole, adriamycin is less cardiotoxic but is more toxic to mucous membranes. Definitive comparative trials would be needed to determine if there is any significant difference in their relative merits.

Cytosine arabinoside
The value of cytosine arabinoside in AML has been amply confirmed but there is still no consensus about its administration. When given intravenously it is cleared from the blood extremely fast so that continuous infusion has been widely adopted to maintain a supposedly necessary concentration in the plasma. In fact, rapid clearance through the liver is counterbalanced by the very rapid uptake in leukaemic cells where phosphorylation to the active triphosphate is an essential step. Harris et al (1979) have shown that according to circumstances, such as rates of cell uptake, of phosphorylation and of incorporation into DNA, the optimal mode of administration, either I.V. bolus or infusion (possibly also subcutaneous injection), varies from one patient to another. There is no easy and generally practical way to predict which is the best for the individual patient. In the light of this variation, it is not surprising that trials have not demonstrated a convincing advantage for either bolus (8 or 12 hourly) or infusion schedules. A new depot-type analogue of Ara-C — Behenoyl Ara-C — may be more convenient to administer (O'Hara et al, 1980) but attempts to augment the chemotherapeutic effect by previous cell synchronisation with Ara-C have not succeeded (Steuber et al, 1978).

Other drugs (Gale, 1979)
Thioguanine is always preferred to mercaptopurine on the basis of clinical trial (Holland et al, 1976); daily or twice daily oral dosage remains the standard.

Vincristine is a component of several AML regimes, but the relative benefits and hazards have yet to be measured. Cyclophosphamide is included in COAP and some other regimes. Azacytidine is undoubtedly an effective drug in AML but its toxicity — especially nausea, vomiting and diarrhoea — has prevented its general adoption.

Of the podophyllotoxins, VP 16213, has been most often employed in AML and can be effective either alone or in combination. Some results have suggested that monocytic types of disease are the most susceptible to this agent, and the response of some histiocytic neoplasms carries a similar implication.

The role of steroid is being closely studied since some prediction of response based either on cell receptors for steroids or on the presence of TdT might be feasible. Regimens which include steroid in the induction combination have not demonstrated a convincing superiority over those without steroid and they carry some hazard of increased susceptibility to infection but possibly cases of AML with known high receptor levels (perhaps M5 variants) or those with high TdT levels should receive corticosteroid.

Non-intensive treatments

Although intensive treatment is more likely to induce a remission in AML than is a gentle treatment, there remain cases for whom it is probably inappropriate. There is a wide boundary zone of cases intermediate between AML and chronic myeloproliferative disease, sometimes designated subacute leukaemia, where conservative treatment, i.e. blood transfusion and treatment of infections, may be a better and more acceptable way of prolonging life and enhancing its quality.

Patients with a prolonged preleukaemic phase and patients developing AML after treatment for other diseases, e.g. Hodgkin's disease, may be similarly placed in that remission is rarely obtained in these circumstances (Preisler & Lyman, 1977).

Chromosome analysis and the choice of treatment

The chromosomes of AML cells are considered in Chapter 11. At this point, it is relevant to question whether particular findings should influence treatment. The absence of normal karyotypes from a leukaemic marrow makes the attainment of a remission unlikely and the same may be true of extreme karyotypic diversity. Conservative treatment or possibly early marrow transplantation would then be preferable. On the other hand, some specific abnormalities, e.g. t(8;21), are associated with relatively long remissions and their presence might favour a decision towards conventional chemotherapy.

Management of AML in remission

The improvement in remission rates in AML has not as yet been matched by much prolongation of the remission. Two objectives can be defined; a general prolongation for which the median remission duration is a useful index and the proportion of cases with long remissions (four years or more) many of whom may have had actual eradication of the leukaemia.

Consolidation and maintenance treatments (Gale, 1979)

The value of chemotherapy after remission has been gained in AML remains entirely undecided. In a few recent and current trials some comparison has been attempted but either the numbers have been small, the treatment possibly suboptimal, or it is too soon to reach conclusions. Furthermore, conclusions from a trial where the initial remission rate was under 50 per cent may be no longer applicable when the remission rate reaches 80 per cent. Also in any evaluation the variables of age, cell type and perhaps other parameters must be taken into account. Age may be particularly important, as the prospects of really long remission (cures ?) may be higher in children and young adults (Oliff & Poplack, 1978). A current trial of the Medical Research Council may indicate whether two or six courses of consolidation chemotherapy are to be preferred. As to the form of chemotherapy, a simple schedule of Ara-C + TG as given by Peterson and Bloomfield (1977) avoids the cardiotoxicity of repeated anthracyclines and has a four-year remission rate of about 20 per cent. On the other hand, the highly complex multidrug regimens of the Memorial Hospital give a similar tale of long remitters (Clarkson et al, 1976). A comparison between these divergent philosophies of treatment with the addition of a no-treatment control arm would be fascinating, but is not likely to be realised.

Other modes of AML treatment
Late intensification of chemotherapy in AML involves the administration of a short course of multiple drug combination before stopping chemotherapy. Characteristically good but controversial results have been claimed at the M. D. Anderson Hospital (Bodey et al, 1976).

A variable proportion of AML patients, especially children, develop disease in the CNS for which irradiation and/or intrathecal Ara-C and methotrexate have been given either as prophylaxis or treatment. The benefit of radiation prophylaxis is more than outweighed by the increased rate of marrow relapse but intrathecal Ara-C may reduce the number of CNS relapses (Choi & Simone, 1976).

Splenectomy has been tried in childhood AML with possibly slight benefit.

Prediction of treatment in acute leukaemia
Variation in the response of leukaemic cells to different drugs and to different combinations of drugs has encouraged the formulation of systems of prediction. These have been based on basic cell characteristics including antigens, enzymes, cell receptors or chromosome abnormality or more definitively, on tests in vitro or in recipient (immunodeficient) mice. For example the most recent of these (Park et al, 1980) depends upon culture in agar after exposure of leukaemic cells to appropriate drugs and might be of some value although, as with many other systems, there is a moderate time lag. Simple rapid and reliable tests have yet to be evolved (but see Preisler, 1980).

Leukaemia specific antigens and the role of immunotherapy
The detailed characterisation of leukaemic cells has shown that in both lympho-blastic and myeloid types of acute leukaemia the cell usually exhibits the phenotype of a normal haemopoietic cell which has been 'frozen' at one stage of its development (see Ch. 10). Efforts to demonstrate leukaemia specific antigens have not succeeded; even the fact that leukaemic myeloblasts can stimulate autologous lymphocytes to proliferate loses its significance in view of the ability of some autologous washed lymphocytes to do the same. Simultaneously, the claims of immunotherapy in human neoplasia have been generally confounded by the negative results of adequate controlled trials (see Terry & Windhorst, 1978). The only well-founded exception seems to be acute myeloid leukaemia where immunotherapy (BCG plus blasts or methanol extracted residue (MER) of BCG and/or neuraminidase-treated blasts) may have given longer remissions or may have facilitated a second remission (Whittaker & Slater, 1977; Harris et al, 1978; MRC, 1978; Whittaker, 1980). Such differences could be attributable to a true immune effect against a leukaemia antigen but might also occur if a nonspecific disturbance of homeostasis, resulting from persistent bombardment with immunotherapy 'soups' favoured the proliferation of normal haemopoietic cells in preference to the leukaemic clone.

There remains the observation that remission marrow cells can stimulate auto-logous lymphocytes when relapse is impending (Baker et al, 1979). This might or might not indicate the presence of leukaemia-specific antigen (see above) but could be of occasional clinical use. With the abandonment of most prejudices and convictions on immunotherapy, the whole subject remains open to further investigation.

REFERENCES

Adamson J W 1979 The New England Journal of Medicine 301: 378–380
Aksoy M 1978 The Lancet 1: 441
Auclerc G, Jacquillat C, Auclerc M F, Weil M, Bernard J 1979 Cancer 44: 2017–2025
Baker M A, Falk J A, Carter W H, Taub R N, the Toronto Leukemia Study Group 1979 The New England Journal of Medicine 301: 1353–1357
Bennett J M, Catovsky D, Daniel M T, Flandrin G, Galton D A G, Gralnick H R, Sultan C 1981 British Journal of Haematology 47: 553–561
Bennett J M, Catovsky D, Daniel M-T, Flandrin G, Galton D A G, Gralnick H R, Sultan C 1976 British Journal of Haematology 33: 451–458
Birch J M, Marsden H B, Swindell R 1979 The Lancet 2: 854–855
Bloomfield C D 1980 Annals of Internal Medicine 93: No. 1 (Pt 1) 133–135
Bloomfield C D, Lindquist L L, Arthur D, McKenna R W, LeBien T W, Peterson B A, Nesbit M E 1981 Cancer Research (in press)
Bodey G P, Freireich E J, Gehan E A, McCredie K, Rodriguez V, Gutterman J, Burgess M A 1976 The Journal of the American Medical Association 235: 1021–1025
Broxmeyer H E, Grossbard E, Jacobsen N, Moore M A S 1979 The New England Journal of Medicine 301: 346–351
Caldwell G G, Kelley D B, Heath C W Jr 1980 American Medical Association Journal 244(14): 1575–1578
Choi S-I, Simone J V 1976 Medical and Pediatric Oncology 2: 119–146
Clarkson B D, Dowling M D, Gee T S, Cunningham I B, Burchenal J H 1975 Cancer 36: 775–795
Craddock C G, Crandall B F, Como R 1975 The American Journal of Medicine 59: 737–743
Craft A Personal Communication
Dym M, Fawcett D W 1970 Biology of Reproduction 3: 308–326
Eaves C J, Eaves A C 1978 Blood 52: 1196–1210
Eden O B 1980 Proceedings of the International Society for Paediatric Oncology (S.I.O.P.) 'Société Internationale de Oncologie Pediatrique'
Eiser C 1979 In: Whitehouse J M A, Kay H E M (eds) CNS Complications of malignant disease, Macmillan Press Ltd, London. Ch 22, p 236–247
Elfenbein G J, Brogaonkar D S, Bias W B, Burns W H, Saral R, Sensenbrenner L L, Tutschka P J, Zaczek B S, Zander A R, Epstein R B, Rowley J D, Santos G W 1978 Blood 52: 627–636
Fialkow P J, Singer J W, Adamson J W, Berkow R L, Friedman J M, Jacobson R J, Moohr J W 1979 The New England Journal of Medicine 301: 1–5
Finch S C 1979 The American Journal of Medicine 66: 899–901
Fisher R I, Kubota T T, Mandell G L, Broder S, Young R C 1978 Annals of Internal Medicine 88: 799–800
Fox R M, Piddington S K, Tripp E H, Dudman N P, Tattersall M H N 1979 The Lancet 2: 391–393
Francis D P, Cotter S M, Hardy, Jr, W D, Essex M 1979 Cancer Research 39: 3866–3870
Freeman J E, Johnston P G B, Voke J M 1973 British Medical Journal 4: 523
Frei III, E, Salian S E 1978 Cancer 42: 828–838
Gale R P 1979 The New England Journal of Medicine 300: 1189–1199
Gallagher R, Collins S, Trujillo J, McCredie K, Ahearn M, Tsai S, Metzgar R, Aulakh G, Ting R, Ruscetti F, Gallo R 1979 Blood 54: 713–733
Garrett T J, Grossbard E, Hopfan S, Koziner B, Clarkson B D, Good R A, O'Reilly R 1980 Cancer 45: 2006–2008
Gee T S, Haghbin M, Dowling, Jr, M D, Cunningham I, Middleman M P, Clarkson B D 1976 Cancer 37: 1256–1264
Golomb H M, Rowley J D, Vardiman J W, Testa J R, Butler A 1980 Blood 55: 253–259
Greaves M F, Janossy G, Peto J, Kay H 1981 British Journal of Haematology 48: 179–197
Green D M, Freeman A I, Sather H N, Sallan S E, Nesbit M E, Cassady J R, Sinks L F, Hammond D, Frei III E 1980 The Lancet 1: 1398–1401
Hanto D, Frizzera G, Gajl-Peezalska K, Purtilo D, Klein G 1980 Proceedings of the VIII International Congress of the Transplantation Society (in press)
Harris A L 1978 British Medical Journal 1: 1169–1171
Harris C C 1979 Journal of the National Cancer Institute 63: 275–277
Harris A L, Potter C, Bunch C, Boutagy J, Harvey D J, Grahame-Smith D G 1979 British Journal of Clinical Pharmacology 8: 219–227
Henderson E S, Scharlau C, Cooper M R, and 21 others 1979 Leukaemia Research 3: 395–407
Holland J F, Glidewell O, Ellison R R, Corey R W, Schwartz J, Wallace H J, Hoagland H C, Wiernik P, Rai K, Beksei J G, Cuttner J 1976 Archives of Internal Medicine 136: 1377–1381
Howell S B, Taetle R, Mendelsohn J 1980 Blood 55: 505–510

Jacquillat C, Weil M, Gemon-Auclerc M F, Izrael V, Bussel A, Boiron M, Bernard J 1976 Cancer 37: 653–659

Jones B, Holland J F, Glidewell O, and 21 others 1977 Medical and Pediatric Oncology 3: 387–400

Kay H E M 1978 U.K. leukaemia clinical trials for children and adults. Leukaemia Research Fund, 13th Annual Guest Lecture, p 20–32

Kay H E M 1979 In: Whitehouse J M A, Kay H E M (eds) CNS Complications of Malignant Disease, Macmillan Press Ltd, London. Ch 26, p 285–291

Kinlen L J, Sheil A G R, Peto J, Doll R 1979 British Medical Journal 2: 1461–1466

Knox G 1964 Applied Statistics 13: 25–29

Koeffler H P, Golde D W, Lippman M E 1980 Cancer Research 40: 563–566

Lawler S D, Summersgil B M, Clink H McD, McElwain T J 1979 The Lancet 2: 853–854

Lyon J L, Klauber M R, Gardner J W, Udall K S 1979 The New England Journal of Medicine 300: 397–402

Magrath I T, Ziegler J L 1980 Leukaemia Research 4: 33–59

Marks S M, Baltimore D, McCaffrey R 1978 The New England Journal of Medicine 298: 812–814

Mauer A M 1980 Blood 56: 1–10

McCulloch E A 1979 Journal of the National Cancer Institute 63: 883–891

Medical Research Council 1977 British Medical Journal 2: 495–497

Medical Research Council 1978a British Medical Journal 1: 334–338

Medical Research Council 1978b British Journal of Cancer 37: 1–14

Mertelsmann R, Thaler H T, to L, Gee T S, McKenzie S, Schauer P, Friedman A, Arlin Z, Cirrincione C, Clarkson B 1980 Blood 56: 5, 773–781

Miller D R, Leikin S et al 1980 Cancer Treatment Reports 64(2–3): 381–392

Mitelman F, Brandt L, Nilsson P G 1978 Blood 52: 1229–1237

Mole R H 1975 British Journal of Radiology 48: 157–169

Najarian T, Colton T 1978 The Lancet 1: 1018–1020

Nesbit M E 1980 Proceedings of the American Society of Clinical Oncology (in press)

Nesbit M E, Robison L L, Ortega J A, Sather H N, Donaldson M, Hammond D 1980 Cancer 45: 2009–2016

Nesbit M E, Robison L L, Ortega J A, Sather H N, Donaldson M, Hammond D 1980 Cancer 45: 2009–2016

Ohara K, Kojima T, Sugihara T, Kamiya O, Hoshino A, Yamazaki K 1980 18th Congr International Society of Haematology. Abstract No 1625

Oliff A, Poplack D 1978 Medical and Pediatric Oncology 5: 219–223

Omura G A, Moffitt S, Vogler W R, Salter M M 1980 Blood 55: 199–204

Park C H, Amare M, Savin M A, Goodwin J W, Newcomb M M, Hoogstraten B 1980 Blood 55: 595–601

Pasmino M, Tonini G P, Rosanda C, Massimo L 1977 The Lancet 1: 608

Peterson B A, Bloomfield C D 1977 The Lancet 2: 158–160

Preisler H D 1980 Blood 56(3): 361–367

Preisler H D, Bjornsson S, Henderson E S, Hryniuk W, Higby D, Freeman A, Naeher C 1979 Medical and Pediatric Oncology 7: 269–275

Preisler H D, Lyman G H 1977 American Journal of Hematology 3: 209–218

Prentice H G, Smyth J F, Goneshagum K, Wonke B, Bradstock K F, Janessey G, Goldstone A H, Hoffbrand A V 1980 Lancet, II: 170–172

Price R A 1979 In: Whitehouse J M A, Kay H E M (eds) CNS Complications of Malignant Disease, Macmillan Press Ltd, London. Ch 1, p 3–15

Price R A, Birdwell D A 1978 Cancer 42: 717–728

Price R A, Jamieson P A 1975 Cancer 35: 306–318

Rieffers J, Reynal F, Broustet A 1980 Cancer 45: 2816–2820

Riehm H, Henze G, Langermann H J, Ritter J, Schellong G The BFM studies 1970/76 and 1976/79 in childhood acute lymphoblastic leukaemia (ALL). Proceedings of Meeting in Hamburg June 1980

Rosenkrantz J G, Wong K Y, Ballard E T, Cox J A, Martin L W 1978 Journal of Pediatric Surgery 13: 753–756

Rowley J D 1980 18th Congr International Society of Haematology, Abstract No 313

Sallan S E, Ritz J, Pesando J, Gelber R, O'Brien C, Hitchcock S, Coral F, Schlossman S F 1980 Blood 55: 395–401

Secker-Walker L M, Lawler S D, Hardisty R M 1978 British Medical Journal 2: 1529–1530

Shalet S M, Beardwell C G 1979 In: Whitehouse J M A, Kay H E M (eds) CNS Complications of Malignant Disease, Macmillan Press Ltd, London. Ch 19, p 202–217

Simone J 1976 British Journal of Haematology 32: 465–472

Smith P G 1978 Cancer 42: 1026–1034

Smith S D, Uyeki E M, Lowman J T 1978 Blood 52: 712–718
Steuber C P, Humphrey G B, McMillan C W, Vietti T J 1978 Medical and Pediatric Oncology 4: 337–342
Storring R A, Jameson B, McElwain T J, Wiltshaw E, Spiers A S D, Gaya H 1977 The Lancet 2: 837–840
Swift P G F, Kearney P J, Dalton R G, Bullimore J A, Mott M G, Savage D C L 1979 In: Whitehouse
    J M A, Kay H E M (eds) CNS Complications of Malignant Disease, Macmillan Press Ltd, London.
    Ch 20, p 218–226
Terry W D, Windhorst D (eds) 1978 Immunotherapy of Cancer: Present Status of Trials in Man. Raven
    Press, New York
Thiry L 1979 In: Tyrell D A J (ed) Aspects of slow and persistent virus infections. New Perspectives in
    Clinical Microbiology 2: 153
Tsiftsoglou A S, Gusella J F, Volloch V, Housman D E 1979 Cancer Research 39: 3849–3855
Twomey J J, Lewis V M, Ford R, Goldstein G 1980 The American Journal of Medicine 68: 377–380
Vaughan W P, Karp J E, Burke P J 1980 Cancer 45: 859–865
Viana M B, Maurer H S, Ferenc C 1980 British Journal of Haematology 44: 383–388
Weinstein H J et al 1980 The New England Journal of Medicine 303: 473–478
Whittaker J A, Slater A J 1977 British Journal of Haematology 35: 263
Zuelzer W W 1978 Johns Hopkins Medical Journal 142: 115–127

9. The chronic leukaemias

D A G Galton

As a result of recent advances in the characterisation of leukaemic cells it is now apparent that the chronic myeloid leukaemias include several distinct entities which differ in their age incidence, clinical and haematological features, cytogenetics, prognosis and response to treatment. There is, as yet, no agreed nomenclature for the variants of CML, and in this account the following terms are used for the five variants:

1. *Chronic granulocytic leukaemia* (CGL): the most common variant; rare below age 5; has characteristic pattern of evolution, course and response to treatment; characteristic blood picture includes essentially normal blood-cell morphology, neutrophil and myelocyte peaks in differential count, high absolute basophil counts, low relative monocyte counts; almost always Philadelphia-chromosome positive (Ph'+); biphasic course; easily controlled in chronic phase: median duration of survival about $3\frac{1}{2}$ years.

2. *Atypical chronic myeloid leukaemia:* rare below age 30; variable pattern of evolution, course, and response to treatment; variable blood picture, merges with acute myeloid and chronic myelomonocytic leukaemia; monocyte counts often increased, basophil counts not increased, morphological abnormalities common; biphasic, but poorly controlled in chronic phase; great majority Philadelphia-chromosome negative (Ph'−); median duration of survival less than 18 months.

3. *Chronic myelomonocytic leukaemia* (CMML): rare below age 60; variable pattern of evolution, absolute neutrophilia and monocytosis common (pure monocytic variant rare), immature forms absent in chronic phase; myelodysplastic features frequent; merges with refractory anaemia with excess blasts (RAEB) when monocyte counts low; Ph'−; biphasic course, chronic phase may exceed 10 years.

4. *Neutrophilic leukaemia:* very rare; rare below age 60; high neutrophil counts, but immature granulocytes not present; high content of alkaline phosphatase in neutrophils; Ph'−; biphasic course.

5. *Juvenile chronic myeloid leukaemia:* very rare; probably does not occur above 5 years; characteristic clinical and haematological picture; origin in fetal stem cell (high Hb-F, fetal red cell enzymes); Ph'−; poor response to treatment.

CHRONIC GRANULOCYTIC LEUKAEMIA (CGL)

Among the chronic myeloid leukaemias, the major advances concern particularly (1) cytogenetics, (2) the analysis of the homeostatic defect responsible for the development of the features of the chronic phase, (3) the characterisation of the stem cell that gives rise to chronic-phase CGL, the various forms of transformed CGL, and of de novo Ph'+ acute leukaemias, and to a lesser extent (4) treatment.

Cytogenetics

Rowley (Ch. 11) reviews the features of the Ph'+ chromosome which have been revealed by banding techniques.

In most CGL patients almost every analysable bone marrow cell metaphase is Ph'+ at the time of diagnosis, even when the diagnosis is made by chance, when the leucocyte count is only moderately raised. This is also the case in patients whose leucocyte counts have been reduced to within the normal range by treatment. Thus it is not likely that early ascertainment accounts for the mixtures of Ph'+ and Ph'− cells that are sometimes found at the time of diagnosis. Indeed such patients often have a particularly benign course (Brandt et al, 1976; Golde et al, 1976; Sakurai et al, 1976), suggesting that the Ph'-bearing stem cells were less than usually active in replacing the normal population, in altering the homeostasis of the granulocytic series, and in increasing the risk of malignant transformation. A few patients, unusually sensitive to busulphan, have, after a phase of marrow hypoplasia, regenerated apparently normal marrow with a normal blood count and a normal blood picture. The marrow, however, contained mixtures of Ph'+ and Ph'− cells with a preponderance of Ph'− cells. The subsequent fate of these patients has varied from those whose marrow became totally replaced with Ph'+ cells between 3 and 7 years later (E K Blackburn, personal communication, and personal observations) to one, originally reported by Finney et al (1972) who remains in remission after 17 years (G A McDonald, personal communication) with no change in the low proportion of Ph'− cells. Thus the Ph'+ stem cells do not invariably have a growth advantage over Ph'− stem cells. Lack of the Y chromosome, found in nearly 10 per cent of male patients, has been associated with longer survival in some (Sakurai & Sandberg, 1976) but not all series (Lawler, 1977). In less than 10 per cent of patients in the chronic phase, additional chromosomal abnormalities are found, especially duplication of the Ph' (which arises secondarily and therefore does not involve a second translocation), and the presence of three no. 8 chromosomes (First International Workshop on Chromosomes in Leukaemia, 1978). These abnormalities do not appear to influence the prognosis (Rowley, Ch. 11).

Cytogenetics of transformed CGL

In 75 to 80 per cent of cases the clinical and haematological events of transformation are associated with a change in the karyotype of the Ph'+ cell population. The changes in karyotype are sometimes found up to a few months before the onset of clinical and haematological evidence of transformation; rarely chronic phase disease continues long after the changes have been found (Hayata et al, 1975). The commonest changes involve gains by reduplication, or rearrangements, while losses are rare. The commonest reduplications involve the Ph' itself, and one of pair no. 8 resulting in trisomy, and the commonest rearrangement involves no. 17 with the production of an isochromosome for the long arm. One or more of these three aberrations are the commonest changes in transformed CGL (Mitelman & Levan, 1978; Rowley, 1980), and it is possible that additional changes depend on the type of treatment administered during the chronic phase (Alimena et al, 1979). Serial analysis may demonstrate the evolution of subclones, a phenomenon already known before the introduction of banding techniques (Grouchy et al, 1968), and when cells from different tissues, for example bone marrow and spleen, are examined serially, the origin of a subclone in one and its spread to others may be demonstrated (Brandt & Mitelman, 1977). New clones originating in the spleen may be eliminated by splenectomy before they have colonised the marrow (Gomez et al, 1975), or having colonised the marrow may fail to establish themselves there as shown by their disappearance from the marrow after splenectomy (Lawler, 1977). The clone that proves lethal is the one that succeeds by virtue of its proliferative advantage and its capacity to disseminate. Clinical and haematological transformation occurs without any additional chromosome changes in less than one quarter of all cases.

CGL as a monoclonal disease

The earliest evidence of monoclonality was the cytogenetic evidence showing that the Ph' was an acquired defect confined to a myeloid stem cell and its descendants, but absent from blood lymphocytes, skin fibroblasts, and marrow fibroblasts. Subsequently, the existence of chromosomal polymorphisms permitted demonstration of monotypy in every Ph'+ cell. Complementary biochemical evidence of monoclonality comes from the study of G6PD polymorphism in the rare female heterozygotes with CGL who have the A and B alleles. The gene is located on the X chromosome. Because of random inactivation of one X chromosome, each allele occurs in one half of the cells of normal tissues. All the Ph'+ myeloid cells however contain the same allele (Fialkow et al, 1977). When G6PD assays were made on the cell populations from individual granulocyte/monocyte colonies plated on agar there was no evidence of any mixed populations (Singer et al, 1979), but this observation needs confirmation in newly diagnosed cases because residual Ph'− stem cells might be selectively destroyed by treatment.

Chronic-phase CGL as a defect of granulocyte homeostasis

Although the Ph' abnormality affects the myeloid-committed stem cell and its erythroid, megakaryocytic, granulocytic and monocytic descendants, the main expression of the abnormality is in the granulocytic series, resulting in the characteristic granulocytic hyperplasia of the bone marrow at the expense of the erythropoietic cells and of the fat cells, and in the exponential rise in the peripheral blood granulocyte count including immature cells. The same granulocytic hyperplasia is seen in the red pulp of the enlarging spleen, and in the sinusoids of the liver. Cytokinetic studies have shown free traffic between the proliferating myeloid cells in the bone marrow, spleen, and peripheral blood (Galbraith & Abu-Zhara, 1972). The progressive expansion of the total myeloid-tissue mass is reflected in the orderly sequence of events whereby the total leucocyte count (TLC) begins to rise only after the increasing cellularity of the marrow, now almost entirely replaced by Ph'+ cells, has led to the disappearance of the fat cells, and the spleen becomes palpable when the TLC is of the order of 100×10^9/l. That granulocyte homeostasis is disturbed rather than lost is shown by the cyclical oscillations in the TLC occasionally found (Galton, 1962; Morley et al, 1967; Vodopick et al, 1972; Gatti et al, 1973). Occasionally, the platelet counts also show cyclical oscillations.

Under normal steady-state conditions, the supply of granulocytes is regulated by an integrated system of stimulatory and inhibitory influences acting on haemopoietic stem cells (Ch. 6). The immediate granulocyte-series precursor stem cell (CFUc) which also gives rise to monocytes and macrophages forms colonies of granulocytes and macrophages in semi-solid media, provided it is supplied with 'colony-stimulating factor' (CSF). The monocyte is a major source of CSF, and must be considered as the principal cell responsible for maintaining the levels of neutrophil counts in conditions other than CGL. Thus Bain & Wickramasinghe (1976) found a constant ratio between the logarithms of the monocyte and neutrophil counts in states of neutrophilia at various levels of neutrophil count except in CGL where, at all neutrophil counts, the corresponding monocyte counts were lower than in other conditions. Crudely, the monocyte/granulocyte ratio is normally maintained by a balance between the production of CSF by the monocytes, and the inhibition of its production and release by a substance with colony-inhibitory-activity (CIA) (Broxmeyer et al, 1977), probably iron-saturated lactoferrin (Broxmeyer et al, 1978), released by neutrophils. When the neutrophil count rises in response to bacterial infection the inhibitory action of CIA is counteracted by monocyte-activating substances of bacterial origin (Broxmeyer and Ralph, 1977), and the monocyte and neutrophil count ratio is maintained. In CGL the release of CIA by the neutrophils was found to be diminished (Broxmeyer et al, 1977), and in addition the production of CSF by CGL monocytes and macrophages was inhibited less by CIA from normal neutrophils than that produced by normal monocytes and macrophages. These observations suggest a functional defect in the CFUc in CGL. The absolute number of CFUc in the marrow is markedly increased in CGL, and in the peripheral blood, where few are normally present, the number in CGL, in relation to the number of nucleated cells plated is hundreds of times greater than in the marrow. As the TLC rises, the proportion of CFUc increases, and Goldman et al (1980) have shown that the proportion of erythropoietic stem-cells (BFUe) in the peripheral blood also increases as the TLC rises but less rapidly than the CFUe. Although the pluripotent stem-cell cannot be assayed quantitatively in man, the rapidity with which haemopoietic reconstitution is established by autografts of cryopreserved peripheral blood leucocytes collected from CGL patients in the chronic-phase (Goldman et al, 1979), shows that they circulate in large numbers when the TLC is high.

The neutrophils in chronic-phase CGL
Although certain abnormalities are present in circulating CGL neutrophils, it is not clear whether these are intrinsic defects or merely a consequence of the abnormal age structure of the circulating neutrophil population due to the disturbed cytokinetics of the greatly expanding total mass of myeloid tissue. Thus in normal conditions, the newly formed granulocyte remains in the bone marrow for several days, and when released into the circulation, the $T\frac{1}{2}$ there is only about 7 hours (Dancey et al, 1976). However, in CGL where the total mass of myeloid tissue has a disproportionately large precursor, especially myelocytic compartment, the mature granulocyte compartment is correspondingly reduced, and cells are released prematurely, to circulate for a longer time ($T\frac{1}{2}$ 26–89 hr) (Athens et al, 1965). Most of the granulocyte properties that are abnormal in CGL when the TLC is high approach normality when the TLC has been lowered by treatment to the normal range.

CGL neutrophils look normal in blood films and by transmission electron microscopy (Ullyott & Bainton, 1974). At high counts a much higher proportion than normal pass through glass bead columns and are poor phagocytes (Brandt, 1965); some efficient phagocytic neutrophils are defective in killing some ingested organisms (Odeberg et al, 1975), and fail to discharge lysosomal enzymes into the phagosomes (El-Maalem & Fletcher, 1976). At normal counts, the killing capacity in some tests may be normal (Goldman & Th'ng, 1973). Apart from alkaline phosphatase, most of the enzymes normally present in neutrophils are functionally normal and present in normal amounts in CGL (Rustin & Peters, 1979). In the few cases reported, the content of lactoferrin, a secondary granule protein, has been variable (Mason, 1977; Rausch et al, 1978) but no systematic survey has yet been made.

The low alkaline phosphatase content of CGL neutrophils (NAP) was described by Wachstein (1946), and is an almost constant feature of Ph'+ CGL. But it is often found in Ph'–CML and in idiopathic myelofibrosis with myeloid metaplasia. In CGL when the TLC has been lowered by treatment, the NAP often increases towards normal, and higher values are obtained during infections, and after operations, especially splenectomy (Spiers et al, 1975). In agar cultures, the neutrophils in colonies from CGL patients have a normal NAP content (Hellmann & Goldman, 1980), as do those grown in liquid cultures (Chiyoda & Kinugasa, 1978) or in diffusion chambers in mice (Chikkappa et al, 1973). When CGL neurophils are transfused into neutropenic recipients they acquire a normal NAP content (Rustin, 1980): NAP is localised to a cytoplasmic organelle, the phosphasome (Rustin et al, 1979). In CGL neutrophils the amount of NAP is only about 13 per cent of normal, but the activity of the NAP present is normal (Rustin & Peters, 1979). The culture and transfusion studies suggest that in CGL the production of NAP is inhibited by an extracellular factor. Two chronic-phase CGL patients who after ablative therapy have received marrow transplants from their identical twins at Hammersmith Hospital now have normal blood counts and Ph'– bone marrow, but their NAP scores are persistently low (J M Goldman, personal communication). This suggests that an abnormality associated with CGL and affecting donor neutrophils has not been eradicated by destroying the Ph'+ stem-cell population.

Transformed CGL cells

The transformation of chronic-phase CGL to a more obviously malignant condition is sometimes an abrupt event in which an acute blast cell crisis (BC) intrudes on an apparently well controlled quiescent chronic phase. More often it is a multistage process, the earliest change being the increased difficulty in maintaining control by previously easily managed treatment. Later minor changes in the differential leucocyte count appear with higher proportions of immature granulocytes, not necessarily blast cells, and the presence of morphologically abnormal granulocytes. In about one-fifth of cases the chronic phase is succeeded, often over a transitional period lasting for many months, by myelosclerotic disease which may prove fatal with or without the appearance of overt BC, while in a minority of cases focal blast cell lesions produce clinical effects, for example compression paraplegia, or localised bone pain, before the onset of any recognisable haematological change. It is, however, the nature of the blast cells in the more acute forms of transformation that has attracted more interest in recent years because the cells can now be characterised with precision by recently introduced techniques. The resulting information has thrown new light on the nature of the stem cell from which CGL arises, and following the recognition of Ph'+ conditions other than CGL, has necessitated re-assessment of the place of CGL among the whole spectrum of Ph'+ leukaemias. CGL-BC cells are best characterised by integrating the results obtained by morphology (light and electron microscopy), light and electron microscope cytochemistry, cytogenetics (see Ch. 11) enzyme assays, especially (TdT) and the use of immunological markers (see Ch. 10). As a result of the application of these methods it is now apparent that the blast cells in an individual case can rarely be characterised accurately by single techniques, although even they may provide useful prognostic information and some guide to treatment. Thus Marmont & Damasio (1973) reported that small non-granular blasts were associated with a better prognosis and response to treatment with prednisone and vincristine than large granular blasts, while Marks et al (1978) found the same association with TdT positivity, independently of morphology. However, the use of several methods has shown that in a majority of cases the blast-crisis cells are of 'myeloid' origin, in about a fifth they have the same range of phenotypes as is found in 'common' acute lymphoblastic leukaemia (ALL), while in the remainder cells of both 'myeloid' and 'lymphoid' phenotypes are found. Rarely the same cells have reacted with anti-ALL serum and with anti-myeloid serum (Roberts, 1979).

'Myeloid' and 'lymphoid' phenotypes cannot safely be recognised from routine morphological examination alone, and mixed phenotypes always require the application of special techniques. Monocytic, myelomonocytic, basophilic and most erythroblastic BC can be recognised morphologically but early megakaryoblastic BC cells often appear undifferentiated and may be identifiable only by seeing platelet demarcation membranes by TEM or by demonstrating the presence of platelet-peroxidase (Breton-Gorius et al, 1978; Marie et al, 1979). The survival of patients with myeloid phenotype BC is very short, and most patients do not respond to treatment with vincristine and prednisone.

Pure lymphoid phenotype BC is more likely to give rise to meningeal infiltration than myeloid phenotype BC, and more likely to respond to treatment with regimens that include vincristine and prednisone (Beard et al, 1976; Woodruff et al, 1977; Chessels et al, 1979). When the BC clone totally replaces the Ph'+ chronic phase stem cell clone and is exquisitely sensitive to vincristine and prednisone, it may be virtually eliminated by the treatment leaving a hypoplastic bone marrow from which, rarely, Ph'− haemopoietic stem cells may regenerate (Janossy et al, 1979). If some Ph'+ myeloid stem cells survive their proliferation will repopulate the marrow with chronic phase CGL cells. Far more often the response to treatment is partial, transient or temporary: nevertheless the median duration of survival is considerably longer in lymphoid than in myeloid-phenotype BC though still measured in months rather than years, and patients who survive after responding to treatment may succumb to one or more blast crises of lymphoid, myeloid or mixed phenotype (Janossy et al, 1979).

The presence of the Ph' in ALL-like BC cells used to be accepted as evidence of their myeloid provenance, but the demonstration that their phenotype was indeed the same as that of common ALL and occasionally of the pre-B phenotype (ALL+, TdT+, Ia+, CyIgM+) (Greaves et al, 1979) as found in nearly one third of cases of de novo ALL in childhood, raised the question of the nature of the stem cell from which CGL arose. This is best considered by examining CGL and CGL-BC in the context of the whole spectrum of the Ph'+ leukaemias.

The Ph'+ leukaemias

Until recently routine chromosome examination was rarely performed in cases diagnosed clinically and haematologically as ALL or AML, and it was too readily assumed that the occasional case of apparently de novo Ph'+ ALL or AML represented CGL that had entered BC at an early stage. This was a reasonable extrapolation from the well known if uncommon cases in which the blast cells co-existed with features usually associated with chronic phase CGL, especially high platelet counts, high neutrophil counts with low NAP score, basophilia, and myelocytes. However, it is now clear that about 2 per cent of all cases of childhood ALL are Ph'+, and considerably more of adult ALL (Catovsky, 1979). Following the successful treatment of the ALL, a tiny minority of the patients go on to develop classical chronic phase CGL, and they may subsequently develop one or more episodes of BC of lymphoid, myeloid, or mixed phenotype. But the majority do not and the course of their disease is that of Ph'− ALL appropriate to their age, though in adults the prognosis of the Ph'+ cases may be particularly bad (Bloomfield et al, 1977). It is therefore clear that Ph'+ ALL can exist as an independent entity and the association with CGL is an inconstant and evidently rare phenomenon. The frequency of de novo Ph'+ AML is more difficult to ascertain because the recognition of CGL-associated features is so uncertain in the haematological context of AML. However, there is little doubt that it occurs (Wayne et al, 1979).

Boggs (1974) and Janossy et al (1976) proposed a pre-lymphoid/pre-mycloid target cell for CGL to account for the occurrence of lymphoid BC, and this is now widely accepted. But it is necessary now to consider the implications of the whole spectrum of the Ph'+ leukaemias in terms of the effect of the Ph'-chromosome on the stem cell bearing it. First, it is clear that the Ph' confers a risk of malignant transformation on the target cell. The magnitude of the risk is impossible to assess in terms of the total number of mitotic divisions in the clone before malignant transformation occurs, but it is likely to be very small, as suggested by the case of Canellos & Whang-Peng (1972) in which a small population of Ph'+ cells was discovered by chance in the marrow and did not increase explosively until the occurrence of terminal blast-cell leukaemia over 5 years later. This case also shows that the descendants of the cells originally affected by the Ph' were unable to undergo further differentiation or maturation for they were not identified in any normal haemopoietic cell lines. The phenotype of the cells of de novo Ph'+ ALL is usually that of the most frequent type of 'common' Ph'− ALL cell, namely ALL+, Ia+, TdT+, believed to be a prelymphoid stem cell, but as more Ph'+ cases are studied, it is possible that the less common phenotypes will be reported. The target cell from which these phenotypes arise is thought to be an earlier prelymphoid/premyeloid stem cell.

To account for the development of chronic-phase CGL and the subsequent development of the more common myeloid-phenotype BC and the less common lymphoid-type BC it is necessary to postulate two phenomena; first, a rare cell in the differentiation-blocked Ph'+ prelymphoid/premyeloid stem cell clone overcomes the block and responds to the stimulus which permits entry into the myeloid differentiation compartment; secondly, the Ph' abnormality affects this myeloid-committed stem cell by disturbing its homeostatic mechanism so that it proliferates, some of its descendants undergo maturation, and the clone replaces the normal myeloid stem cell population with the development, as an epiphenomenon, of all the events of chronic-phase CGL. The Ph'+ myeloid stem cells, now outnumbering the dormant prelymphoid/premyeloid stem cell population from which they arose, are at risk of undergoing malignant transformation because of the effect of the Ph', and may therefore, at any time give rise to the events of myeloid-phenotype BC. The smaller number of prelymphoid/premyeloid stem cells accounts for the lower risk of lymphoid phenotype BC. The occurrence of occasional cases of BC with the pre-B phenotype (Greaves et al, 1979) indicates that Ph'+ cells from the undifferentiated clone that have entered the lymphoid differentiation pathway retain the risk of malignant transformation. Only two cases of BC with cells showing features of thymocyte differentiation have so far been recorded; in one the cells were TdT+, Ia−, ALL−, and reacted weakly with antithymocyte serum (Janossy et al, 1979), in the other the cells formed E rosettes, but no other tests were done (Forman et al, 1977).

The treatment of CGL

The chronic phase (for acute phase see Ch. 8)
There has been no significant recent advance in the management of chronic phase CGL. It is still not known whether conventional busulphan therapy at low daily dosage is more effective if administered continuously throughout the chronic phase, or in courses started when the leucocyte count rises to some arbitrary level, and there is no evidence that treatment administered to symptomless patients whose disease has been diagnosed by chance at a relatively early stage is beneficial. The administration of single large doses of busulphan at intervals of several weeks controls the chronic phase as effectively as conventional treatment (Sullivan et al, 1977; Douglas & Wiltshaw, 1978; Vicariot et al, 1979) but there is no evidence of any long-term advantage.

With conventional busulphan therapy, it is customary to aim to maintain the TLC at approximately 10×10^9/l. It is not possible to stabilise the count at lower levels with busulphan because of the risk of inducing long-standing hypoplasia. However, it is possible to maintain levels around 5×10^9/l by giving busulphan at a daily dose of 2 mg in combination with mercaptopurine or thioguanine at a daily dose of 80 mg for up to 5 days per week (Allen et al, 1978). The possibility that the stabilisation of the TLC at 5×10^9/l by this method may prolong the chronic phase is being tested in a current MRC trial.

Evidence that early splenectomy might prolong the duration of the chronic phase by removing an organ where malignant clones were frequently generated led to several trials of elective splenectomy, a retrospective survey of 26 cases having suggested possible benefit (Spiers et al, 1975). None of the trials has shown any evidence that elective splenectomy prolongs the chronic phase (Ihde et al, 1976; Italian Cooperative Study Group, 1978; Parish & Cuckle, 1980). In the MRC trial data were collected to discover whether the quality of life was better after transformation for patients who had undergone splenectomy, compared with those who had not, but no difference was found.

It might be supposed that if the entire population of Ph'+ cells could be destroyed, regeneration of normal marrow would ensue and a complete remission result. The rare instances have been referred to above in which this has been brought about by the disease itself, with replacement of the entire chronic phase stem cell population by lymphoid phenotype BC, itself eliminated by treatment with vincristine and prednisone. Deliberate attempts have been less successful.

In the largest trial (Cunningham et al, 1979), only transient or temporary conversion to Ph'-negativity was achieved after intensive therapy in 12 out of 37 cases. The survival of the 12 patients whose marrow regenerated Ph'− cells was superior to that of the remaining patients, but since all received essentially the same treatment the authors considered that the treatment had merely selected a group with a more favourable prognosis. A logical extension of the effort to eliminate the Ph'+ clone is the use of totally ablative therapy following which no stem cells could survive to repopulate the marrow: repopulation would be accomplished by marrow transplantation. In the first trial, the donors were identical twins, which avoided the complications of graft-versus-host disease (GVHD). Since the first report (Fefer et al, 1979) with the longest follow-up of 31 months, eight patients have been treated. After a maximum follow-up of 4 years, seven patients remain Ph'−, only one having relapsed (A Fefer, personal communication). The marrow ablative therapy administered was the 'standard' schedule of high dose cyclophosphamide followed by whole body irradiation to 1000 rads. Because the median survival of conventionally treated CGL is still only about $3\frac{1}{2}$ years, it would seem that marrow ablative therapy followed by marrow transplantation from an identical twin may be the best treatment for chronic-phase CGL, unfortunately available for only a select few. The extension to a larger number of patients by accepting matched siblings as donors must be considered in the light of the high frequency of serious, often fatal GVHD. However, initially, while experience was being gained, some form of selection of recipients might be used, for example, younger patients with poor prognostic features at presentation (Jacquillat et al, 1976; Monfardini et al, 1973; Parish & Cuckle, 1980) whose leucocyte count after an initial course of busulphan therapy increased with a short doubling time, because it is known that long doubling time is associated with a better prognosis (Bergsagal, 1967).

THE CHRONIC LYMPHOID LEUKAEMIAS

The recent application to the lymphoid leukaemias of new methods for identifying specific markers for different lymphocyte populations has shown that much of the well known clinical variability is due to the existence of distinct entities that were formerly unrecognised. Each form of leukaemia is considered to represent the proliferation of a target cell that might belong to any one of several subsets of lymphocytes, in either the B or T differentiation pathways, maturation being arrested at different stages in different conditions. It is certain that as the methods for identifying particular phenotypes are improved, simplified and adapted for routine use, a much higher proportion of cases will be accurately typed than is now possible. A wide range of immunological markers is already available and the introduction of commercially available monoclonal antibodies against specific cell components will permit the characterization of cells from individual cases with a precision that is still limited to specialist laboratories. It is important to emphasise, however, that the process of integrating the results of marker studies with cytomorphological, ultra-structural, histological, cytogenetic, cytochemical and biochemical information on the one hand, and epidemiological, clinical, treatment response, and survival patterns, on the other is still in progress, and the current trend towards characterising more 'entities' seems likely to continue, with clinical usefulness as the pragmatic criterion for their ultimate acceptance. The most likely development in the next few years will be improvement in the general characterisation of the T-cell leukaemias and it is probable that particular clinical and haematological features will come to be associated with different subsets of T lymphocytes. At present, therefore, any classification of the chronic lymphoid leukaemias must be regarded as provisional and subject to refinement or revision.

For the present account the following classification is offered:

B-cell chronic lymphoid leukaemias

Chronic lymphocytic leukaemia (B-CLL): the most common chronic lymphoid leukaemia; rare below age 40; rare in the Far East; increased incidence in first degree relatives; regular pattern of clinical and haematological evolution; target cell an early B lymphocyte with characteristic morphology and ultrastructure, monoclonal surface membrane immunologlobulin (SmIg) (M, D, or both) at low density, and receptor for mouse erythrocytes on a high proportion of cells; lymph-node histology that of small-cell lymphocytic lymphoma. Disease may be static for long periods.

Prolymphocytic leukaemia (B-PLL): rare; exceptional below age 60; early splenic enlargement; lymph nodes not enlarged, or minimally enlarged except terminally; target cell a later B lymphocyte with characteristic morphology and ultrastructure, monoclonal SmIg at high density and mouse erythrocyte receptor on low proportion of cells. Disease always progressive.

Hairy cell leukaemia (B-HCL): probably less uncommon than PLL; occurs from third decade onwards; early marrow infiltration and splenic enlargement; lymph-node enlargement uncommon; target cell a later B lymphocyte than that of PLL with characteristic morphology and ultrastructure; tartrate-resistant acid phosphatase positivity characteristic though not entirely specific; the cells secrete SmIg with the same light chain but sometimes more than one heavy chain including A or G; they are weakly phagocytic. Disease may be static for long periods, and may remit spon-taneously.

T-cell chronic lymphoid leukaemias

Small cell chronic lymphocytic leukaemia (T-CLL): all ages, including first two decades; early splenic enlargement, lymphocytosis high in proportion to marrow infiltration; skin lesions common; characteristic morphology and ultrastructure of Tγ lymphocyte with cytoplasmic acid-phosphatase-positive granules and parallel tubular arrays. Variable course, may be static or slowly progressive for several years.

Prolymphocytic leukaemia (T-PLL): clinical features and cytomorphology indis-tinguishable from B-PLL but lymph-node involvement probably more frequent;

transmission electron microscopy shows cytoplasmic granules in some cells; acid-phosphatase reactivity variable, and localised to granules; localised acid α-naphthyl acetate esterase positivity favours Tμ origin.

Pleomorphic cell leukaemia (Japanese adult T-cell leukaemia): in Japan largely confined to persons above age 40 born on Kyushu island; sporadic elsewhere; subacute course; some features merge with those of cutaneous T-cell lymphoma; target cell a large pleomorphic cell with Tγ features.

Hairy cell leukaemia (T-HCL): very rare; clinically resembles B-HCL but target cells have T-cell features.

B-CELL CHRONIC LYMPHOCYTIC LEUKAEMIA

Features of prognostic significance

In the past, authors stressed the great variability of CLL and the consequent difficulty in arriving at a policy of treatment that would suit all patients. Some part of the variability is accounted for by the inclusion of cases that would now be regarded as examples of follicular lymphoma, diffuse lymphomas with lymphocytosis and marrow infiltration, hairy cell leukaemia, prolymphocytic leukaemia, Waldenström's macro-globulinaemia and the allied IgG- and IgA-secreting lymphoplasmacytoid lymphomas, as well as the T-cell leukaemias and lymphomas. This problem should be largely solved in current clinical trials such as that of the Medical Research Council (MRC), in which the diagnosis in every case is supported by comprehensive morphological, cytochemical and immunological marker findings. However, most of the variability results from two features; first, patients present at different stages in the evolution of a very chronic disease; and secondly, the rate of progression at all stages may be either so slow as to be essentially static even though complications arising from autoimmune phenomena, hyersplenism, bone-marrow failure, or immunodeficiency, cause serious illness with a downhill course in what is basically essentially static disease, or the disease itself may progress relentlessly. Two methods have been used in attempts to identify groups of patients with differing prognosis. Both rely on simply obtained clinical and haematological data, the first by arranging the items empirically in the attempt to identify the stage of the disease (the staging systems of Rai et al (1975), Binet et al (1977), Rundles & Moore (1978)), the second by using multivariate analysis of many features recorded at presentation so permitting the recognition of major features of independent prognostic significance which can be combined to define groups of good and poor risk patients (Binet et al, 1980).

The first staging system of Rai et al is the best known and its original form was as follows:

Stage 0	lymphocyte count $>15 \times 10^9/l$ and lymphocytes >40 per cent of bone marrow cells
Stage I	as above with enlarged lymph nodes
Stage II	as 0 or I with enlarged liver, spleen or both
Stage III	as 0, I, or II but haemoglobin concentration $<10\,g/dl$
Stage IV	as 0, I, II or III but platelet count $<100 \times 10^9/l$

When applied to four series of 125, 83, 152 and 167 cases (Rai et al, 1975; Boggs et al, 1966; Hansen, 1973; Phillips et al, 1977) this staging system gave median durations of survival of 150 to 180 months for stage 0, 60 to 130 for stage I, 47 to 108 for stage II, 9 to 26 for stage III, and 19 to 42 for stage IV. Although there is a clear trend for shorter survival with advancing stage, there is wide overlap between I and II, and no prognostic discrimination in III and IV. Binet et al found the same general pattern by applying all three staging systems to two series of 86 and 169 patients followed up for 120 and 42 months. Better prognostic discrimination was, however, obtained by using the three following prognostic groupings arrived at by multivariate analysis:

Group A (good prognosis) Hb > 10 g/dl, platelet count > 100×10^9/l, fewer than three sites of palpable organ enlargement.

Group C (poor prognosis) Hb ⩽ 10 g/dl or platelets ⩽ 100×10^9/l.

Group B (intermediate prognosis) Hb and platelets as A but three or more sites of palpable organ enlargement. A 'site of organ enlargement' means palpable enlargement of the spleen or liver, or of nodes in the neck, or axillae, or groins.

The three staging systems and the prognostic groupings of Binet et al are simple to apply and it is to be hoped that their relative merits will be assessed in prospective clinical trials with the possibility of further improvement. None of the systems incorporates a means of assessing whether the disease is static or progressive. In the past many physicians have been reluctant to treat patients with static disease regardless of its apparent stage of advancement. However, it is possible that the duration of survival might be influenced by treatment in static disease, but to discover whether this is so in a prospective trial it is necessary to be able to discriminate between static and progressive disease. In the current MRC Trial progressive disease is defined as follows for Rai stages I and II (patients in the later stages are assumed to have progressive disease although as described above 'progression' in some cases may be secondary in character): a persistent downward trend in either haemoglobin or platelet count towards the values which define stages III and IV, accompanied by one or more of the following, or any two if the haemoglobin and platelets are not falling: (1) a significant increase in physical signs; (2) a consistent upward trend in the lymphocyte count, doubling within 12 months; (3) constitutional symptoms (for example, weight loss, sweating, malaise). In individual cases of static disease, the activity of the disease may change after months or years of observation, and from then on the course will be progressive. On the other hand the course in a case of progressive disease has not been observed to change to a static character.

It should be noted that attempts to determine the possible prognostic significance of certain features considered in isolation may be potentially misleading unless allowance is made for the major determinants of prognosis such as those used in the Binet groupings. For example, in one study large cells were associated with good prognosis (Peterson et al, 1975), but in two others (Gray et al, 1974; Dubner et al, 1978) with poor prognosis. In a follow-up of the first study, the favourable prognostic significance of large cells disappeared when clinical stage was taken into account (Peterson et al, 1980).

The biology of the B-CLL lymphocyte

B-CLL is now accepted as a monoclonal proliferation of an early B lymphocyte whose descendants perpetuate its immunological immaturity but are markedly defective in undergoing further immunological maturation when activated by the stimulus to which their normal counterparts respond. They are long-lived cells and some of their properties may reflect their age rather than those of their normal counterpart. The evidence for monoclonality is largely immunological. Thus, in many cases the maturation arrest is not absolute, and subclones of cells proceed to synthesise and secrete free light chains with appear in the urine; these are always monoclonal (Brouet & Seligmann, 1977). Occasionally monoclonal paraproteins appear in the serum. Rarely, the cytoplasm of some of the lymphocytes contains amorphous or crystalline inclusions that have been proved to consist of monoclonal Ig (Cawley et al, 1973; Clark et al, 1973; Neis et al, 1976), often with K light chains in the amorphous (Smith et al, 1977) and λ chains in the crystalline inclusions (Cawley et al, 1976). The heavy chains of the SmIg on B-CLL lymphocytes have been shown to be homogeneous in respect of their subclass, Gm allotype, and idiotypic specificity of the variable region (Froland et al, 1972; Fu et al, 1974; Salsano et al, 1974; Schroer et al, 1974). In rare cases the idiotypic identity of the variable regions of both light and heavy chains has been shown by the antibody specificity of the SmIg, for example anti-Forssmann activity against sheep erythrocytes (Brouet & Prieur, 1974) or rheumatoid factor activity against IgG (Preud'homme & Seligmann, 1972).

B-CLL lymphocytes appear to migrate and recirculate in an orderly manner, accumulating in the bone marrow, blood, lymph nodes, spleen, and hepatic portal tracts, and they enter lymph nodes through the high-endothelium of the post-capillary venules (Manaster et al, 1973), leaving via the thoracic duct, though more slowly than normal B-lymphocytes (Flad et al, 1973; Bremer et al, 1978). They proliferate more slowly than normal lymphocytes, but when the total lymphocyte mass (TLM) is very large, the total production rate is higher than normal (Theml et al, 1973; Stryckmans et al, 1977). Measurements of the DNA content of the individual cells in large populations of both peripheral blood and bone-marrow lymphocytes by flow cytometric analysis has confirmed the results of cytokinetic measurements, indicating a diploid content for all but a tiny minority of the cells (Andreff et al, 1980).

Morphologically, by light and electron microscopy, intact B-CLL cells are indistinguishable from normal B-lymphocytes, but, characteristically, a variable, sometimes high proportion of peripheral blood lymphocytes form smudge cells in films; marrow lymphocytes in the same case, however, often show little or no tendency to form smudge cells. Other evidence also suggests that the cells in different tissues have different properties. Thus, a high proportion of peripheral blood lymphocytes in B-CLL form rosettes when incubated with mouse erythrocytes (Stathopoulos & Davies, 1976; Catovsky et al, 1979), but a lower proportion of those from the spleen and fewer still from the bone marrow and lymph nodes do so (Catovsky et al, 1979; Cherchi & Catovsky, 1980). Perhaps these differences indicate the retention by CLL lymphocytes of the capacity to respond to signals that direct the migration and recirculation of their normal counterparts. However, no subset of normal B lymphocytes has yet been found in which all the recorded features are the same as in B-CLL cells. Some B-CLL cells in the spleen and lymph nodes appear to undergo further immunological maturation than do those in the blood, as shown by the presence of SmIgG (Catovsky et al, 1979).

The size distribution of B-CLL cells in the peripheral blood may be accurately determined by cell volume measurement on the Coulter ZB1 counter linked to a channelyser (Costello et al, 1980). B-CLL lymphocyte populations prove to be remarkably homogeneous in size. The homogeneity has also been demonstrated by equilibrium centrifugation on linear density gradients of polysucrose-metrizoate (Huber et al, 1978). B-CLL cells have a high buoyant density, and are distinct from the low buoyant density follicular centre B cells.

Unlike normal peripheral blood B lymphocytes, a high proportion of B-CLL cells are retained when passed through a polystyrene-bead column, and they are ultrasensitive to destruction when exposed to colchicine at high dilution (10^{-6} M) (Thompson et al, 1972; 1974). Their content of some but not all plasma-membrane enzyme is very low, suggesting that an unbalanced age distribution alone does not account for the findings. The values for alkaline phosphatase and alkaline phosphodiesterase I were found to be normal (Kramers et al, 1978), whereas those for L-γ-glutamyl-transpeptidase, maltase, trehalase, leucine aminopeptidase, and 5'-nucleotidase were very low (Kramers et al, 1978; La Mantia et al, 1977; Kramers & Catovsky, 1978). Ramot et al (1976) have shown that the activity of several lymphocyte enzymes exhibits circadian rhythm. In B-CLL, the rhythm is retained but with a variable phase shift, each patient showing an individual pattern of activity.

The fluidity of the plasma membrane lipids as shown by fluorescence polarisation and the fluorescent lifetime of the probe 1:6 diphenyl-hexatriene has been found to be the same in normal and B-CLL lymphocytes (Johnson & Kramers, 1978). Nevertheless the mobility of the mannosyl binding sites for the lectin concanavalin A (Con-A) in the plasma membrane is markedly reduced in CLL cells, as well as in those of other lymphoproliferative diseases, as shown by the impaired capping when the cells are exposed to fluorescent Con-A (Ben-Bassat et al, 1974; 1980). The receptors for other mitogens thought to activate B lymphocytes (anti-β_2-microglobulin, sepharose-bound protein A, anti-F(ab^1)$_2$ Ig serum) also cap poorly, and the cells transform poorly (Godal et al, 1978). However, Autio et al (1978) found that CLL cells would respond normally to *Staphylococcus aureus* protein A if they were cultured in the presence of fetal calf serum. Normal lymphocytes exposed to Sendai virus release interferon; CLL lymphocytes release significantly less (Chisholm & Cartwright, 1978).

The overall surface marker profile of the B-CLL lymphocyte is that of a B-cell at an early stage of immunological maturation. The B-CLL cell has lost the cytoplasmic IgM of the pre-B cell, and has just begun to synthesise SmIgM, or SmIgM and D. In about 20 per cent of cases SmIg is undetectable by routine methods, and occasionally only light chains are demonstrable (Jayaswal et al, 1977; Catovsky et al, 1978). The B-CLL cell possesses receptors for one portion of the third component of complement C3d, and receptors for mouse erythrocytes (Catovsky et al, 1979; Stathopoulos & Elliott, 1974) the expression of which appears to be confined to a short phase during normal B-cell maturation (Forbes & Zalewski, 1976; Gupta et al, 1976).

The CLL clone accumulates because its members are incapable of, or have a severely restricted capacity for, undergoing further maturation in response to physiological stimuli. Many of the defects summarized earlier are likely to be acquired as a result of the prolonged survival of these unresponsive cells; the fundamental defect remains unknown.

The accumulation of long lived B lymphocytes accounts for most of the features of static CLL, and the proliferative element appears to be minimal. In progressive disease however, the proliferative element dominates as shown by the rapid enlargement of involved organs, the short doubling time of the lymphocyte counts, and the speed of progression towards bone-marrow failure. In some cases acceleration of the tempo of the disease is accompanied by an increasing proportion of large anaplastic pleomorphic lymphocytes often with prominent nucleoli: these 'prolymphocytoid' cells bear the same immunological markers as the population of small lymphocytes among which they appear, and must not be confused with the more homogeneous populations of large lymphoid cells of prolymphocytic leukaemia (PLL) which carry different immunological markers (Enno et al, 1979).

Circulating T-lymphocytes in B-CLL
As the monoclone of B lymphocytes expands during the evolution of CLL the proportion of T-cells falls (Foa et al, 1979). However, the absolute number is increased in 30 to 80 per cent of cases (Fernandez et al, 1975; Mellstedt et al, 1978; Foa et al, 1979) and may reach $20 \times 10^9/l$. The increase is evidently confined to the Tγ (suppressor) subset of T lymphocytes (Lauria et al, 1980), and may represent a response to the increasing numbers of B cells. The absolute numbers of Tμ (helper) cells in B-CLL blood is normal, but Chiorazzi et al (1979) have reported a helper-cell defect in CLL. It is possible that the increase in Tγ cells may play a part in the falling concentrations of serum Ig as the disease progresses because following splenic irradiation in a case of B-CLL the reversed Tγ/Tμ ratio became normal and the serum Ig concentrations increased towards the normal range (Catovsky et al, 1980).

B-prolymphocytic leukaemia (B-PLL)
B-PLL is a rare variant of B-CLL most likely to be found in elderly subjects (Galton et al, 1974). The disease is apparently always progressive and usually presents at an advanced stage, with splenic enlargement but little or no peripheral lymph-node enlargement, and impaired marrow function. The leucocyte counts are typically very high, occasionally up to $1000 \times 10^9/l$, due to the presence of the characteristic PLL cell.

B-PLL Cells
In peripheral blood films PLL cell populations appear homogeneous in any one case, but in different cases, the cells vary in size from slightly to considerably larger than the small lymphocytes of B-CLL. In contrast to B-CLL, PLL cells show little tendency to smudge. The nuclei are slightly to moderately larger than those of B-CLL, and there is usually relatively more cytoplasm. The chromatin is condensed, though less coarsely in the cases with larger cells, but in all cases the striking feature is the presence in almost every cell of a large conspicuous nucleolus. This, and the absence of smudge cells are the chief distinguishing features in the small-cell cases. In the large-cell cases the nucleus may be irregular in shape, or deeply notched. All of these features are clearly demonstrable by electron microscopy (Costello et al, 1980). The homogeneity of size of the cells of PLL populations, and their larger modal size

as compared with CLL are shown by cell-volume measurements (Costello et al, 1980b).

The migration routes and homing pattern of B-PLL cells differ from those of B-CLL: in both conditions the blood and bone-marrow are involved at an early stage, but whereas in CLL, lymph-node enlargement usually precedes splenic enlargement, often by many years, in PLL splenic enlargement appears early, while lymph-node enlargement if it occurs at all, is a late event. The histological pattern of early lymph node involvement is therefore not known, and the single case in which the follicular mantle-zone involvement was prominent may not be characteristic (Palleson et al, 1979). The pattern of splenic involvement is similar in PLL and CLL with dense often bizonal accumulation of lymphocytes in the white pulp, and diffuse infiltration of the red pulp (Bearman et al, 1978; Lampert et al, 1980). In both conditions the bone marrow infiltrates are primarily central or intramedullary and not paratrabecular (Lampert et al, 1980).

The surface membrane properties on which migration routes and homing patterns depend are unknown. However, B-PLL lymphocytes differ markedly from B-CLL cells in their SmIg content and in their capacity to form mouse red cell rosettes. In standard fluorescence tests for SmIg, PLL cells fluoresce strongly, CLL cells weakly or not at all (Catovsky et al, 1979), while measurements of the number of SmIg sites per cell have shown 6 or more times as many sites on PLL as on CLL cells (Dighiero et al, 1980). Whereas CLL cells readily form rosettes with mouse red cells, PLL cells do not in most cases (Catovsky et al, 1979). A paraprotein is found in the urine or serum in a higher proportion of cases of B-PLL than in B-CLL. Thus the B-PLL target cell appears to be at a more advanced stage of immunological maturation than the B-CLL cell.

Hairy-cell leukaemia

Hairy-cell leukaemia (HCL) is now generally accepted as a B-lymphoproliferative disease (Catovsky, 1977; Burns et al, 1977; Cawley et al, 1979), although rare cases with T-cell features have been recorded (Cawley et al, 1978; Advani et al, 1976; Hernandez et al, 1976; Saxon et al, 1978). Although the characteristic hairy cells are so distinctive by light microscopy (LM), by scanning (SEM) and transmission electron microscopy (TEM) and in their enzyme and immunological features, their normal counterpart is unknown. HCL is commoner in males, and occurs in the third and fourth decades as well as at older ages. Clinically it is characterized by progressive splenomegaly associated with hypersplenism, progressive impairment of bone-marrow function leading to marrow failure, the appearance in the blood and bone marrow of hairy cells, and monocytopenia is characteristic (Catovsky et al, 1974; Golomb et al, 1978; Turner & Kjeldsberg, 1978).

Hairy cells

The morphology of hairy cells as seen by LM, SEM, and TEM is now well known (Catovsky, 1977; Sweet et al, 1977). Hairy cells are on average considerably larger than small lymphocytes, and histograms made from cell volume channelyser measurements also show a greater variability than do cell populations in other B-lymphoproliferative conditions (Costello et al, 1980b). In most but not all cases (Catovsky, 1977), the cells contain the tartrate-resistant isoenzyme 5 of acid phosphatase but this property, though characteristic, is not specific for HCL and has been found in occasional cases of B-PLL (Buskard et al, 1976), T-PLL (Löffler et al, 1977), and T-CLL (Catovsky et al, 1979). A characteristic crescentic pattern of granular positivity to α-naphthyl butyrate esterase has been reported for hairy cells (Higgy et al, 1978), and the reaction is not fluoride-sensitive. In this reaction, the proportion of positive mononuclear cells is higher than that of cells identifiable as hairy cells in Romanowsky-stained films.

Hairy cells share some properties with monocytes but they lack the major characteristics of monocytes (Catovsky, 1977; Golom et al, 1978). They adhere to glass, are feebly phagocytic, and possibly bactericidal, and they possess strong Fc receptors for IgG (Rieber et al, 1976). However, their dominant features are those of B cells. They bear SmIg with a single light chain, though often with more than one heavy-chain isotype (Catovsky, 1977; Burns et al, 1978; Jansen et al, 1979; Rieber et al, 1979), and occasionally a paraprotein appears in the serum (Cawley et al, 1979). The SmIg has been shown to be secreted by the hairy cells and is not extrinsic Ig bound to the Fc receptors (Rieber et al, 1976; Burns et al, 1978). Hairy cells form rosettes with mouse red cells, though less avidly than do CLL cells (Catovsky et al, 1979).

T-CELL CHRONIC LYMPHOID LEUKAEMIAS

The T-cell chronic leukaemias are very uncommon and full descriptions of their characteristics are therefore accumulating only slowly. 'New' diseases are always first differentiated from similar diseases by their more extreme variants, and it is therefore not surprising that at present T-CLL and more especially the Japanese pleomorphic T-cell leukaemia seem to possess distinctive features. However, T-PLL and the even more uncommon T-HCL appear clinically and haematologically similar to the commoner B-cell diseases. Skin involvement appears to be a feature in a high proportion of cases in all types of chronic T-cell leukaemias as it is in the T-cell lymphomas, while lymph-node enlargement as well as splenomegaly appears to be a feature of T-PLL.

T-CLL

T-CLL is very uncommon, but until immunological characterisation of the chronic lymphoid leukaemias becomes routine it would be premature to quote an incidence rate. Published reports (Sumiya et al, 1973; Yodoi et al, 1974; Brouet et al, 1975; Uchiyama et al, 1977; Saxon et al, 1979) and experience in the MRC Leukaemia Unit indicate a variable clinical presentation, but a pattern is emerging. Unlike B-CLL, T-CLL has been recorded in the first three decades of life as well as in older subjects. It has been diagnosed by chance following routine blood tests, and in some of these cases the course has been similar to that of Stage 0 B-CLL. Splenomegaly tends to be a prominent feature, skin lesions are common, and the extent of lymphocytic infiltration of the bone marrow is less than would be expected from the lymphocyte count.

T-CLL lymphocyte populations have a homogeneous appearance in stained blood films and there are few smudge cells. Their nuclei resemble those of B-CLL cells, but the cells are slightly larger because there is usually a wider rim of grey-blue cytoplasm and unlike the cytoplasm of B-CLL cells, that of T-CLL cells contains azurophilic granules varying in number and size, the larger ones sometimes being irregular in shape. These granules on transmission electron microscopy have been shown to contain acid phosphatase which is tartrate sensitive except in rare cases (Catovsky et al, 1979). At TEM parallel tubular arrays (Brunning & Parkin, 1975), which are thought to be confined to Tγ cells, are a common feature (McKenna et al, 1977; Costello et al, 1980a) and can be identified with the large irregular azurophilic granules of LM (Costello et al, 1980a). T-CLL cells are also rich in β-glucuronidase, alkaline phosphatase, N-acetyl-β-glucosaminidase, and α-L-fucosidase, in all of which B-CLL cells are deficient (Brouet et al, 1975; Crockard et al, 1979). T-CLL cells (Catovsky & Costello, 1979) usually do not show the strong localised positivity for acid α-naphthyl-acetate esterase found in Tμ cells (Grossi et al, 1978), while their frequent capacity to form EA (IgG) rosettes and their poor growth in culture (Catovsky et al, 1979) also suggest that they are usually Tγ cells. However in one case (Saxon et al, 1979) both Tγ and Tμ cells were identified suggesting origin from an uncommitted precursor.

T-PLL

In contrast to the extreme rarity of T-CLL in relation to B-CLL, about one fifth of all PLL patients appear to have T-PLL (Catovsky, 1980). They include a higher proportion of patients under age 70 than is found in B-PLL and the prognosis of T-PLL appears to be even worse than that of B-PLL (Catovsky, 1980). Otherwise the clinical and haematological features are similar, though enlarged lymph nodes are sometimes found in T-PLL.

T-PLL cells resemble B-PLL cells in Romanowsky-stained films, and may possess the strong localised acid α-naphthyl-acetate esterase positivity characteristic of Tμ cells (Catovsky & Costello, 1979). T-PLL cells lack the parallel tubular arrays seen by TEM in T-CLL cells.

Pleomorphic T-cell leukaemia (PTL)

Japanese authors have characterised a form of T-cell leukaemia in which almost all the patients were born in and around Kyushu (Hanaoka et al, 1979), unlike the other T-cell leukaemias in which no particular geographical distribution was recorded. It is not clear whether PTL is a disease that has recently appeared or the incidence of which has recently increased, or whether it was simply not recognised as an entity before it was possible to characterise lymphocytes immunologically.

Clinically, PTL affects adults from the third decade onwards, mostly beyond the fifth decade, with a moderate preponderance of males. A high proportion of the patients have skin lesions, enlargement of peripheral lymph nodes, spleen and liver, but mediastinal enlargement has not been recorded. The disease is refractory to treatment and most patients have died within 1 year of the time of diagnosis.

PTL cells are highly pleomorphic large cells with markedly contorted, deformed, irregularly segmented or lobed nuclei with several nucleoli. As in other chronic T-cell leukaemias they form rosettes with sheep red cells, and those tested have had features of Tγ cells (Broder et al, 1979).

Although the epidemiological significance of Japanese PTL is not yet apparent, it appears to be a distinctive syndrome. Nevertheless in some cases the features overlap with those of cutaneous T-cell lymphoma and with T-cell lymphomas in general, and it remains to be seen whether sporadic cases of typical PTL will be found in other parts of the world.

TREATMENT OF THE CHRONIC LYMPHOID LEUKAEMIAS

The evaluation of the effects of treatment in CLL has, as already discussed, always been hampered by the great variability of the disease and the lack of agreed criteria for recording the response. The availability of staging systems or prognostic groupings that are easy to apply, and in an increasing number of centres, of facilities for characterising the different types of chronic lymphoid leukaemia opens the way for designing and carrying out controlled trials of different methods of treatment. It should thus be possible to discover (1) whether the traditional view that treatment is not indicated for static, symptomless CLL without evidence of impaired marrow function is wise, or whether, as claimed by Osgood (1964) the chance of long survival is increased by long-term treatment from the time of diagnosis, (2) whether different forms of treatment are required at different stages, (3) whether the capacity to respond to treatment is inherent in the disease or whether, in particular cases, the disease may respond differently to different treatments. It is already known that the survival of patients who respond to treatment is better than those who do not, and this suggests that efforts to obtain a response may improve survival. Traditionally, there has been understandable reluctance to apply toxic, inconvenient and sometimes potentially dangerous treatment to patients who might survive for many years without treatment, but it should now be possible to assess the value of treatments with more confidence. It may also become possible to develop laboratory tests to predict the likelihood of response to particular agents. For example Bloomfield et al (1980) have shown that steroid responsiveness is associated with the presence of steroid receptors in lymphoma cells.

Unfortunately no new forms of treatment with a clear advantage have been introduced in recent years. It is possible that short courses of chlorambucil at high dosage in combination with prednisone are somewhat superior to continuous low-dose chlorambucil therapy (Sawitsky et al, 1979), and there may be some advantage in the vincristine-cyclophosphamide-prednisone combination (Liepman & Votaw, 1978). The M-2 protocol of Phillips et al (1977) involves the use of vincristine, BCNU (bis-chloroethylnitrosourea), cyclophosphamide, melphalan and prednisone; early results were encouraging but long term results are not yet available. The place of radiation therapy is uncertain. Neither whole-body irradiation (Johnson, 1977) nor mediastinal irradiation (Richards et al, 1978) has become popular, but there appears to be a case for reevaluating splenic irradiation as is being done in one arm of the current MRC Council trial where 10 fractions, each of 100 rad, are administered at weekly intervals. The rationale for this method, developed in Padua (M Fiorentino, personal communication to D Catovsky), is that the long interval between treatments allows time for the replacement of a high proportion of the splenic lymphocyte population by recirculation between treatments thus increasing the absolute number of cells killed at each exposure and reducing the likelihood of irradiating many cells already killed by the previous treatment.

In comparison with B-CLL, information on the treatment of the other chronic lymphoid leukaemias is scanty. PLL responds poorly to conventional chemotherapy,

though a few patients have responded well to doxorubicin or CHOP (cyclophosphamide, hydroxydaunorubicin, vincristine, and prednisone in combination) administered in short courses (König et al, 1979; Sibbald & Catovsky, 1979) and a higher
proportion of patients appear to respond to splenic irradiation than was formerly
reported (Catovsky, 1980); the role of splenectomy remains to be evaluated. In HCL
the indications for splenectomy have become clarified (Catovsky, 1977). In principle
the operation can help only in the presence of at least some functional bone marrow.
In planning treatment the waxing and waning character of HCL must always be
remembered: the activity of the disease may decline for long periods, and Slater et al
(1979) have reported a case in which the disease appears to have died out after many
years.

At the present time there is no solid information on the response to treatment of the
T-cell leukaemias, though the Japanese pleomorphic T-cell disease appears to be
largely refractory to treatment (Hanaoka et al, 1979).

REFERENCES

Advani S H, Talwalkar G V, Nadkarni J S, Nadkarni J J, Sirsat S M, Srinivasan V 1976 Indian Journal of
    Cancer 13: 283–287
Alimena G, Brandt L, Dallapiccola B, Mitelman F, Nilsson P G 1979 Cancer Genetics and Cytogenetics
    1: 79–85
Allan N C, Duvall E, Stockdill G 1978 The Lancet ii: 523
Andreeff M, Darzynkiewicz Z, Sharpless T K, Clarkson B D, Melamed M R 1980 Blood 55: 282–293
Athens J W, Raab S O, Haab O P, Boggs D R, Ashenbrucker H, Cartwright G E, Wintrobe M M 1965
    Journal of Clinical Investigation 44: 765–777
Atkinson K R, Kay H E M, Lawler S D, Wells D G, McElwain T J 1975 Cancer 35: 529
Autio K, Turunen O, Lundqvist C, Schröder J 1978 Clinical and Experimental Immunology 34: 188–192
Bain B J, Wickramasinghe S N 1976 Acta Haematologica 55: 89
Beard M E J, Durrant J, Catovsky D, Wiltshaw E, Amess J L, Brearley R L, Kick B, Wrigley P M F,
    Janossy G, Greaves M F, Galton D A G 1976 British Journal of Haematology 34: 169
Bearman R M, Pangalis G A, Rappaport H 1978 Cancer 42: 2360–2372
Ben-Bassat H, Goldblum N, Manny N, Sachs L 1974 International Journal of Cancer 14: 367
Ben-Bassat H, Penchas S, Polliack A, Mitrani-Rosenbaum S, Naparstek E, Matzner Y, Kedar A, Shouval
    D, Eldor A, Prokocimer M, Goldblum N 1980 Blood 55: 205–210
Binet J L, Auquier A, Dighiero G, Chastang C, Piguet H, Goasguen J, Vaugier G, Potron G, Colona P,
    Oberling F, Thomas M, Tchernia G, Jacquillat C, Boivin P, Lesty C, Duault M T, Gremy F 1981
    Cancer (in press)
Binet J-L, Leporrier M, Dighiero G, Charron D, d'Athis Ph, Vaugier G, Merle Beral H, Natali J C,
    Raphael M, Nizet M G, Follezou J Y 1977 Cancer 40: 855–864
Bloomfield C D, Smith K A, Peterson B A, Hildebrandt L, Zaleskas J, Gajl-Peczalska K J, Frizzera G,
    Munck A 1980 The Lancet i: 952–956
Boggs D R 1974 Blood 44: 449
Boggs D R, Sofferman S A, Wintrobe M M, Cartwright G E 1966 American Journal of Medicine 40: 243
Brandt L 1965 Scandinavian Journal of Haematology 2: 126
Brandt L, Mitelman F, Panani A, Lenner H C 1976 Scandinavian Journal of Haematology 16: 321–325
Bremer K, Engeset A, Fröland S S 1978 Lymphology 11: 231–237
Breton-Gorius J, Reyes F, Vernant J P, Tulliez M, Dreyfus B 1978 British Journal of Haematology
    39: 295–303
Broder S, Uchiyama T, Waldmann T A 1979 American Journal of Clinical Pathology, supplement,
    72: 724–731
Brouet J-C, Flandrin G, Sasportes M, Preud'homme J-L, Seligmann M 1975 The Lancet ii: 390
Brouet J-C, Prieur A M 1974 Clinical Immunology and Immunopathology 2: 481
Brouet J-C, Seligmann M 1977 In: Galton D A G (ed) The Chronic Leukaemias. Clinics in Haematology,
    vol 6. W B Saunders, London p 169–184
Broxmeyer H E, Mendelsohn N, Moore M A S 1977 Leukemia Research 1: 3
Broxmeyer H E, Moore M A S, Ralph P 1977 Experimental Hematology 5: 87
Broxmeyer H E, Ralph P 1977 Cancer Research 37: 3578

Broxmeyer H E, Smithyman A, Eger R R, Meyers P A, de Sousa M 1978 Joural of Experimental Medicine 148: 1052
Brunning R D, Parkin J 1975 American Journal of Pathology 78: 59
Burns G F, Cawley J C, Barker C R, Goldstone A H, Hayhoe F G J 1977 British Journal of Haematology 36: 71
Burns G F, Cawley J C, Worman C P, Karpas A, Barker C R, Goldstone A H, Hayhoe F G H 1978 Blood 52: 1132–1147
Buskard N A, Catovsky D, Okos A, Goldman J M, Galton D A G 1976 Hämatologie und Bluttransfusion 18: 237–253
Canellos G P, Whang-Peng J 1972 The Lancet ii: 1227.
Catovsky D 1977 In: Galton D A G (ed) Clinics in haematology. The Chronic Leukaemias. W B Saunders, London pp 245–268
Catovsky D 1979 British Journal of Haematology 42: 493–498
Catovsky D 1980 In: Gunz F W & Henderson E S (eds) Leukemia. Grune and Stratton, New York
Catovsky D, Cherchi M, Galton D A G, Hoffbrand A V, Ganeshaguru K 1978 In: Clarkson B, Marks P A, Till J E (eds) Differentiation of normal and neoplastic hematopoietic cells. Cold Spring Harbor Laboratory, p 811–822
Catovsky D, Costello C, O'Brien M, Cherchi M 1979 In: Neth R, Gallo R C, Hofschneider P-H, Mannweiler K (eds) Modern trends in human leukemia III. Springer, Berlin, p 107–113
Catovsky D, Lauria F, Matutues E, Foa R, Mantovani V, Tura S, Galton D A G 1980 Submitted to British Journal of Haematology
Catovsky D, Pettit J E, Galetto J, Okos A, Galton D A G 1974 British Journal of Haematology 26: 29–37
Catovsky D, Pittman S, O'Brien M, Cherchi M, Costello C, Foa F, Pearce E, Hoffbrand A V, Janossy G, Ganeshaguru K, Greaves M F 1979 American Journal of Clinical Pathology 72: (supplement) 736–745
Cawley J C, Barker C R, Britchford R D, Smith J L 1973 Clinical and Experimental Immunology 13: 407
Cawley J C, Burns G F, Bevan A, Worman C P, Smith J L, Gray L, Barker C R, Hayhoe F G J 1979 British Journal of Haematology 43: 215–221
Cawley J C, Burns G F, Nash T A, Higgy K E, Child J A, Roberts B E 1978 Blood 51: 61–69
Cawley J C, Smith J, Goldstone A H, Emmines J, Hamblin J, Hough L 1976 Clinical and Experimental Immunology 23: 78
Cherchi M, Catovsky D 1980 Clinical and Experimental Immunology 39: 411–415
Chessells J M, Janossy G, Lawler S D, Secker Walker L 1979 British Journal of Haematology 41: 25–41
Chikkappa G, Boecker W R, Carsten A L, Cronkite E P, Ohl S 1973 Journal of Clinical Investigation 52: 18a (Proceedings of the Annual Meeting of the American Society for Clinical Investigation, Atlantic City)
Chiorazzi N, Fu S M, Montazeri G, Kunkel H G, Rai K, Gee T 1979 Journal of Immunology 122: 1087–1090
Chisholm M, Cartwright T 1978 British Journal of Haematology 40: 43–50
Chiyoda S, Kinugasa K 1978 Acta Haematologica Japonica 41: 564–566
Clark C, Rydell R E, Kaplan M E 1973 New England Journal of Medicine 289: 113
Costello C, Catovsky D, O'Brien M, Galton D A G 1980a British Journal of Haematology 44: 389–394
Costello C, Wardle J, Catovsky D, Lewis S M 1980b British Journal of Haematology 45: 209–214
Cunningham I, Gee T, Dowling M, Chaganti R, Bailey R, Hopfan S, Bowden L, Turnbull A, Knapper W, Clarkson B 1979 Blood 53: 375–395
Dighiero G, Bodega E, Mayzner R, Binet J L 1980 Blood 55: 93–100
Dancey J T, Deubelbeiss K A, Harker L A, Finch C A 1976 Journal of Clinical Investigation 58: 705
Douglas I D C, Wiltshaw E 1978 British Journal of Haematology 40: 59
Dubner H N, Crowley J J, Schilling R F 1978 American Journal of Hematology 4: 337–341
El-Maalem H, Fletcher J 1976 British Journal of Haematology 34: 95–103
Enno A, Catovsky D, O'Brien M, Cherchi M, Kumaran T O, Galton D A G 1979 British Journal of Haematology 41: 9–18
Fefer A, Cheever M A, Thomas E D, Boyd C, Ramberg R, Glucksberg H, Buckner C D, Storb R 1979 The New England Journal of Medicine 300: 333–361
Fernandez L A, MacSween J M, Langley G R 1975 Immunology 28: 231–241
Fialkow P J, Jacobson R J, Papayannopoulou T 1977 American Journal of Medicine 63: 125
Finney R, McDonald G A, Baikie A G, Douglas A S 1972 British Journal of Haematology 23: 283–288
Flad G D, Huber C, Bremer K, Menne H D, Huber H 1973 European Journal of Immunology 3: 688–693
Foa R, Catovsky D, Brozovic M, Marsh G W, Ooyirilangkumaran T, Cherchi M, Galton D A G 1979 Cancer 44: 483–487
Forbes I J, Zalewski P D 1976 Clinical and Experimental Immunology 26: 99

Froland S S, Natvig J B, Stavem P 1972 Scandinavian Journal of Immunology 1: 351
Fu S M, Winchester R J, Feizi T, Walzer P D, Kunkel H G 1974 Proceedings of the National Academy of
    Science 71: 4487–4490
Gahrton G, Lindsten J, Zech L 1974 Blood 43: 837–840
Galbraith P R, Abu-Zhara H T 1972 British Journal of Haematology 22: 135–143
Galton D A G 1962 In: The Scientific Basis of Medicine Annual Reviews. Athlone Press, London.
    p 152–171
Galton D A G, Goldman J M, Wiltshaw E, Catovsky D, Henry K, Goldenberg G J 1974 British Journal of
    Haematology 27: 7
Gatti R A, Robinson W A, Deinard A S, Nesbit M, McCullough J J 1973 Blood 41: 771
Godal T, Henriksen A, Iversen J-G, Landaas T, Lindmo T 1978 International Journal of Cancer
    21: 561–569
Golde D W, Bersch N L, Sparkes R S 1976 Cancer 37: 1849–1852
Goldman J M, Catovsky D, Hows J, Spiers A S D, Galton D A G 1979 British Medical Journal
    1: 1310–1313
Goldman J M, Shiota Faith, Th'ng K H, Orchard Kin 1980 British Journal of Haematology 46: 7–13
Goldman J M, Th'ng K H 1973 British Journal of Haematology 25: 299–308
Golomb H M, Catovsky D, Golde D W 1978 Annals of Internal Medicine 89: 677–683
Gomez G, Hossfeld D K, Sokal J E 1975 British Medical Journal 1: 421
Gray J L, Jacobs A, Block M 1974 Cancer 33: 1169–1178
Greaves M F, Verbi W, Reeves B R, Hoffbrand A V, Drysdale H C, Jones L, Sacker L S, Samaratunga I
    1979 Leukaemia Research 3: 181–191
Grossi C E, Webb S R, Zicca A, Lydyard P M, Moretta L, Mingari M C, Cooper M D 1978 Journal of
    Experimental Medicine 147: 1405
Grouchy J de, Nava C de, Feingold J, Bilsky-Pasquier G, Bousser J 1968 European Journal of Cancer
    4: 481–492
Gupta S, Good R A, Siegal F P 1976 Clinical and Experimental Immunology 26: 204
Hanaoka M, Sasaki M, Matsumoto H, Tankawa H, Yamabe H, Tomimoto K, Tasaka C, Fujiwara H,
    Uchiyama T, Takatsuki K 1979 Acta Pathologica Japonica 29: 723–738
Hansen M M 1973 Chronic lymphocytic leukaemia. Scandinavian Journal of Haematology supplement 18
Hayata I, Sakurai M, Kakati S, Sandberg A A 1975 Cancer 36: 1177–1191
Hellmann A, Goldman J M 1980 Scandinavian Journal of Haematology 24: 237–242
Hernandez D, Cruz C, Carnot J, Dorticos E, Espinosa E 1978 British Journal of Haematology 40: 504
Higgy K E, Burns G F, Hayhoe F G J 1978 British Journal of Haematology 38: 99
Huber C, Zier K, Michlmayr G, Rodt H, Nilsson K, Theml D, Lutz D, Braunsteiner H 1978 British
    Journal of Haematology 40: 93–103
Ihde D C, Canellos G P, Schwartz J H, De Vita V T 1976 Annals of Internal Medicine 84: 17-21
Italian Cooperative Study Group on Chronic Myeloid Luekemia 1978 Bolletino dell'Istituto Sieroterapico
    Milanese 47: 360
Jacquillat Cl, Chastang Cl, Tanzer J, Briere J, Weil M, Pereira-Neto M, Gemon-Auclerc M F, Schaison G,
    Domingo A, Boiron M, Bernard J 1978 Bolletino dell'Istituto Sieroterapico Milanese 57: 237–246
Janossy G, Roberts M, Greaves M F 1976 The Lancet ii: 1058–1061
Janossy G, Woodruff R K, Pippard M J, Prentice G, Hoffbrand A V, Paxton A, Lister T A, Bunch C,
    Greaves M F 1979 Cancer 43: 426–434
Jansen J, Schuit H R E, Van Zwet Th L, Meijer C J L M, Hijmans W 1979 British Journal of Haematology
    42: 21–33
Jayasawal U, Roath S, Hyde R D, Chisholm D M, Smith J L 1977 British Journal of Haematology 37: 207
Johnson R E 1977 In: Galton D A G (ed) Clinics in Haematology. The Chronic Leukaemias. W B Saunders
    Company Ltd, London. Vol 6, no 1, p 237
Johnson S M, Kramers M 1978 Biochemical and Biophysical Research Communications 80: 451–457
König E, Meusers P, Brittinger G 1979 British Journal of Haematology 42: 487–488
Kramers M T C, Catovsky D 1978 British Journal of Haematology 38: 453–462
Kramers M T C, Catovsky D, Foa R 1978 British Journal of Haematology 40: 111–118
La Mantia K, Conklyn M, Quagliata F, Silber R 1977 Blood 50: 683–689
Lampert I, Catovsky D, Marsh G W, Child J A, Galton D A G 1980 Histopathology 4: 1–17
Lauria F, Foa R, Catovsky D 1980 Scandinavian Journal of Haematology 24: 187–190
Lawler S D 1977 In: Galton D A G (ed) Clinics in haematology. The Chronic Leukaemias. W B Saunders,
    London. Vol 6, p 55–75
Liepman M, Votaw M L 1978 Cancer 41: 1664–1669
Manaster J, Frühling J, Stryckmans P 1973 Blood 41: 425
Manusow D, Weinerman B H 1975 American Medical Association Journal 232: 267–269
Marie J P, Vernant J P, Dreyfus B, Breton-Gorius J 1979 British Journal of Haematology 43: 549–558

Marks S M, Baltimore D, McCaffrey R 1978 The New England Journal of Medicine, 298: 812–814
Marmont A M, Damasio E E 1973 Acta Haematologica 50: 1–8
Mason D Y 1977 Journal of Clinical Pathology 30: 541–546
Mellstedt H, Pettersson D, Holm G 1978 Acta Medica Scandinavica 204: 485–589
Mitelman F, Levan G 1978 Hereditas 89: 207–232
Monfardini S, Gee T, Fried J, Clarkson B D 1973 Cancer 31: 492
Morley A A, Baikie A G, Galton D A G 1967 The Lancet ii: 1320–1323
McKenna R W, Parkin J, Kersey J H, Gajl-Peczalska K J, Peterson L, Brunning R D 1977 American
    Journal of Medicine 62: 588
Neis K M, Marshall J, Oberlin M A, Halpern M S, Brown J C 1976 American Journal of Clinical Pathology
    65: 948
Odeberg H, Olofsson T, Olsson I 1975 British Journal of Haematology 29: 427–441
Osgood E E 1964 Journal of Nuclear Medicine 5: 139
Pallesen G, Madsen M, Pedersen B B 1979 Scandinavian Journal of Haematology 22: 407–416
Parish S, Cuckle H 1980 Report to the Medical Research Council's Annual Review Meeting on Leukaemia
    Trials (April)
Peterson L C, Bloomfield C D, Brunning R D 1980 British Journal of Haematology 45: 563–567
Peterson L C, Bloomfield C D, Sundberg R D, Gajl-Peczalska K J, Brunning R D 1975 The American
    Journal of Medicine 59: 316–322
Phillips Elizabeth A, Kempin S, Passe Sharon, Mike Valerie, Clarkson B 1977 In: Galton D A G (ed)
    Clinics in Haematology. The Chronic Leukaemias. W B Saunders Company, London vol 6, no 1, p 203
Preud'homme J L, Seligmann M 1972 Blood 40: 777
Rai K R, Sawitsky A, Cronkite E P, Chanana A D, Levy R N, Pasternack B S 1975 Blood 46: 219–234
Ramot B, Brok-Simoni F, Chweidan E, Ashkenazi Y E 1976 British Journal of Haematology 34: 79
Rausch P G, Pryzwansky K B, Spitznagel J K, Herion J C 1978 Blood Cells 4: 369–376
Richards F, Spurr C L, Feree C, Blake D D, Raben M 1978 American Journal of Medicine 64: 947–
    954
Rieber E P, Hadam M R, Linke R P, Saal J G, Riethmüller G, Von Heyden H W, Waller H D 1979 British
    Journal of Haematology 42: 175–188
Rieber E P, Saal J G, Riethmüller G, von Heyden H W, Waller H D 1976 Zeitschrift für
    Immunitätsforschung 151: 282–288
Roberts M M 1979 Maturation linked expression of antigens of normal and leukaemic cells of the human
    haemopoietic system. PhD Thesis, University of London
Rundles R W, Moore J O 1978 Cancer (suppl.) 42: 941–945
Rustin G 1980 British Journal of Haematology 45
Rustin G J S, Peters T J 1979 British Journal of Haematology 41: 533–543
Rustin G J S, Wilson P D, Peters T J 1979 Journal of Cell Science 36: 401–412
Sakurai M, Hayata I, Sandberg A A 1976 Cancer Research 36: 313–318
Sakurai M, Sandberg A A 1976 Cancer 38: 762–769
Salsano F, Froland S S, Natvig J B, Michaelsen T E 1974 Scandinavian Journal of Immunology 3: 841
Sawitsky A, Rai K R, Glidewell O, Silver R T, and participating members of CALGB 1977 Blood
    50: 1049–1059
Saxon A, Stevens R H, Golde D W 1978 Annals of Internal Medicine 88: 323–326
Saxon A, Stevens R H, Golde D W 1979 The New England Journal of Medicine 300: 700–704
Schroer K R, Briles D E, Van Boxel J A, Davie J M 1974 Journal of Experimental Medicine 140: 1416
Sibbald R, Catovsky D 1979 British Journal of Haematology 42: 488–490
Singer J W, Fialkow P J, Steinmann L, Najfeld V, Stein S J, Robinson W A 1979 Blood 53: 264–268
Smith J L, Gordon J, Newell D G, Whisson M 1977 British Journal of Haematology 37: 217
Spiers A S D, Baikie A G, Galton D A G, Richards H G H, Wiltshaw E, Goldman J M, Catovsky D,
    Spencer J, Peto R 1975 British Medical Journal 1: 175
Spiers A S D, Liew A, Baikie A G 1975 Journal of Clinical Pathology 28: 517–523
Stathopoulos G, Davies A J S 1976 The Lancet i: 1078
Stathopoulos G, Elliott E V 1974 The Lancet i: 600
Stryckmans P A, Debusscher L, Collard E 1977 In: Galton D A G (ed) The Chronic Luekaemias. Clinics in
    Haematology. W B Saunders, London, vol 6, p 21–40
Sullivan J R, Hurley T H, Bolton J H 1977 Cancer Treatment Reports 61: 43
Sumiya M, Mizoguchi H, Kosaka K, Miura Y, Takaku F, Yata J I 1973 The Lancet ii: 910
Sweet D L, Golomb H M, Ultmann J E 1977 In: Galton D A G (ed) Clinics in Haematology. The Chronic
    Leukaemias. W B Saunders, London, Vol 6, p 141–157
Theml H, Trepel F, Schick P, Kaboth W, Begemann H 1973 Blood 42: 723–736
Thomson A E R, O'Connor T W E, Wetherley-Mein G 1972 Scandinavian Journal of Haematology
    9: 231–247

Thomson A E R, O'Connor T W E, Wetherley-Mein G 1974 In: Proceedings of Eighth Leukocyte Culture Conference, New York. Academic Press, New York, p 655–671

Turner A, Kjeldsberg C R 1978 Medicine 57: 477–499

Uchiyama T, Yodoi J, Sagawa K, Takatsuki K, Uchino H 1977 Blood 50: 481–492

Ullyott J L, Bainton D F 1974 Blood 44: 469

Vicariot M, Goldman J M, Catovsky D, Galton D A G 1979 European Journal of Cancer 15: 559–563

Vodopick H, Rupp E M, Edwards C L, Goswitz F A, Beauchamp J J 1972 New England Journal of Medicine 286: 284–290

Wachstein M 1946 Journal of Laboratory and Clinical Medicine 31: 1

Wayne A W, Sharp J C, Joyner M V, Sterndale H, Pulford K A F 1979 British Journal of Haematology 43: 353–360

Woodruff R K, Malpas J S, Wrigley P F M, Lister T A, Paxton A M, Janossy G 1977 British Medical Journal 2: 1375–1376

Yodoi J, Takatsuki K, Masuda T 1974 New England Journal of Medicine 290: 572–573

10. Leukaemia and lymphoma: recent immunological and biochemical developments

G Janossy K Ganeshaguru A V Hoffbrand

INTRODUCTION

The purpose of this review is to give a 'bird's eye view' of the development of biological markers in leukaemia and lymphoma during the last four years. In 1977, a clear classification of acute lymphoblastic leukaemia (ALL) into two major groups, common non-T, non-B ALL (c-ALL) and thymic ALL (T-ALL or Thy-ALL) had already been established. The existence of rare cases with B markers (B-ALL) had also been noted (Catovsky, 1977). A highly absorbed rabbit antiserum to c-ALL was found to react not only to the vast majority of childhood non-T, non-B ALL and approximately 50 per cent of adult cases (Greaves et al, 1975) but also with 'lymphoid' blast crisis (BC) of Ph' positive chronic granulocytic leukaemia (CGL; Janossy et al, 1976; reviewed by Galton, 1977). The finding of a nuclear enzyme, terminal deoxynucleotidyl transferase (TdT) in ALL (McCaffrey et al., 1973) as well as in 'lymphoid' BC (reviewed by Wu & Gallo, 1977) had already cast some light on the further developments summarized here.

    Why do two diseases with different presentation, course, chromosome change and prognosis (i.e. the Ph'− cALL and the lymphoid BC of Ph'+ CGL) express both the c-ALL antigen and TdT (Hoffbrand et al, 1977)? A common viral pathogenesis is unlikely and there is no evidence that viruses induce the expression of TdT. A plausible explanation is that the blasts in these two diseases show the same phenotype (c-ALL+ and TdT+ but negative with T and B markers) because they express the characteristics of a normal cell type involved in both diseases. This is analogous to other diseases with different chromosome abnormalities such as acute promyelocytic leukaemia (Ch. 8) and promyelocytic blast crisis of CGL which also involve the same cell type — the promyelocyte. The difference between the two situations is that the normal promyelocyte is known, while the normal c-ALL+, TdT+ bone marrow (BM) cell has until recently been hypothetical (Greaves & Janossy, 1978). This cell's exact origin, function and developmental options are indeed still unknown.

    During the course of these recent studies, three advances have been made. First, a similar panel of membrane markers (conventional antisera standardized after absorptions) and enzyme assays have been established in a number of laboratories for leukaemia analysis (Table 10.1). By combining the study of nuclear TdT (labelled with anti-TdT serum, Bollum, 1979) and membrane markers in double colour immunofluorescence tests, the immunoenzymatic analysis of individual single cells has become feasible (Fig. 10.1). The method is simple, and double marker assays of this kind prove useful in the analysis of new specific 'monoclonal' antibodies (McAbs) on minute lymphohaemopoietic cell subpopulations.

    The second major advance has been the introduction of McAbs for leukaemia diagnosis and BM analysis. These reagents are produced in large quantities by

Table 10.1   Panel of reagents for leukaemia diagnosis*

Antibody to	Made in	References below and availability
Terminal deoxynucleotidyl transferase (TdT)	Rabbit**	1, 2; Bethesda Research Labs
Ia-like (p 28, 33)	Rabbit	3, 4, 5; Alpha-Gamma Labs, USA
	Chicken	2
	Monoclonal (mouse & rat)	6; Sera Labs, UK and other firms
Common ALL (cALL) antigen	Rabbit	7, 8
	Monoclonal (mouse)	9
Human T/thymic lymphocyte antigen (HuTLA)	Rabbit	2, 3, 10 and other laboratories
	Monoclonal (mouse)	11, 12
Human thymocyte antigen	Monoclonal (mouse)	12, 13; Sera Labs, UK
Human IgM	Goat**	3, 14 and other laboratories

* Due to lack of space only some of the relevant references are shown.
** These reagents are pure antibodies eluted from the relevant immunoadsorbent column.
(1) Bollum F J 1975 Proc Natl Acad Sci USA, 72: 4119. (2) Janossy G et al 1979 J Immunol 123: 1525. (3) Schlossman S F et al 1976 Proc Natl Acad Sci USA 73: 1288. (4) Billing R et al 1976 J Exp Med 144: 167. (5) Winchester R J et al 1977 Proc Natl Acad Sci USA 74: 4012. (6) Charron D et al 1979 Blood 54 (Suppl. 1): 82a. (7) Greaves M F & Janossy G 1978 Biochem Biophys Acta 516: 193. (8) Billing R et al 1978 J Natl Cancer Inst 61: 423. (9) Ritz J et al 1980 Nature 283: 583. (10) Touraine J I et al 1974 Clin Exp Immunol 16: 503. (11) Kung P C et al 1979 Science 206: 347. (12) Reinherz E et al 1980 Proc Natl Acad Sci 77: 1588. (13) McMichael A J et al 1979 Eur J Immunol 9: 205. (14) Gathings W E et al 1972 Eur J Immunol 7: 804.

'immortal' clones of mouse (or rat) hybrids which are each descendants of a single hybrid cell. This is formed by the fusion of an antigen stimulated B lymphocyte and a continuously growing myeloma cell (Köhler & Milstein, 1975). 'Wanted' clones are selected by screening of hundreds of clones according to the reactivity of the secreted homogeneous antibody; these react with given antigenic determinants and do not require absorption. During the last two years McAbs have confirmed the major acute leukaemia subgroups identified by conventional antisera but revealed additional heterogeneity in each group. Further comparisons between leukaemic cells and their normal equivalent cells have also been made and positive and negative selection of cells reactive with McAbs has also become possible.

The third development has been the realization that a better understanding of the antigenic and enzymatic makeup (particularly in purine metabolism) of leukaemic cells, may lead to highly selective methods of treatment.

CELLS IN NORMAL BONE MARROW

Terminal transferase positive (TdT⁺) cells

The major phenotypic groups of acute leukaemia cells are shown in Table 10.2. With the notable exception of thymic (Thy-)ALL (see below) all types seem to have corresponding cells in the normal bone marrow. The typical leukaemic blast cells in common ALL and lymphoid BC of CGL express three markers concommitantly: c-ALL and Ia-like membrane antigens and TdT in the nucleus (c-ALL⁺, Ia⁺, TdT⁺). A few cells with this phenotype can be found in normal BM (Fig. 10.2).

These antigens are now chemically defined. The c-ALL antigen is a glycosylated peripheral membrane protein, MW 100 000 (Sutherland et al, 1979), which can be modulated: on incubation with the antibody the cells temporarily lose c-ALL antigen

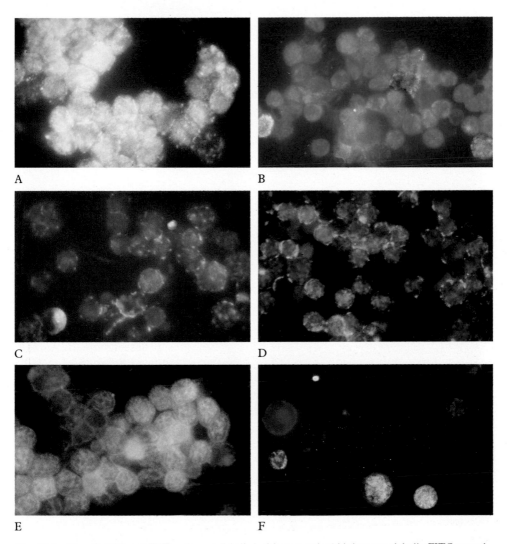

Fig. 10.1 Use of rabbit anti-TdT antiserum (labelled with goat anti-rabbit immunoglobulin-FITC second layer; green nuclear staining) in combination with other antisera for the immunological diagnosis of acute leukaemias. Figures (A), (B) and (C) were stained with the anti-TdT/anti-Ia-like antigen combination (chicken anti-human Ia and sheep anti-chicken-Ig-TRITC second layer; red membrane staining). (A) shows a case of acute undifferentiated leukaemia with the non-T, non-B ALL phenotype (TdT$^+$, Ia$^+$); (B) is a Thy-ALL (TdT$^+$, Ia$^-$) with two residual Ia$^+$, TdT$^-$ cells which probably do not belong to the leukaemic clone; (C) is an AML (TdT$^-$, Ia$^+$). Figure (D) is again a Thy-ALL. The staining is for T lymphoid antigen (HuTLA) using rabbit anti-HuTLA and goat anti-rabbit Ig-TRITC (red). The HuTLA$^+$, TdT$^+$ cells are normally absent from the bone marrow and this reagent combination can be used to monitor residual Thy-ALL blasts in treated patients. The anti-HuTLA serum is unreactive with blasts of non-T, non-B ALL phenotype. Figures (E) and (F) are stained for cytoplasmic IgM (goat anti-human IgM-TRITC: red). (E) is a pre-B ALL with the majority (but not all) of cells expressing the TdT$^+$, CyIgM$^+$ phenotype. (F) depicts a normal bone marrow sample with a typical pre-B cell (CyIgM$^+$, TdT$^-$ on the left) and two typical TdT$^+$ lymphoid precursor cells (TdT$^+$, CyIgM$^-$). The double labelled cell (TdT$^+$, CyIgM$^+$) is a very rare pre-B cell in normal marrow. This is a larger cell; some other normal TdT$^+$, CyIgM$^-$ cells (approximately 10 per cent of all TdT$^+$ cells) also have intermediate to large size (not shown). From Janossy et al,(1980a.).

Table 10.2   Markers and leukaemia phenotypes

Markers	Common non-T, non-B ALL and lymphoid blast crisis of CGL	Thy-ALL	B-CLL, B lymphomas B-ALL	AML, AMML, AMoL and myeloid blast crisis of CGL
Anti-ALL serum	+	−	−	−
Terminal transferase	+	+	−	−
Anti-Ia serum	+	−	+	+ or ±
E rosettes	−	+	−	−
Anti-T serum	−	+	−	−
Anti-immunoglobulin	−	−	+	−
Anti-myeloid serum	−	−	−	+

(Ritz et al, 1980). The Ia-like molecules consist of two polypeptides (MW 28 000 and 33 000), analogues to Ia-antigens in mice. Their synthesis is governed by the HLA-DR region of the major histocompatible locus on chromosome 6; these molecules are widely expressed on B cells, immature myeloid and erythroid cells and are thought to play an important role in immunoregulation.

The c-ALL$^+$, Ia$^+$, TdT$^+$ normal cells are present in the highest numbers in juvenile BM (1 to 20 per cent). Non-T, non-B cells, c-ALL$^+$, Ia$^+$ are also present in foetal liver and foetal BM (Greaves & Janossy, 1978) although they do not contain detectable TdT. In contrast, in adult bone marrow TdT$^+$, Ia$^+$ cells are easily detectable (0.5 to 3 per cent) but are c-ALL$^-$ (Bradstock et al, 1981a). These cell types appear to belong to the same family of BM precursor cells which undergo age-related changes. These patterns reflect the dominant phenotype of the malignant non-T, non-B ALL blasts in the similar age groups (Hoffbrand et al, 1979; Greaves et al, 1980; Bradstock et al, 1981a). These TdT$^+$ cells in normal BM are rather unremarkable small lymphocytes with approximately 10 per cent larger blast forms (Fig. 10.1). Their features in regenerating BM are similar although their proportion

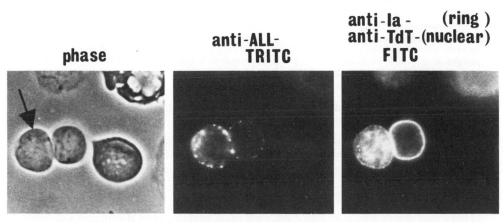

phase   **anti-ALL-TRITC**   **anti-Ia-(ring) anti-TdT-(nuclear) FITC**

Fig. 10.2   Small cells of lymphoid morphology in the normal bone marrow express the phenotype of cALL leukaemia. This preparation was stained for cALL antigen (TRITC; patchy membrane staining), Ia-like antigen (FITC; ring membrane staining) and TdT (FITC; nuclear staining). The cell with arrow is cALL$^+$, Ia$^+$, TdT$^+$. From Janossy et al, 1979.

can be higher. High numbers are also seen in some babies with 'neonatal leukaemoid' reactions accompanied by moderate anaemia and infections (Greaves & Janossy, 1978).

A number of new McAbs react with these cells (Fig. 10.3). Two (J-5 and BA-2) react with bone marrow TdT+ cells only, J-5 with the c-ALL antigen p100 (Ritz et al, 1980) and BA-2 with a new marker (Kersey & Greaves; personal communication). The antigens detected by other McAbs are expressed not only on BM TdT+ cells but also on early cells in differentiation lineages such as thymocytes, BM B-cells and myeloid precursors (Fig. 10.3).

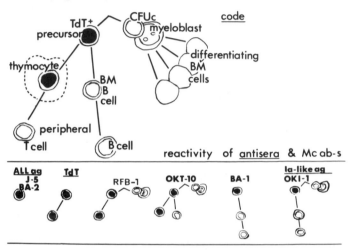

Fig. 10.3 Immunological characterization of human bone marrow precursor cells. The reagents shown include monoclonal antibodies (McAbs) and conventional antisera (underlined). These reagents are used for membrane staining (with TRITC; red) in combination with nuclear TdT staining (on BM precursor cells and cortical thymocytes; depicted by full nucleus), with human T lymphoid antigen (HuTLA) staining (on thymocytes and T cells) or with surface membrane Ig staining (SmIg; on B cells). Myeloblasts can be recognized by their strong staining with Ia-like antigen and morphology (large blasts with multiple nucleoli and minimal cytoplasmic granulation). Myeloid colony forming cells can be studied in cultures (CFUc) after labelling the BM cells with the given antibody and separating the antibody reactive (positive) and unreactive (negative) populations on the cell sorter for cultivation in vitro (Crawford et al, 1981). The reactivity of J-5, BA-1 and BA-2 is based on observations made in other laboratories. The abbreviations refer to the following McAbs: J-5 (Ritz et al, 1980; Greaves et al, 1981); BA-2 (Kersey et al, personal communication); OKT-10 (Reinherz et al, 1980a; Janossy et al, 1981); BA-1 (Le Biem et al, 1981); OKI-1 (Reinherz et al, 1980d). From Bodger et al (1981).

Other antisera detect differentiation antigens on the different lineages but do not react with TdT+ cells (Tables 10.1 and 10.2). Thus, the composite phenotype of BM TdT+ cells is c-ALL+, J-5+, BA-2+, RFB-1+, OKT-10+, BA-1+, Ia+, OKIa-1+ while negative with T lineage markers (E-rosetting, HuTLA, OKT-4, 5, 6, 8 and 11; Fig. 10.5), B lineage markers (SMIg, FMC-1) and anti-myeloid antisera. The phenotype of non-T, non-B ALL is the same in most cases (Ritz et al, 1980; Abramson et al, 1980; Brooks et al, 1980; Bodger et al, 1981; Greaves et al, 1981).

There is evidence that BM TdT+ cells are early precursors of B-lymphocytes (pre-B cells; summarized now) and of thymocytes (prothymocytes; see later). A few TdT+ cells express cytoplasmic immunoglobulin μ chain (Fig. 10.1). These CyIgM+, TdT+ cells represent only about 1.5 per cent of all TdT+ cells and about 2 per cent of all

CyIgM$^+$ pre-B cells in the normal BM. All these are negative for surface Ig (SmIg$^-$; Janossy et al, 1979). Approximately 30 per cent of cases of non-T, non-B ALL also show blasts which are CyIgM$^+$ (pre-B ALL; Vogler et al, 1978; Greaves et al, 1979). Many of these leukaemic populations contain variable mixtures of CyIgM$^-$ and CyIgM$^+$ blasts (Janossy et al, 1980a). Another piece of evidence is the observation that seven of eight cases of non-T, non-B ALL analysed for Ig gene structure showed rearrangements of the immunoglobulin heavy chain μ gene characteristic of B-lymphoid precursors. This μ rearrangement can be clearly distinguished from the germ line μ configuration found in fibroblasts, thymocytes and Thy-ALL blast cells. Thus, Ig gene probes indicate that non-T, non-B ALL, in the majority of cases, is a pre-B malignancy (Korsmeyer et al, 1981).

All these cells are immature and require further differentiation steps before they can give rise to B lymphocytes. The Ig gene probes quoted above show that the non-T, non-B ALL cases studied rarely 'managed' to arrange their light chain genes into a proper B lymphocyte configuration (Korsmeyer et al, 1981), and mixed leukaemias with non-T, non-B blasts and SmIg$^+$ B-ALL blasts are very rare. Similarly, mixtures of c-ALL blasts and Thy-ALL blasts are very rarely detected in laboratories where the stringent methods for the classification of these diseases (shown in Fig. 10.1 and Table 10.2) have been adopted.

B lymphoid bone marrow precursors

The first stages of B cell differentiation occur in environments (such as fetal liver and both fetal and childhood BM) which are relatively free of exogenous antigens and overt T cell influence. In the developing clones of B cells the diversity of antigen specific recognition sites (i.e. the variable regions of Ig heavy and light chains) and that of heavy chain expression are generated (reviewed by Williamson, 1979; Korsmeyer et al, 1981). The first pre-B cells appear which contain cytoplasmic μ chain only (see above). The progeny of pre-B cells are smaller B lymphocytes expressing surface IgM (SIgM, heavy plus light chain). The antigen-recognition sites of Ig molecules (i.e. the light chain and the variable part of heavy chain) can also become attached to other heavy chain constant regions (δ, γ and α) and surface Ig molecules of IgD, IgG and IgA class (SIgD, SIgG and SIgA) appear. It has originally been thought that these isotypes appear in a regular M→D→G→A sequence (Gathings et al, 1977); in human BM, B cells mostly express only SIgM and some SIgD. Recent studies on human lymphoid lines and leukaemias, however, indicate that occasionally pre-B cells with cytoplasmic γ chain only may also be generated (Vogler et al, 1981).

Relatively little is known about the distinctive features of human BM B lymphocytes: they respond poorly to nonspecific stimulants, such as pokeweed mitogen (even when blood borne T lymphocytes are added to 'help' these cultures). The small amount of Ig synthesized is almost exclusively IgM contrasting with peripheral B cell cultures which synthesize IgM, IgG and IgA (De Gast & Platts-Mills, 1978). One difficulty in analysing BM B cells is that the currently used B lymphocyte subset markers (e.g. C3 and Fc receptors) are expressed on B cells as well as myeloid cells (Ross et al, 1977; see also below). Four McAbs have already been reported to show reaction with B lymphocytes: two, FMC-1 (Brooks et al, 1980) and B-1 (Stashenko et al, 1980) probably react with SmIg$^+$ B cells only although their reactivity with pre-B cells is still unknown. Another McAb, BA-2, reacts with TdT^+ cells as well as with B lymphocytes (Abramson et al, 1980). OKT-10 seems to distinguish BM B lymphocytes ($OKT-10^+$) from peripheral B-cells which are mostly $OKT-10^-$ (Janossy et al, 1981). The reactivity of OKT-10 with various B cell malignancies including B leukaemias and lymphomas is currently being studied.

Myeloid precursors

New enzyme tests have been developed. For example, the identification of platelet peroxidase in the perinuclear cysternae of 'undifferentiated' blasts can establish that the cells are megakaryocyte precursors (Breton-Gorius et al, 1979). The analysis of membrane phenotypes of myeloid precursors is a relatively recent additional development. Blasts reacting with highly absorbed anti-myeloid antisera (Roberts & Greaves, 1978; Sagawa & Minowada, 1981) together with antisera to Ia-like antigens (Winchester et al, 1977; Janossy et al, 1978) are likely candidates of early myeloid precursors (Table 10.2). These observations do not, however, give direct information about the function and differentiation level of these cells which is provided in colony forming assays (Chs. 5 and 6). Separation of cells by a combination of immunological and physical criteria (e.g. reactivity with fluorescence labelled antiserum and light scatter) on the fluorescence activated cell sorter (FACS) has allowed both antibody reactive and unreactive populations to be cultured in various colony forming assays (Janossy et al, 1978; Sieff et al, 1980). Elimination of certain populations by antibodies and cytolytic complement allows analysis of one subpopulation (Cline & Billing, 1977); and these techniques can be used in various permutations with more than one antibody to give increasingly informative data (Beverley et al, 1980). Furthermore, selection of positive and negative cells in immunoabsorbent columns also represents a satisfactory analytic technique.

Two examples of the efficacy of this new combined technology are mentioned. Analysis of rat bone marrow cells on the FACS on the basis of reactivity with anti-Thy-1 antibody is shown in Figure 10.4. Cells which form spleen colony forming units (CFUs) in vivo in the rat show the strongest Thy-1 positivity. TdT^+ cells react marginally weaker. By a combination of fluorescence intensity and scatter, pure populations of various precursor cells can be separated; e.g. the purity of TdT^+ populations can be as high as 87 per cent. It remains to be seen whether similar analytical purity can be achieved with human BM cells using OKT-10 or RFB-1 McAbs (Fig. 10.3). The other example is the remarkable enrichment of human haemopoietic precursor cells (including TdT^+ and CFUc cells) by the elimination of lymphoid and mature myeloid cells using combinations of antilymphoid and anti-granulocyte McAbs (Beverley et al, 1980).

On the basis of these observations it appears that myeloid CFUc cells are indeed TdT^-, $c-ALL^-$ and Ia^+ to a variable degree and react with conventional rabbit anti-myeloid sera prepared against ML-1 or HL-60 myeloid cell lines (Sagawa & Minowada, 1980). The BFUe cells are also Ia^+ (Sieff et al, 1980). No McAb has as yet been described which selectively reacts with myeloblasts; so far McAbs made against myeloid cells have only detected differentiated myeloid cells (from myelocytes onwards; Beverley et al, 1980; Zola et al, 1981).

The reactivity of human pluripotential cells (corresponding to CFUs in mice and rats) is more controversial; these cells, according to observations by Moore et al (1980)

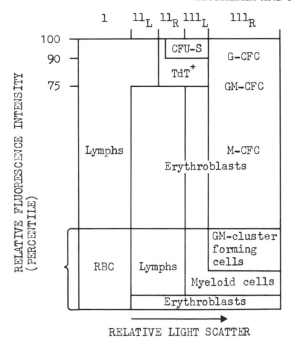

Fig. 10.4   Gated analysis of rat bone marrow cell subsets according to relative low-angle light scatter (size) and relative fluorescence intensity for Thy-1 antigen on the FACS. Composite diagram based on data from Goldschneider et al (1980). 'Fractions' (abscissa) refers to gated fractions separated according to relative light scatter. 'Percentile' (ordinate) refers only to gated fractions of Thy-1$^+$ (fluorescing) cells. Abbreviations: CFUs, in vivo spleen colony forming unit; TdT$^+$: TdT$^+$ cells, these fractions contain astonishingly pure (87 to 92 per cent) TdT$^+$ cells; G-CFC: granulocyte colony forming cells; GM-CFC: granulocyte-monocyte colony forming cell; M-CFC: monocyte CFC; lymphs: lymphocytes; RBC: red cells. From Goldschneider et al (1980).

might be Ia$^-$. Furthermore, if one can extrapolate from observation on rats (see Fig. 10.4 and Vines et al, 1980) these cells are likely to be TdT$^-$.

The myeloid antigen$^+$, Ia$^+$, TdT$^-$ phenotype attributed to normal CFUc cells (Janossy et al, 1978; Sagawa & Minowada, 1980) is the dominant phenotype in most cases of acute myeloid leukaemia (AML). The lack of Ia-like antigens on acute promyelocytic leukaemic blasts (Janossy et al, 1977a; McVerry et al, 1979) is in line with the differentiation linked loss of Ia on normal maturing myeloid cells (Winchester et al, 1977). Many cases of AML are, however, Ia$^-$ and it is difficult to interpret the derivation of these cases without additional studies.

CELLS OF THE HUMAN T LYMPHOID DIFFERENTIATION PATHWAY

Immature cells

The analysis of normal and leukaemic cells of the human thymus has progressed in three stages. In the first, conventional technology was used. Rosette formation with sheep erythrocytes (E-rosettes) is a marker for human Thy-ALL cell lines (e.g. MOLT-4) and for normal thymocytes and T lymphocytes. Specific antisera reacting with human thymocyte/T cell antigens were also made (anti-HuTLA; Mills et al, 1975; Schlossman et al, 1976; Balch et al, 1977; Janossy et al, 1977b). TdT is restricted, in all mammals including man (reviewed by Bollum, 1979 and Janossy et al, 1980c) to cortical immature thymocytes and is absent from medullary mature thymocytes and all peripheral T lymphocytes. Taken together, these studies have demonstrated that the phenotype of cortical thymocytes is E+, HuTLA+, human thymocyte antigen+, TdT+ and Ia−; the phenotype of blasts in most cases of Thy-ALL is identical (Greaves & Janossy, 1978; Table 10.2). Although these results suggested that Thy-ALL may derive from cortical thymocytes, they did not exclude the possibility that at least some cases originate from rare bone marrow cells (prothymocytes). This suggestion is relevant because some Thy-ALL cases with HuTLA+, TdT+, Ia− phenotype fail to form E-rosettes and express c-ALL weakly (Minowada et al, 1978).

In the second stage conventional antisera were used in combinations. In humans, HuTLA+, TdT+, Ia− cells were found to be restricted to the thymus and were absent from the normal or regenerating BM. In the BM HuTLA+ cells were found to be TdT−, Ia− (peripheral T lymphocytes); while TdT+ cells were HuTLA−, Ia+ (Janossy et al, 1979a; Bradstock et al, 1981a). These results support the view that Thy-ALL derives from the thymus and not from the BM. They also show that the HuTLA-TdT staining combination (Fig. 10.1) is specific for normal immature thymocytes which are 'alien' to normal BM or other tissues such as peripheral blood, cerebrospinal fluid or testis. Thus monitoring of residual Thy-ALL blasts is feasible at a single cell level in the BM and elsewhere. Only extensively absorbed anti-HuTLA antisera are useful for this purpose.

In the third stage, thymocyte differentiation (Fig. 10.5) and leukaemia (Reinherz et al, 1980a; Bradstock et al, 1980a) were studied with McAbs. These studies have

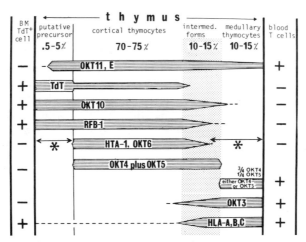

Fig. 10.5 Scheme of human thymocyte differentiation based on the reactivity of cells with monoclonal antibodies. Positivity of a cell population is shown by horizontal bars; dotted lines indicate barely detectable or very weak positivity on a few cells. Cells expressing HTA-1 and OKT6 appear to be the same cortical thymocyte population and are depicted together. These cells simultaneously express both OKT4 and OKT5. HTA-1− cells (separated by the elimination of HTA-1+ cells on immunoabsorbent columns); are clearly heterogenous (see asterisks). The large TdT+ blasts are likely to be the earliest thymic precursors because in many respects they resemble bone marrow TdT+ cells which are also OKT10+, RFB-1+ (see Fig. 10.3). The phenotype of these blasts is similar to that of most cases of Thy-ALL (Bradstock et al, 1980a; Reinherz et al, 1980a). There are a number of identifiable intermediate forms (see shaded area) between cortical and medullary thymocytes. From Tidman et al (1981).

confirmed the above observations by demonstrating that a series of reagents (OKT11, OKT6, NA1/34, OKT4, OKT5, OKT8 and OKT3) reacted exclusively with thymocytes and/or peripheral T cells according to the differentiation pattern shown in Figure 10.5, but not with TdT⁺ cells in the BM (Janossy et al, 1981). In addition, in the infant thymus a large blast cell type has been defined showing dark blue cytoplasm and an oval nucleus which stains particularly strongly with anti-TdT antiserum and has one to two prominent nucleoli. As this blast cell shows a 'transitional' phenotype between TdT⁺ cells in the BM and TdT⁺ cortical thymocytes (Fig. 10.5) it might be a putative thymic precursor which derives from BM TdT⁺ cells.

Animal experiments support this possibility. TdT⁺ BM cells from athymic mice can be induced in vitro to express Ly-1,2,3 antigens (which are thought to be thymocyte/T cell specific markers) during a brief incubation with thymosin or its purified α_1 peptide form (Goldschneider et al, 1981). Furthermore, a specific antiserum reacting with membrane antigen(s) on rat TdT⁺ BM cells also label the blast cells in the subcapsular region of the thymus. These subcapsular blast cells probably correspond to the human thymic blast (Goldschneider, I, personal communication).

These studies have to be interpreted with some caution. Experiments using thymic factors on purified human TdT⁺ BM cells have not yet been performed and the induction of bona fide thymocyte markers (as defined by the new McAbs; Fig. 10.5) on these cells has not been proven. Also leukaemias of typical non-T, non-B ALL type do not seem to develop into Thy-ALL blasts except extremely rare cases (Koike et al, 1978) but frequently express pre-B features (see above).

Thy-ALL blasts
Two facts have emerged from the comparative analysis of normal thymocytes and acute Thy-ALL blast cells. First is that the malignant cells frequently reflect the phenotype of the large thymic blast cells (putative precursors) and less frequently show the exact features of typical cortical thymocytes (Bradstock et al, 1980a; Reinherz et al, 1980a). Thy-ALL cases reflecting the phenotype of medullary or peripheral T cell types are rare. The second observation is that the similarity between Thy-ALL blasts and their probable 'normal equivalent' cells is not always absolute. Leukaemic cells in 10 to 15 per cent of Thy-ALL cases show various 'scrambled' phenotypes which cannot be easily allocated to any defined position in the hypothetical normal differentiation scheme shown in Figure 10.5 (Reinherz et al, 1980; Greaves et al, 1981). This indicates an aberrant control of normal gene products in a low proportion of leukaemias. Furthermore many Thy-ALL blast cells express OKT9 antigen and large amounts of HLA-A,B,C (Reinherz et al, 1980a; Bradstock et al, 1980b; Greaves et al, 1981b; Tidman et al, 1981) whilst single cell assays by fluorescence show that less than 3 per cent of TdT⁺ thymic blast cells and typical TdT⁺ cortical thymocytes express OKT9 (Tidman et al, 1981) or large amounts of HLA-A, B, C (Bradstock et al, 1980b). OKT9 is a fascinating reagent which probably recognizes antigenic determinants on activated cells only (Greaves et al, 1981), and the exact interpretation of these observations is not yet clear. One possibility is nevertheless that these changes are epiphenomena of the leukaemic transformation in Thy-ALL. As more than 99 per cent of TdT⁺ cells in the normal BM are OKT9⁻, the

OKT9-TdT staining combination can also be useful for identifying residual Thy-ALL blasts in the BM (OKT9$^+$, TdT$^+$; Tidman et al, 1981).

Peripheral T lymphocytes

T cells in blood and peripheral lymphoid organs form E-rosettes and react with anti-T lymphocyte antisera but are TdT$^-$ (Bollum, 1979). In man, two main T cell subsets (i.e. T cells of 'inducer' and 'suppressor-cytotoxic' phenotypes) are generated during late stages of thymocyte development and form distinct subsets on the periphery (Reinherz et al, 1980a).

In earlier studies 'inducer' (also referred to as 'helper') T cells were recognized by their ability to form rosettes with ox erythrocytes coated with IgM antibody (Tμ cells; Moretta et al, 1977). These cells have strong localized enzyme staining for alpha-naphthol acid esterase (dot-like ANAE$^+$; Grossi et al, 1978). More recently a McAb OKT4 has been shown to detect 'inducer' T cells which help the activation of B lymphocytes (to develop into plasma cells in pokeweed stimulated cultures) and also help the other T subset to develop into cytotoxic T cells (see below and Reinherz et al, 1979a). Although Tμ and OKT4$^+$ cells may not represent exactly the same population (Reinherz et al, 1979a, b) the existence of a distinct inducer subset is beyond doubt. It has been shown that OKT4$^+$ cells predominate in T cell traffic areas and in lymphoid tissues around specialized macrophages expressing large amounts of Ia-like antigens (e.g. in thymic medulla, lymph node paracortex and the lamina propria of gut; Janossy et al, 1980e).

The other T cell subset includes suppressor and cytotoxic T lymphocytes. At least some of these can be recognized by erythrocytes coated with IgG (Tγ cells) and show weak diffuse ANAE positivity (ANAE$^\pm$). These cells are therefore distinct from ANAE$^+$ Tμ cells and also from typical monocytes (which, in contrast to Tγ cells, show very strong ANAE staining throughout the cytoplasm; Grossi et al, 1978). More recently a T cell subset has been defined using a horse antibody to TH$_2$ antigen (Reinherz et al, 1979b) and two similar but not exactly identical McAbs: OKT5 and OKT8 (Reinherz et al, 1980a, b). The TH$_2$$^+$, OKT5$^+$, OKT8$^+$ cell population includes suppressor T cells which inhibit the induction of Ig synthesis in B lymphocytes, and also contain the cytotoxic T cells and their precursors. These cell populations might be involved in defence against viral infections; many OKT8$^+$ blast cells circulate in the blood of patients with infectious mononucleosis (Crawford et al, 1981). OKT8$^+$ cells are predominant in the normal T cell population of bone marrow (Janossy et al, 1980e) and the gut epithelium (intraepithelial lymphocytes; Selby et al, 1980). Both the inducer and cytotoxic-suppressor T cell populations can express small to medium amounts of Ia-like antigens when activated by antigenic or mitogenic stimulation in vitro (Fu et al, 1978) or by bacterial or viral infections in vivo (Reinherz et al, 1979c). These activated T lymphocytes are nevertheless always TdT$^-$.

These membrane and enzyme markers are useful for the analysis of chronic T cell leukaemias and cutaneous T cell lymphomas. These disorders are TdT$^-$ and can be classified into OKT4$^+$, OKT8$^-$ malignancies of 'inducer' cell type and OKT8$^+$, OKT4$^-$ malignancies of suppressor-cytotoxic cell type. The former group is clinically heterogenous: it includes cases of T-CLL, prolymphocytic leukaemia of T cell type, Sezary syndrome and mycosis fungoides (Reinherz et al, 1979d; Kung et al, 1980). In earlier studies these types of malignant T cells have been shown to exhibit helper functions (Broder et al, 1976). The second group includes a few cases of T-CLL (Pandolfi et al, 1981; Rambotti et al, 1981) which should not be confused with reactive T cell responses seen in viral infections (e.g. infectious mononucleosis) or with rare cases of immunoregulatory disorders where very high numbers of OKT8+ cells express variable amounts of Ia-like antigens and are frequently accompanied by symptoms of bone marrow dysfunction (Callard et al, 1981; Webster et al, 1981).

ANALYSIS OF PERIPHERAL B LYMPHOCYTES

Salmon & Seligmann (1974) pointed out that B lymphoid malignancies are heterogenous for two main reasons. First, some malignant populations are capable of undergoing differentiation and develop into plasma cells (monoclonal gammopathies: Waldenström macroglobulinaemia and multiple myeloma) while other B lymphoid malignancies seem to be 'frozen' at a lymphoid differentiation stage. Second, these malignancies may originate from different B lymphocyte subpopulations (i.e. 'virgin' B lymphocytes or memory B cells). The analysis of these questions is not possible without the exact understanding of normal B cell differentiation and without the availability of precise markers for the different B subsets similar to those shown for T lineage cells in Figure 10.5. It is very likely, however, that chronic lymphocytic leukaemias of B cell type and lymphomas in adults originate from peripheral lymphoid organs.

As has been pointed out above, during the last few years the B cell differentiation schemes have been mainly based on Ig isotype expression (Cooper et al, 1977; De Gast & Platts-Mills, 1979), on the analysis of receptors for C3 components (C3d and C3b) and for the Fc part of IgG (EA) or IgM. Only a few attempts have been made to 'map' the phenotypic characteristics of malignant B cells into the schemes of normal differentiation (Stein et al, 1978; Habeshaw, 1979) but these suggestions are interesting. It seems that immature B lymphocytes express C3d receptors only, while more mature B cells in the lymph node germinal centre and follicular mantle have both C3d and C3b receptors. B lymphocytes seed from the germinal centres into the marginal cortex and into the medulla. During this process B cells differentiate into plasma cells (Nieuwenhuis & Keuning, 1974) and lose the C3d receptors but retain C3b (Stein et al, 1978). It is tempting to speculate that these stages are reflected in the malignant phenotypes: 80 per cent of CLL cases are C3d+, C3b− (immature B ?), most follicular lymphomas are C3d+, C3b+ (mature or memory B ?) and cases of macroglobulinaemia are C3b+, C3d− (plasmacytoid; Ross & Pooley, 1975; Stein et al, 1978). (A similar sequence of complement receptor expression is observed during granulocyte differentiation; Ross et al, 1978).

During the last two years concensus has been reached on a number of issues in the diagnosis of non-Hodgkin lymphomas. Previously, the immunological studies of malignant lymphomas have been carried out either in suspensions of cells prepared from the involved nodes or in tissue sections of formalin fixed samples. In the first case, membrane marker analysis is informative and sensitive (Habeshaw et al, 1979), the tissue organization is, however, disrupted. In contrast, in formalin fixed samples the staining of cell membranes is not feasible and only the cytoplasmic or nuclear antigens are preserved. Recently it has been shown that sections of frozen biopsies can give excellent membrane staining of the various lymphoid populations (Levy et al,

1977; Warnke et al, 1978; Stein et al, 1980; Janossy et al, 1980d) and with careful handling the tissue preservation is also acceptable (Stein et al, 1980).

It has also become clear that the histological and immunological characterization of cells in non-Hodgkin lymphomas of B cell type is complementary. The aim of the histological analysis is to study normal tissue organization in lymphoid organs as well as the pattern of the disruption of these normal tissues by the lymphoma. This conventional technique is adequate for diagnosis in most cases, but is not a suitable method to assess minimal malignant involvement and for analysis of the type of the individual cells. In contrast, the aim of immunological studies is the identification of individual cells and the definition of exact cellular composition of different cell types in the various tumours. Thus the immunological methods are of importance in analysing the exact cellular derivation of tumours, the presence of residual normal cells (e.g. regulatory T cells), the early stages of lymphoma development and the cases in which the diagnosis is particularly difficult and the histopathological observations show equivocal results (Janossy et al, 1980d).

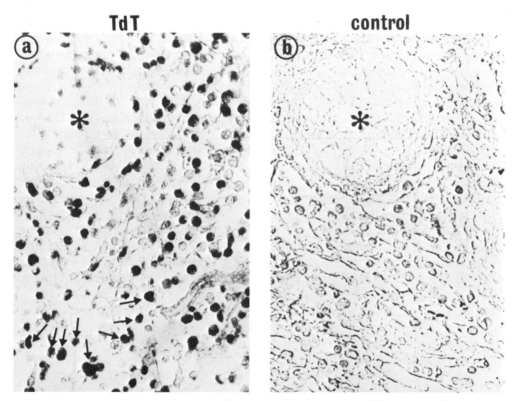

Fig. 10.7 Demonstration of nuclear terminal deoxynucleotidyl transferase (TdT) in lymphoid leukaemic blast cells infiltrating the testis. Rabbit anti-TdT antibody was labelled with peroxidase anti-peroxidase (PAP) method in paraffin embedded, dewaxed and DNA-ase-treated sections (A). Infiltrating acute lymphoblastic leukaemia cells are stained for nuclear TdT (arrows point to some of the TdT⁺ cells). Second layer (PAP only) shows minimal staining (B). The fields were photographed with phase contrast to visualize unstained cells. (*) Seminiferous tubule. From Janossy et al (1980d). We find it difficult to standardize DNA-ase digestion. We have therefore recently used frozen biopsies. These are cut and fixed (with 10% buffered formalin at −20°C) in the cryostat. The morphology is excellent and no DNA-ase is required for optimal TdT staining. (Thomas J. A. et al submitted to Blood).

The range of cases in which this additional immunological information is clinically useful is increasing. It is well known that non-Hodgkin lymphomas of B type consist of cells which derive from one single B lymphocyte carrying either $\varkappa$ or λ light chain. Thus the combined staining for $\varkappa$ or λ can establish whether the B lymphoid infiltration is malignant (predominantly $\varkappa$ or λ) or rather a reactive non-malignant population (2:1 mixture of $\varkappa:\lambda$ cells; Fig. 10.6). In addition a characteristic network pattern of Ig distribution is detectable within the germinal centres in normal nodes and in benign reactive hyperplasia but is not seen in neoplastic follicles (Braylan & Rappaport, 1973). This simple test might be used in combination with a recently developed McAb which detects normal follicular dendritic cells as well as the residual follicular dendritic cells in the malignant follicles (Stein et al, 1981a). These reagents, when used together, yield informative combinations which discriminate lymphoid hyperplasia from malignancy.

As McAbs work well in sections of frozen tissue biopsies, the scene is now set for opening a new chapter in the study of normal B lymphocyte differentiation and lymphoma diagnosis. Antibodies with wide reactivity against lymphoid cells (Pizzolo et al, 1981) and B lymphocytes (Brooks et al, 1980; Stashenko et al, 1980) can be used to discriminate lymphomas from anaplastic carcinomas. Further reagents against B cell subsets are nevertheless required. One of the potentially useful reagents (FMC-7; Zola et al, 1980) is already in clinical use. Furthermore, a specific rabbit antiserum to Reed-Sternberg cells may open up new possibilities in the study of the derivation of this peculiar cell as well as in the early diagnosis of Hodgkin disease (Stein et al, 1981).

Finally, recent studies have clearly established that lymphomas of the younger age groups show different immunological phenotypes from adult non-Hodgkin lymphomas and can be 'typed' effectively with the reagents used for leukaemia diagnosis (Habeshaw, 1980; Bernard et al, 1979). In particular, lymphoblastic lymphomas of convoluted type derive from thymic blasts and some other cases show non-T, non-B ALL phenotype. These malignancies contain TdT which can be detected in tissue section of formalin fixed samples using anti-TdT antibodies and peroxidase label (Fig. 10.7).

BIOCHEMICAL ASPECTS

It is now possible to detect a wide range of enzymes histologically, cytochemically, biochemically or immunologically and analyse differences in concentrations or iso-enzyme pattern between different leukaemic or lymphoma cell populations and normal tissues. These studies have recently revealed characteristic patterns, e.g. for acid-phosphatase in Thy-ALL, hexoseaminidase isoenzymes in c-ALL and platelet peroxidase in megakaryoblastic leukaemia (see reviews Catovsky, 1977, 1980). In this chapter, however, we wish to concentrate on four enzymes (adenosine deaminase, purine nucleotide phosphorylase, 5' nucleotidase and TdT) which are of particular current interest in the diagnosis and treatment of lymphoblastic leukaemias (Blatt et al, 1980a).

Adenosine deaminase (ADA) (E.C. 3.5.4.4)

Clinical interest in ADA began when two patients with combined immune deficiency were found to be ADA deficient (Giblett et al, 1972). ADA catalyses the conversion of adenosine to inosine and deoxyadenosine to deoxyinosine (Fig. 10.8). The enzyme is present in most human tissues but the highest levels are found in the thymic cortex (Barton et al, 1979). Thymic medullary cells and peripheral T cells show lower levels than thymic cortical cells but nevertheless higher than in B lymphocytes or myeloid cells.

Accumulation of adenosine, deoxyadenosine and compounds derived from them occurs in the cells of ADA deficient patients and two mechanisms of toxicity for ADA deficiency to lymphocyte precursors have been proposed (Fig. 10.8). Accumulation of dATP in thymocytes may inhibit the enzyme ribonucleotide reductase and thus cause starvation of the other DNA precursors dATP, dCTP and dGTP which rely on ribonucleotide reductase for their formation (Cohen et al, 1978). Alternatively accumulation of adenosine has been shown to lead to a build up of S-adenosyl homocysteine (SAH) and this in turn causes a fall in cell S-adenosyl methionine (SAM) concentration leading to inhibition of methylation reactions in protein and RNA synthesis which depend on SAM as methyl donor (Johnston & Kredich, 1978; Hershfield & Kredich, 1980). Other biochemical differences between DNA synthesis in thymic derived cells and other cell types may also be relevant (Piga et al, 1981).

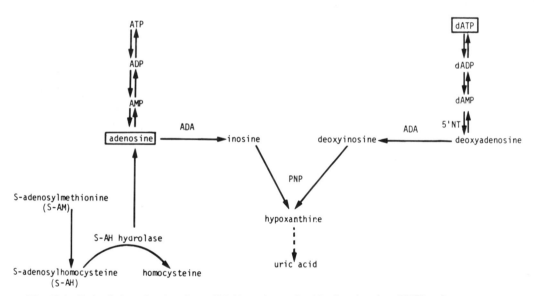

Fig. 10.8   Role of adenosine deaminase (ADA), purine nucleotide phosphorylase (PNP) and 5'nucleotidase (5'NT) in purine degradation. A = adenosine, d = deoxyribose, MP, DP, TP = mono-, di- and tri-phosphate respectively. PNP is also concerned in degradation of deoxyguanosine and guanosine to guanine.

The explanation why thymocytes are selectively destroyed in ADA deficiency is probably due to their relative inability to degrade deoxyadenosine and its derivatives. Thus T-cells and their precursors are less able to degrade dATP than B cells or other body cells (Carson et al, 1979; Wortmann et al, 1979). They have a particularly low level of 5' nucleotidase (5'NT), a membrane associated degradative enzyme, and Thy-ALL cells have been found less effective than B cells or myeloid cells in degrading dTTP or dATP. Moreover most cells are able to functionally compartmentalize DNA precursors into a high concentration small sized pool at the DNA replication fork, and a low concentration, larger sized pool which is largely degraded (Reddy & Pardee, 1980; Taheri et al, 1981). In immature T-cells virtually 100 per cent of the immediate DNA precursors seem destined for DNA synthesis and a functionally separated, degradative system is not present. The absence of such an escape route may make these cells particularly vulnerable to accumulation of a DNA precursor, e.g. of dATP as in ADA deficiency (or of dGTP in purine nucleoside phorphorylase deficiency). Moreover, T-cells have an active kinase which enables them to accumulate dAMP effectively from deoxyadenosine. T-cells also have lower levels of thymidine phosphorylase (Fox et al, 1979) and of SAH-hydrolase than B cells. These biochemical differences may account for the suceptibility of immature T-cells to deoxyadenosine when ADA is absent. Recent studies using the ADA inhibitor deoxycoformycin to treat patients with Thy-ALL have suggested that it is the rise in dATP rather than inhibition of SAH hydrolase that most closely parallels killing of the blast cells (Russel et al, 1981). On the other hand, in vitro studies suggest that toxicity to mature lymphocytes of ADA deficiency or inhibition is more likely to be due to SAH accumulation (Hershfield & Kredich, 1980; Lee et al, 1981).

ADA levels in leukaemia
In acute leukaemia the highest ADA levels are found in Thy-ALL. There is nevertheless a considerable overlap in values between Thy-ALL and non-B, non-T ALL whether or not this is positive for the c-ALL antigen (Coleman et al, 1978; Smyth et al, 1978; Ben-Bassat et al, 1980; Ganeshaguru et al, 1981). ADA levels are also raised above normal peripheral bood or bone marrow in about 50 per cent of patients with AML. In B-ALL, the levels are below normal (Ben-Bassat et al, 1980). The enzyme can be detected antigenically in serum or in cell extracts as well as by the more widely used biochemical assay. The two techniques show a good correlation (Chechik et al, 1980). The antigenic assay of serum ADA offers a possible test of whether Thy-ALL blasts remain in the body in apparent remission judged on the basis of marrow morphology.

In contrast to the results in acute leukaemia, in B-cell CLL, ADA levels are less than those in normal peripheral blood lymphocytes (Silber et al, 1976; Ramot et al, 1977). In chronic T-cell CLL and prolymphocytic leukaemias, however, ADA levels may be midly raised. Among the lymphomas, the highest levels are again found in the immature T-cell tumours with intermediate values in Hodgkin's disease the lowest values being found in B-cell tumour tissue (Ganeshaguru et al, 1981).

Use of the ADA inhibitor (Deoxycoformycin) in therapy
Inhibition of ADA in vivo with deoxycoformycin (dCF) has been found to selectively kill Thy-ALL cells, even in patients whose leukaemic cells are resistant to other drugs (Prentice et al, 1980; Mitchell et al, 1980; Siaw et al, 1980). Similar responses have not been found in c-ALL or AML (Koller & Mitchell, 1979; Grever et al, 1981, Prentice et al, 1981a).

Although dCF inhibits ADA in Thy-ALL cell lines in vitro providing concentrations of 10^{-6} M or higher are used, the cells remain viable even after 12 hours incubation. If deoxyadenosine (dA) 10^{-4} M is also added in vitro, however, toxicity with loss of cell viability occurs within a few hours (Lee et al, 1981). Presumably, in vivo deoxyadenosine (dA) accumulates in serum when dCF therapy is given and this dA potentiates the toxicity to Thy-ALL cells.

Purine nucleoside phosphorylase (PNP, E.C. 2.4.2.1)

This enzyme is concerned sequentially with ADA in purine interconversion catalysing the reversible phosphorolysis of deoxyinosine and inosine to hypoxanthine and of deoxyguanosine and guanosine to guanine (Fig. 10.8). Its distribution in lymphoid organs is in reciprocal relation to ADA, however, the highest concentrations being found in spleen and bone marrow with lower concentrations in lymph node and thymus (Barton et al, 1980). In the thymus, the enzyme is greater in medullary than cortical cells. Although the enzyme activity is higher in mature T than B cells (Nishida et al, 1979) the variation in concentration between lymphocyte populations does not simply reflect T and B cell proportions since there is heterogeneity in enzyme activity within various peripheral-T and B-cell populations (Barton et al, 1980).

Partial or complete deficiency of the enzyme is associated with T cell immunodeficiency (Giblett et al, 1975) and this has been ascribed to the accumulation of deoxyguanosine and dGTP in T-cells and their precursors (Carson et al, 1977). Deoxyguanosine is selectively toxic to T lymphoblasts compared with B lymphoblasts in vitro (Ochs et al, 1979). This may be partly due to the higher concentration of deoxycytidine kinase in T precursors, this enzyme phosphorylating deoxyguanosine to dGMP, which is then further phosphorylated to dGTP.

PNP levels measured biochemically or histochemically are lower in Thy-ALL than in c-ALL (Blatt et al, 1980b) and in B-CLL compared to normal peripheral blood lymphocytes (Borgers et al, 1978). Studies in chronic T-cell leukaemias and in lymphomas have not yet been reported. In AML, PNP levels have been found similar to normal blood leukocytes (Mejer & Nygaard, 1979).

5'Nucleotidase (E.C. 3.1.3.5.)

This enzyme is localized to the cell membrane and catalyses the dephosphorylation of 5'-nucleotides to the corresponding nucleosides. In contrast to ADA and PNP, 5'NT activity is greater in peripheral B than T cells. The concentration is particularly low in thymocytes (Edwards et al, 1979) and this may partly explain why these cells are peculiarly liable to toxicity in the face of nucleoside excess. The enzyme is low in

Table 10.3 Reactivity of monoclonal antibodies used for the analysis of Thy-ALL and chronic T cell leukaemias

Designation	Reactivity	Ig class	Ref.[†]
Monoclonal antibodies:			
OKT11	thymocytes + T cells	IgG$_1$, IgG$_2$	1
OKT6 and NA1/34	cortical thymocytes (CT)	IgG$_1$, IgG$_2$	1, 2
OKT4	thymocytes + inducer T cells	IgG$_2$	3
OKT8	thymocytes + suppressor/cytotoxic T cells	IgG$_2$	4
OKT3	peripheral T cells	IgG$_2$	5
OKT9	activated cells (not specific for T cells)	IgG$_1$	6

[†]References: (1) Kung et al, 1980; (2) McMichael et al, 1979; (3) Reinherz et al, 1980a; (4) Reinherz et al, 1980b; (5) Kung et al, 1979; (6) Reinherz et al, 1980b.
For further details about additional interesting McAbs see Figure 10.3.

Thy-ALL and B-CLL and other chronic B-cell tumours (B-PLL, hairy cell leukaemia and macroglobulinaemia) compared to normal circulating lymphocytes but is raised in c-ALL (see reviews Blatt et al, 1980a; Catovsky, 1980).

Terminal deoxynucleotidyl transferase (TdT, E.C. 2.7.7.31)

This enzyme catalyses the polymerization of a single-stranded DNA to the free 3-OH' end of a primer which can be RNA or DNA or an oligonucleotide sequence. The enzyme can be detected biochemically or by immunofluorescence (see earlier and Bollum, 1979). The usual biochemical assay uses ^{3}H-dGTP as substrate and poly(dA) as primer. Although purification of each sample by DEAE cellulose chromatography has been used by some groups for biochemical assay (Srivastava et al, 1980), there is no evidence that this gives more reliable diagnostic information than an assay of a crude cell homogenate. The enzyme TdT is found in only two normal human tissues, thymus and bone marrow (see above). The function of TdT remains unknown but the recent report (Landreth et al, 1981) that a strain of mice ('motheaten') suffering from extensive breakdown of immune homeostasis with multiple autoimmune diseases lack TdT$^+$ cells in bone marrow or thymus may be a clue to the functional role of TdT in the normal generation of the lymphoid system. These mice are known to have a single gene defect on chromosome 6 and to show both T and B cell functional disorders.

Acute leukaemias

TdT is raised in over 90 per cent of cases of c-ALL including pre-B cases (Vogler et al, 1978; Greaves et al, 1979) with a wide range, values more than 100 units/10^6 cells rarely occurring in other leukaemias (Hoffbrand et al, 1977, 1979; Hutton et al, 1979) (Table 10.4). The rare c-ALL$^+$ TdT$^-$ cases tend to be very young children or neonates. Measurement of the enzyme is particularly valuable in adults when c-ALL antigen is often absent from the blast cells. In our experience TdT$^+$ acute undifferentiated leukaemias respond well to vincristine and prednisolone therapy whereas TdT$^-$ cases do not. There is no evidence, however, that response to treatment in c-ALL in children is related to the degree to which the blasts are TdT$^+$. Neither the biochemical nor the immunofluorescent assays for TdT have proved capable of

Table 10.4   Terminal deoxynucleotidyl transferase (TdT) in leukaemia and lymphoma*

Diagnosis	No. studied	No. (%) + ve
non-B, non-T ALL	452	430 (95)
pre-B ALL	35	23 (67)
Thy-ALL	63	59 (94)
CGL-Blast Transformation	158	61 (39)
AML	255	16 (6.3)
acute undifferentiated leukaemia	55	28 (51)
non-Hodgkin's lymphoma†		
B cell (SIg$^+$)	96	0 (0)
Immature T-cell (thymocyte)	36	34 (94)
Mature T-cell	23	2 (8.7)

*Results are taken from large series published between 1973 and 1979. For detailed analysis see Hoffbrand et al, 1979.
†Hodgkin's disease, B-CLL and hairy cell leukaemia are invariably TdT negative.

distinguishing normal TdT[+] BM precursors from residual c-ALL blast cells (see above). On the other hand, TdT[+] cells are not found in extramedullary sites (except thymus). Tests on cerebrospinal fluid or testis by immunofluorescent or immunoperoxidase techniques have proved superior to conventional morphology for detecting small numbers of c-ALL blasts at these sites (Bradstock et al, 1980c; Janossy et al, 1980d).

Thy-ALL blasts also usually (more than 90 per cent of cases) contain TdT. In most studies the mean concentration has been somewhat lower than in c-ALL and Thy-ALL cells rarely show levels more than 100 units/10^8 cells. Thiel et al (1980) describe a pre-T-ALL, which is both c-ALL[+], and anti-HuTLA[+] and this is also usually TdT[+] but in our experience this is a rare combination; this difference may relate to the specificity of the antisera against c-ALL antigen being used.

Since TdT[+], HuTLA[+] cells do not occur in normal marrow (Janossy et al, 1979a) the finding of a single cell positive with this combination of markers implies a Thy-ALL blast cell in the marrow. Thus, immunological monitoring of the bone marrow in Thy-ALL can be useful for detecting residual leukaemia cells in much smaller proportion (e.g. 1 in 10 000) than can be identified morphologically.

In AML, TdT is usually normal. About 6 per cent of cases, however, are TdT[+] (Table 10.4). Immunological studies have shown that the proportion of TdT[+] blasts in these cases ranges from 10 to 90 per cent (Bradstock et al, 1981b). In some, TdT must be aberrantly expressed in myeloblasts in view of cytochemical and electron microscopic observation that over 50 per cent of the cells are myeloblasts and, indeed, some clearly myeloblastic cells (containing granules) are TdT[+] by immunofluorescence. In other cases (Ph'−) there may be mixed cell populations of myeloblasts and lymphoblasts. Whether these arise from a single progenitor or represent two clones is unclear. The response to treatment whether for lymphoblastic or myeloblastic leukaemia is usually poor in these mixed cases, who tend to be older than is usual with AML (Bradstock et al, 1981b). In some studies, the TdT[+] AML cases have shown a myelomonocytic morphology (Srivastava et al, 1980).

Chronic leukaemia and lymphoma
In the chronic phase of Ph' + CGL, TdT is negative by both immunofluorescent and biochemical techniques in marrow and peripheral blood. On the other hand, 20 to 30 per cent of cases in blast transformation are TdT[+]. The TdT[+] blasts usually show lymphoblastic or undifferentiated morphology. In some of these cases mixed populations of TdT[+] lymphoblasts and TdT[−] myeloblasts are present. This transformation occurs mostly in Ph' + CGL but lymphoblastic transformation of Ph' − CGL is also seen (Hughes et al, 1981). TdT[+] lymphoblastic transformation is associated with a response to vincristine and prednisolone and an improved overall survival compared with myeloblastic transformation (Marks et al, 1977; Janossy et al, 1979b).

B-cell tumours, whether CLL, B-ALL or B-cell non-Hodgkin's lymphomas are invariably TdT[−], so are tumours of mature T-cells, e.g. T-CLL, T-prolymphocytic leukaemia and Sezary's disease. A few lymphomas show TdT[+] cells. These are of poorly differentiated or undifferentiated diffuse histology and where immunological markers have been tested, usually of thymocyte origin (Donlon et al, 1977; Habeshaw et al, 1979).

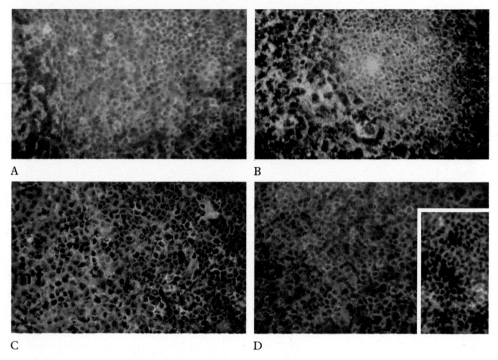

A   B

C   D

Fig. 10.6 Analysis of lymphoid tissues and lymphomas in sections of frozen tissues with combinations of antisera. Figures (A) and (B) are from normal tonsil; Figures (C) and (D) are from three cases of malignant lymphoma. In (A) and (C) T lymphocytes are stained with anti-HuTLA and FITC conjugated second layers. This shows green membrane staining (e.g. on T cells dominating in the paracortical area on the left of Figure (A). In the same picture, immunoglobulin is stained with TRITC conjugated anti-IgM and shows red membrane associated staining on B lymphoid cells and deposits of Ig complexes in the normal germinal centre HH (left).

(B) shows a germinal centre with a B lymphocyte corona (T cell area was not photographed on this figure). Both (B) and (D) have been stained for kappa light chain (TRITC; red) and lambda light chain (FITC; green). In the tonsil the middle of the GC contains Ig complexes which is surrounded by normal lymphocyte corona consisting of mixtures of B cells which either express kappa or lambda light chains. This mosaic-like pattern is typical of normal lymphoid tissue. (Normal $\varkappa : \lambda$ ratio: 2 : 1). In contrast, in the malignant tissue only a few residual T cells are present (in Figure B) and the malignant B cell population homogenously stains with anti-kappa-TRITC or, in the other case of lymphoma shown in the insert, with anti-kappa-FITC (in Figure D). From Janossy et al, (1980d).

A NEW CONTRIBUTION TO THERAPY?

Chemotherapy has improved the survival in acute leukaemia. Remission induction is successful in most patients but many relapse. Effective chemotherapy is often toxic for normal BM and this limits its use. Additional therapy which is selective to leukaemic cells with minimal additional myelotoxicity is still required. Selectivity can be achieved using immunological manipulations with antibodies (directed against membrane antigens). Selectivity may also be achieved by specifically inhibiting enzymes which are required only in certain stages of lymphoid development. During the last few years progress has been made in both areas.

Antibodies to membrane antigens

Antibodies may be of value in both autologous and allogeneic BM transplantation. During this procedure the BM cells can be incubated with antibodies in vitro prior to reinfusion into the heavily treated patients. The injection of antileukaemic antibodies into the patients in vivo is not likely to be of value because these antibodies may not reach a substantial subpopulation of sessile malignant cells.

An obvious role can be suggested for specific antibodies during *autologous* transplantation in lymphoid leukaemias and lymphomas. Specific reagents can be made which bind to the leukaemic cells but do not react with normal BM precursors. The best examples are Thy-ALL and B cell malignancies (e.g. B-ALL) which are antigenically different from myeloid precursors; the common form of ALL might also be amenable for this approach (Netzel et al, 1980). Clearly, the best chance for success with this kind of therapy is to bring the patient into at least temporary good second remission, obtain copious autologous BM suspension and treat it with selective antibody. Then the 'cleansed' BM is reinfused following ablative therapy.

The prevention of graft versus host disease (GvHD) which frequently complicates *allogeneic* BM transplantation should be the primary aim in AML and related diseases. This is because antisera which could effectively distinguish the clonogenic myeloid leukaemic cells from the normal myeloid precursors have, so far, not been produced. Antibodies specifically reacting with peripheral T cells (i.e. the cells responsible for GvHD) are nevertheless already available. It is logical that clinical experimentation with antibodies should start with the assessment of the efficacy of GvHD prevention in allogeneic BM transplantation (Rodt et al, 1980).

The first question is the preparation and specificity of antisera. Apparently successful attempts have been made to prevent GvHD as well as to remove residual leukaemic cells using absorbed conventional rabbit antisera (Rodt et al, 1980; Netzel et al, 1980). It is nevertheless difficult to prepare sufficient quantities of these reagents for clinical trials, although standardization of the absorption protocols (using large amounts of cells from continuously growing lymphoid cell lines) has recently been suggested (Anderson et al, 1981).

An obvious new alternative is the use of McAbs. These reagents do not require absorption and can be made in large amounts. The salient points about the standardization of McAbs for BM transplantation are as follows. A simple analysis of the antibody reactivity against human pluripotent stem cells (from which the BM regenerates) is not yet feasible. There are, however, three relatively simple tests which can establish the antibody reactivity on closely related BM precursors: the TdT$^+$ cells (putative lymphocyte precursors), cells forming myeloid or erythroid colonies in vitro (CFUc and BFUe respectively) and morphologically recognizable immature myeloblasts (Janossy et al, 1981). On this basis a whole range of McAbs can be classified as reagents which react with human BM precursor cells (Fig. 10.3). In contrast, other McAbs can be shown to detect membrane antigens exclusively restricted to thymocyte and T lineage cells (Table 10.3). Of these, McAb OKT3 might be suitable for the prevention of GvHD (since it reacts with all peripheral T lymphocytes; Kung et al, 1979; Janossy et al, 1981; Chang et al, 1981). Two other McAbs, OKT11 and Lyt-3 might also be suitable, in addition, for the removal of Thy-ALL blast cells from autologous BM. These reagents bind to the sheep erythrocyte (E) receptor which is expressed on most cases of Thy-ALL blasts as well as on normal thymocytes and T cells (Kung et al, 1980; Kamoun et al, 1980). Suitable additional McAbs reacting against Thy-ALL and B lymphoid malignancies are still required. Frequently, individual McAbs react only with a proportion of leukaemic cells. Thus mixtures of McAbs would be necessary for the effective removal of all residual leukaemic cells from the BM.

Given the appropriate McAbs, reactive cells may be removed by opsonization. Opsonization is the removal of antibody coated cells by the reticuloendothelial system in the liver and spleen. When OKT3 (an anti-T McAb of IgG_2 class) was injected intravenously as an 'anti-lymphocyte serum' into patients in order to prevent acute kidney rejection the level of circulating T cells dramatically dropped 10 to 15 minutes after the injection of the McAb and lymphopenia developed (Cosimi et al, 1981). It is therefore possible that a relatively simple 'coating' with OKT3 in vitro may result (after the reinfusion of BM) in similar opsonization in vivo. This may lead to the elimination of BM born T lymphocytes. Of the first three evaluable patients who received allogeneic fully matched BM preincubated with OKT3 two developed no acute GvHD and showed an excellent 'take' of the transplanted BM while the third has delayed GvHD (Prentice et al, 1981b). These preliminary results show that the immunological techniques using carefully standardized specific McAbs do not damage BM stem cells. Further studies may be needed to establish more sophisticated methods for removing Ab coated cells (e.g. cytolysis in vitro using rabbit complement, immunoabsorbent columns, McAbs coupled to toxins, drugs or isotopes).

Standardization of enzyme inhibitors for therapy

The types of leukaemia and lymphoma sensitive to dCF in vivo are becoming apparent. Metabolic side-effects of ADA inhibition with this drug, e.g. renal and hepatic damage, are also being noted. Whether the drug alone or in combination with deoxyadenosine can selectively kill residual Thy-ALL blasts in BM in vitro during autologous BM transplantation and leave normal stem cells intact or whether additional deoxyadenosine should be given with dCF in vivo to obtain maximum tumour toxicity remains to be studied. Inhibitors of other enzymes in purine metabolism, e.g. of PNP or 5'NT are also available and their value used alone or in combination with nucleosides for in vitro removal of Thy-ALL cells (in autologous transplantation) or of mature T-cells (for GvHD prevention in allogeneic transplantation) remain to be assessed.

CONCLUSIONS

This review may reflect the selected and perhaps idiosyncratic view of one single laboratory. It also illustrates the speed with which this particular branch of haematology has been developing during the last four years. The improvement of diagnostic methods used for the analysis of leukaemias have led to a new classification and also to a more exact definition of the various prognostic factors on large patient groups (Greaves et al, 1981). Most of the phenotypes observed in leukaemic cells can be placed into stages of normal cell differentiation. The flood of new McAbs is likely to continue during the next few years. These precise analytical reagents will, without doubt, be used for separation of various early normal precursor cells for subsequent functional and biochemical analyses. Thus this development could lead to a detailed description of the functional and phenotypic stages of stem cell differentiation.

A similar kind of development is also likely in the analysis of B lymphocyte differentiation where new subset markers may soon replace the more cumbersome rosette assays. This will enable us to study the tissue distribution and anatomical localization of B cell subtypes and their relation, in normal and pathological conditions, to T lymphoid and non-lymphoid (macrophage/histiocyte) subsets. Some pathologists have already discounted the 'immunological classification' of lymphomas as irrelevant and superficial (Nathwani, 1979); in our view the relevant immunohistological investigations have just begun (Stein, 1980; Stein et al, 1981). Clearly, classical histology remains the most important single method for non-Hodgkin's lymphoma diagnosis. The different histological patterns however could well reflect origin from different B cell subsets (Habeshaw, 1979). It would therefore be not altogether surprising if a well chosen panel of new McAbs against these putative B lymphocyte subsets would provide, together with the already established methods for monoclonality testing (see above), a new and prognostically important tool.

Immunological and enzyme studies have already led to suggestions, and to a few promising clinical experiments, for the introduction of a new type of selective therapy. This approach could be potentially extended to the treatment of at least some younger patients with B lymphomas. Finally it seems that the final aim of the studies which attempt to prevent graft versus host disease by eliminating mature T lymphocytes (and perhaps also BM prothymocytes? Müller-Ruchholz et al, 1978) is to render the transplantation of haplo-identical BM reasonably safe. Removal of BM T cells (with McAbs) combined with preventative cyclosporin A therapy (Ch. 7) might possibly be used to this end. Animal experiments show that this approach may work. Prevention of GvHD in this situation could then dramatically increase the number of patients with otherwise incurable leukaemia who could benefit from BM transplantation (see Ch. 7).

ACKNOWLEDGEMENTS

We are indebted to Drs G. Goldstein and P. C. Kung, Ortho Pharmaceutical Company, Raritan, USA, and to Dr F. J. Bollum for stimulating discussions and supply of monoclonal and anti-TdT antibodies, to Dr H. G. Prentice of the Royal Free Hospital for clinical advice, to Dr M. F. Greaves, Imperial Cancer Research Fund, London, Dr J. Kersey, University Hospital, Minneapolis, USA and Dr T.

Waldman, National Institute of Health, Bethesda, USA for allowing us to see their unpublished manuscripts. We would also like to thank Dr C. Milstein for his encouragement and interest and the Leukaemia Research Fund for generous financial support.

REFERENCES

Abramson C S, Kersey J H, LeBien T W 1980 Journal of Immunology 126: 83–88
Anderson M, Müller-Ruchholtz W, Deljeschlager H 1981 Journal of Cancer Research and Clinical Oncology (in press)
Balch C M, Dougherty P A, Dagg M K, Diethelm A G, Lawton A R 1977 Cancer Immunology and Immunotherapy 8: 448
Barton R, Martiniuk F, Hirschhorn R, Goldschneider I 1979 Journal of Immunology 122: 216–220
Barton R, Martiniuk F, Hirschhorn R, Goldschneider I 1980 Cellular Immunology 49: 208–214
Ben-Bassat I, Simoni F, Holtzman F, Ramot B 1980 Israel Journal of Medical Science 15: 925–927
Beverley P C L, Linch D, Delia D 1980 Nature 287: 332–333
Blatt J, Reaman G, Poplack D G 1980a New England Journal of Medicine 303: 918–922
Blatt J, Reaman G H, Levin N, Poplack D G 1980b Blood 56: 380–382
Bodger M P, Thomas J A, Granger S, Tidman N, Janossy G, Francis G E, Delia D 1981 (in press)
Bollum F J 1979 Blood 54: 1203–1215
Borgers M, Verhaegen H, De Brabander M, DeCree J, DeCock W, Thone F, Geuens G 1978 Blood 52: 886–895
Bradstock K F, Janossy G, Pizzolo G, Hoffbrand A V, McMichael A, Pilch J R, Milstein C, Beverley P, Bollum F J 1980a Journal of the National Cancer Institute 65: 33–42
Bradstock K F, Janossy G, Bollum F J, Milstein C 1980b Nature 284: 455–457
Bradstock K F, Papageorgiou E S, Janossy G, Hoffbrand A V, Willoughby M L, Roberts P D 1980c Lancet i: 1144
Bradstock K F, Janossy G, Hoffbrand A V, Ganeshaguru K, Llewellin P, Prentice H G, Bollum F J 1981a British Journal of Haematology 47: 121–132
Bradstock K F, Hoffbrand A V, Ganeshaguru K, Llewellin P, Patterson K, Wonke B, Prentice H G, Bennett M, Janossy G 1981b British Journal of Haematology 47: 133–143
Braylan R C, Rappaport H 1973 Blood 42: 579–589
Breton-Gorius J, Reyes F, Vernant J P, Tullier M, Dreyfus B 1978 British Journal of Haematology 39: 295–303
Broder L, Edelson R L, Lutzner M A, Nelson D L, MacDermott R O, Waldmann T A 1976 Journal of Clinical Investigation 58: 1297–1306
Brooks D A, Beckman I, Bradley J, McNamara P J, Thomas M E, Zola H 1980 Clinical and Experimental Immunology 39: 477–485
Brown G, Hogg N, Greaves M F 1975 Nature 258: 454–456
Callard R E, Smith C M, Worman C, Linch D, Cawley J C, Beverley P C L 1981 Clinical and Experimental Immunology 43: 497–505
Carson D A, Kaye J, Seegmiller J E 1977 Proceedings of the National Academy of Science 74: 5677
Carson D A, Kaye J, Matsumoto S, Seegmiller J E, Thompson L 1979 Proceedings of the National Academy of Science 76: 2430–2433
Catovsky D 1977 In: Hoffbrand A V, Brain M C, Hirsch J (eds) Recent advances in haematology, 2nd edn. Churchill Livingstone, Edinburgh, p 201–218
Catovsky D 1980 In: Roath S (ed) Topical reviews in haematology, 1st edn. Wright, Bristol, p 157–185
Chang T W, King P C, Gingras S P, Goldstein G 1981 Proceedings of the National Academy of Science, USA 78: 1805–1808
Chechik B E, Rao J, Greaves M F, Hoffbrand A V 1980 Leukaemia Research 4: 343–349
Cline M J, Billing R 1977 Journal of Experimental Medicine 146: 1143–1145
Cohen A, Hirshorn R, Horowitz S, Rubenstein A, Polmar S, Hong R, Martin D W 1978 Proceedings of the National Academy of Science, USA 75: 472–476
Coleman M S, Greenwood M F, Hutton J J, Holland P, Lampkin B, Krill C, Kastelic J E 1978 Blood 52: 1125–1131
Cosimi B A, Colvin R, Goldstein G, Kung P C, Burton R, Delmomico F L, Russell, P S 1981 International Journal of Immunopharmacology (in press)
Crawford D H, Francis G, Edwards A E, Janossy G, Hoffbrand A V, Prentice H G, Secker D, Kung P C, Goldstein G 1981 British Journal of Haematology (in press)
Crawford D H, Brickell P, Tidman N, Janossy G, McConnell I, Hoffbrand A V 1981 Clinical and Experimental Immunology 43: 291–297

de Gast G, Platts-Mills T A E 1979 Journal of Immunology 122: 285–290

Donlon J A, Jaffe E S, Braylan R C 1977 New England Journal of Medicine 297: 461–464

Edwards N L, Gelfand E W, Burk L, Dosch H-M, Fox I M 1979 Proceedings of the National Academy of Science USA 76: 3474–3476

Fox R M, Piddington S K, Tripp E H, Dudman N P, Tattersall M H N 1979 Lancet ii: 391–393

Fu S M, Chiorazzi N, Wang C Y, Montazeri G, Kunkel H G, Ko H S, Gottlieb A B 1978 Journal of Experimental Medicine 148: 1423–1428

Galton D A G 1977 In: Hoffbrand A V, Brain M C, Hirsh J (eds) Recent Advances in Haematology, 2nd edn. Churchill Livingstone, Edinburgh, p 219–242

Ganeshaguru K, Lee N, Llewellin P, Prentice H G, Hoffbrand A V, Catovsky D, Greaves M F, Robinson J, Habershaw J A 1981 Leukaemia Research 5: 215–222

Gathings W E, Lawton A R, Cooper M D 1977 European Journal of Immunology 7: 804–810

Giblett E R, Anderson J E, Cohen F, Pollara B, Meuwissen H J 1972 Lancet ii: 1067–1069

Giblett E R, Ammann A J, Wara D W, Sandeman R, Diamond L K 1975 Lancet ii: 1010–1013

Goldschneider I, Ahmed A, Bollum F J, Goldstein A 1981 Proceedings of the National Academy of Science, USA 78: 2469–2475

Goldschneider I, Metcalf D, Battye F, Mandel T 1980 Journal of Experimental Medicine 152: 419–437

Greaves M F 1981 In: Knapp W (ed) Leukemia Markers, Academic Press, London, p24–32

Greaves M F, Brown G, Rapson N T, Lister T A 1975 Immunopathology 4: 67–84

Greaves M F, Delia D, Janossy G, Rapson N, Chessells J, Woods M, Prentice H G 1980 Leukaemia Research 4: 15–32

Greaves M F, Janossy G 1978 Biochimica et Biophysica Acta, 516: 193–230

Greaves M F, Roberts M, Janossy G, Peto J, Kay H E M 1981a British Journal of Haematology 48: 179–197

Greaves M F, Verbi W, Rao J, Catovsky D, Kung P C, Goldstein G 1981b (submitted for publication)

Greaves M, Verbi W, Vogler L, Cooper M, Ellis R, Ganeshaguru K, Hoffbrand A V, Janossy G, Bollum F J 1979 Leukaemia Research 3: 353–362

Grever M R, Siaw M F E, Jacob W F, Neidhart J A, Coleman M S, Hutton J J, Balcerzak S P 1981 Blood 57: 406–417

Grossi C E, Webb S R, Zicca A, Lydyard P M, Moretta L, Mingari M C, Cooper M D 1978 Journal of Experimental Medicine 147: 1405–1417

Habeshaw J A 1979 Cancer Immunology & Immunotherapy 7: 37–42

Habeshaw J 1980 In: Pochedly C, Graham-Pole J (eds) Non-Hodgkin lymphoma in children. Masson Publishing Co., USA

Habeshaw J A, Catley P F, Stansfeld A G, Brearley R L 1979 British Journal of Cancer 40: 11–34

Habeshaw J A, Catley P F, Stansfeld A G, Ganeshaguru K, Hoffbrand A V 1979 British Journal of Cancer 39: 566–569

Hershfield M S, Kredich N M 1980 Proceedings of National Academy of Science USA 77: 4292–4296

Hoffbrand A V, Ganeshaguru K, Janossy G, Greaves M F, Catovsky D, Woodruff R K 1977 Lancet ii: 520–523

Hoffbrand A V, Ganeshaguru K, Llewellin P, Janossy G 1979 In: Gross R, Hellriegel K-P (eds) Recent results in cancer research, Springer Verlag, Berlin, p 25–39

Hughes A S B, McVerry B A, Walker H, Bradstock K F, Hoffbrand A V, Janossy G 1981 British Journal of Haematology 47: 563–569

Hutton J J, Coleman M S, Keneklis T P, Bollum F J 1979 Advances in Medical Oncology, Research and Education 4: 165–175

Jäger G, Hoffman-Ferer G, Rodt H, Huha D, Thiel E, Thierfelder S 1977 In: Immunological diagnosis of leukaemias and lymphomas, Springer Verlag, Berlin, Heidelberg, New York, p 109–116

Janossy G, Roberts M, Greaves M F 1976 Lancet ii, 1058–1060

Janossy G, Goldstone A H, Capellaro D, Greaves M F, Kulenkampff J, Pippard M, Welsh K 1977a British Journal of Haematology 37: 391–402

Janossy G, Greaves M F, Sutherland R, Durrant J, Lewis C 1977b Leukemia Research 1: 289–300

Janossy G, Francis G, Capellaro D, Goldstone A H, Greaves M F 1978 Nature 276: 176–178

Janossy G, Bollum F J, Bradstock K F, McMichael A, Rapson N, Greaves M F 1979a Journal of Immunology 123: 1525–1529

Janossy G, Wodruff R K, Pippard M J, Prentice G, Hoffbrand A V, Paxton A, Lister T A, Bunch C, Greaves M F 1979b Cancer 43: 426–434

Janossy G, Bollum F J, Bradstock K F, Ashley J 1980a Blood 56: 430–441

Janossy G, Hoffbrand A V, Greaves M F, Ganeshaguru K, Pain C, Bradstock K, Prentice H G, Kay H E M 1980b British Journal of Haematology 44: 221–234

Janossy G, Thomas J A, Bollum F J, Mattingly S, Pizzolo G, Bradstock K F, Wong L, Ganeshaguru K, Hoffbrand A V 1980c Journal of Immunology 125: 202–212

Janossy G, Thomas J A, Pizzolo G, Granger S, McLaughlin J, Habeshaw J, Stansfield A G, Sloane J 1980d British Journal of Cancer 42: 224–242

Janossy G, Tidman N, Selby W S, Thomas J A, Granger S, Kung P C, Goldstein G 1980e Nature
    287: 81–84
Janossy G, Tidman N, Papageorgiou E S, Kung P C, Goldstein G 1981 Journal of Immunology 126:
    1608–1631
Johnston J M, Kredich N M 1979 Journal of Immunology 123: 97–103
Kamoun M, Martin P J, Hansen J A, Brown M A, Nowinski R C 1981 Journal of Experimental Medicine
    153: 207–211
Koike T, Tsukada T, Tamada T, Aoyagi T, Sakai T, Shibata A 1978 Clinical Haematology (Japan)
    19: 1690–1698
Köhler G, Milstein C 1975 Nature 256: 495–497
Koller C A, Mitchell B S, Grever M R, Mejias E, Malspeis L, Metz E N 1979 Cancer Treatment Reports
    63: 11–12
Korsmeyer S, Hieter P, Ravetch J, Waldmann T, Leder P 1981 In: Knapp W (ed) Leukemia Markers
    Academic Press, London, p85–98
Kung P C, Berger C L, Goldstein G, Logarfo P, Edelson R L 1980 Blood 57: 261–266.
Kung P C, Goldstein G, Reinherz E L, Schlossman S F 1979 Science 206: 347–350
Kung P C, Talle M A, DeMaria M, Butler M, Lifter J, Goldstein G 1980 Transplantation Proceedings 12
    (Suppl.): 141–146
Landreth K S, McCoy K, Clagett J, Bollum F J, Rosse C 1981 Nature 290: 409–411
LeBien T, McKenna R, Abramson C, Gajl-Peczalska K, Nesbit M, Coccia P, Bloomfield C, Brunning R,
    Kersey J 1981 Cancer Research (in press)
Lee N, Russel N H, Ganeshaguru K, Jackson B F A, Piga A, Prentice H G, Hoffbrand A V 1981 (in
    preparation)
Levy R, Warnke R, Dorfman R F, Haimovich J 1977 Journal of Experimental Medicine 145: 1014–1028
McCaffrey R, Smoler D F, Baltimore D 1973 Proceedings of the National Academy of Science USA 70: 521
McMichael A J, Pilch J R, Galfre G, Mason D Y, Fabre J W, Milstein C 1979 European Journal of
    Immunology 9: 205–210
McVerry B A, Goldstone A H, Janossy G 1979 Scandinavian Journal of Haematology 22: 53–56
Marks S M, Baltimore D, McCaffrey R 1978 New England Journal of Medicine 298: 812–814
Mejer J, Nygaard P 1979 Leukaemia Research 3: 211–216
Mills B, Sen L, Borella L 1975 Journal of Immunology 115: 1038–1044
Minowada J, Janossy G, Greaves M F, Tsubota T, Srivastava B I S, Morikawa S, Tatsumi E 1978 Journal
    of the National Cancer Institute 60: 1269–1277
Mitchell B S, Killer C A, Heyn R 1980 Blood 56: 556–559
Moore M A S, Broxmeyer H E, Sheridan A P C, Meyers P A, Jacobsen N, Winchester R J 1980 Blood
    55: 682–690
Moretta L, Webb S R, Grossi C E, Lydyard P M, Cooper M D 1977 Journal of Experimental Medicine
    146: 184–200
Müller-Ruchholz W, Wottge H U, Müller-Hermelink H K 1980 In: Thierfelder S, Rodt H, Kolb H J (eds)
    Immunobiology of bone marrow transplantation, Springer Verlag, Berlin, Heidelberg, New York
Nathwani B N 1979 Cancer 44: 347–384
Netzel B, Haas R J, Rodt H, Kolb H J, Thierfelder S 1980 Lancet i: 1330–1332
Nieuwenheus P, Kenning F J 1974 Immunology 26: 509
Nishida Y, Okudaira K, Tanimoto K, Akaoka I 1980 Experimental Hematology 8: 593–598
Ochs U H, Chen S-H, Ochs H D, Osborne W R A, Scott C R 1979 Journal of Immunology 122: 2424–2429
Pandolfi F, Strong D M, Slease R B, Quinti I, Aiuti F 1981 Journal of Immunology 126: 2205–2208
Piga A, Ganeshaguru K, Lee N, Breatnach F, Prentice H G, Hoffbrand A V 1981 British Journal of
    Haematology (in press)
Pizzolo G, Sloane J, Beverley P, Thomas J A, Bradstock K F, Mattingly S, Janossy G 1980 Cancer:
    2640–2647
Prentice H G 1981 In: Besser M, Compston N, Dawson A N (eds) Recent Advances in Medicine, Vol 18,
    Churchill Livingstone, Edinburgh
Prentice H G, Smyth J F, Ganeshaguru K, Wonke B, Bradstock K F, Janossy G, Goldstone A H,
    Hoffbrand A V 1980 Lancet ii: 170–172
Prentice H G, Russell N H, Lee N, Piga A, Ganeshaguru K, Blacklock H, Smyth J F, Hoffbrand A V 1981
    (submitted)
Prentice H G, Janossy G, Hoffbrand A V, Blacklock H, Lopez E, Kung P C, Goldstein G 1981b
    (in preparation)
Rambotti P, Evans R, Lopez C, Osfand M E, Smith M, Estren S, Siegal F P 1981 (in press)
Ramot B, Brok-Simoni F, Barnea N, Bank I, Holtzmann F 1977 British Journal of Haematology 36: 67–70
Reddy G P V, Pardee A B 1980 Proceedings of the National Academy of Science USA 77: 3312–3316
Reinherz E L, Kung P C, Goldstein G, Schlossman S F 1979a Journal of Imunology 123: 2894–2896
Reinherz E L, Kung P C, Goldstein G, Schlossman S F 1979b Journal of Immunology 123: 83–86

Reinherz E L, Kung P C, Pesando J M, Ritz J, Goldstein G, Schlossman S F 1979c Journal of Experimental Medicine 150: 1472–1482

Reinherz E L, Kung P C, Goldstein G, Levey R H, Schlossman S F 1980a Proceedings of the National Academy of Sience, USA 77: 1588–1592

Reinherz E L, Moretta L, Roper M, Breard J M, Mingari M C, Cooper M D, Schlossman S F 1980b Journal of Experimental Medicine 151: 969–974

Reinherz L E, Nadler L M, Rosenthal D S, Moloney W C, Schlossmann S 1979d Blood 53: 1066

Ritz J, Pesando J M, Notis-McConarty, Lazarus H, Schlossman S F 1980 Nature 283: 583

Roberts M, Greaves M F 1978 British Journal of Haematology 38: 439–452

Rodt H, Kolb H J, Netzel B et al 1980 Transplantation Proceedings 13: 257–261

Ross G D, Jarowski C I, Rabellino E M, Winchester R J 1978 Journal of Experimental Medicine 147: 730–744

Ross G D, Polley J 1976 Scandinavian Journal of Immunology 5: 99–111

Russell N, Prentice H G, Lee N, Piga A, Ganeshaguru K, Smyth J F, Hoffbrand A V 1981 British Journal of Haematology (in press)

Sagawa K, Minowada J 1981 (personal communication)

Salmon S E, Seligmann M 1974 Lancet ii: 1230–1233

Schlossmann S F, Chess L, Humphreys R E, Strominger J L 1976 Proceedings of the National Academy of Science, USA 73: 1288

Selby W S, Janossy G, Goldstein G, Jewell D P 1981 Clinical and Experimental Immunology 44: 453–458

Siaw M F E, Mitchell B S, Kollev C A, Coleman M S, Hutton J J 1980 Proceedings of the National Academy of Science, USA 77: 6157–6161

Sieff C, Robinson J, Greaves M F 1980 Nature (in press)

Silber R, Quagliata F, Conklyn N, Gottesman J, Hirschorn R 1976 Journal of Clinical Investigations 57: 756

Smyth J F, Poplack D G, Holiman B J, Leventhal B G, Yarbro G 1978 Journal of Clinical Investigation 57: 710–712

Srivastava B I S, Khan S A, Minowada J, Henderson E S, Rakowski I 1980 Leukemia Research 4: 209–215

Stashenko P, Nadler L M, Hardy R, Schlossman S F 1980 Journal of Immunology 125: 1678–1685

Stein H 1980 Journal of Histochemistry and Cytochemistry 28: 746–756

Stein H, Mason D Y, Gerdes J, Ziegler A, Naiem M, Wernet P, Lennert K 1981 In: Knapp W (ed). Leukemia Markers. Academic Press, London p. 99–108

Stein H, Siemssen U, Lennert K 1978 British Journal of Cancer 37: 520–529

Sutherland D R, Smart J, Greaves M F 1978 Leukemia Research 1: 115–126

Taheri M R, Wickremasinghe R G, Hoffbrand A V 1981 Biochemical Journal 196: 225–235

Thiel E, Rodt H, Huhn D, Netzel B, Gross-Wilde H, Ganeshaguru K, Thierfelder S 1980 Blood 56: 759–772

Tidman N, Janossy G, Bodger M, Granger S, Thomas J A, Kung P C, Goldstein G 1981 Clinical and Experimental Immunology 45 (in press)

Verbi W, Greaves M F, Koubek K, Janossy G, Kung P C, Goldstein G European Journal of Immunology (in press)

Vines R L, Coleman M S, Hutton J J 1980 Blood 56: 501–509

Vogler L B, Crist W M, Bockman D E, Pearl E R, Lawton A R, Cooper M D 1978 New England Journal of Medicine 298: 872–878

Vogler L B, Preudhomme J L, Seligmann M, Gathings W E, Crist W M, Cooper M D, Bollum F J 1981 Nature 290: 339–341

Warnke R, Pederson M, Williams C, Levy R 1978 American Journal of Clinical Pathology 70: 867–875

Webster A D B, Platts-Mills T A E, Janossy G, Morgan M, Asherson G L 1981 Journal of Clinical Immunology (in press)

Williamson A R 1979 Journal of Clinical Pathology 32: Suppl 13, 76–84

Winchester R J, Ross G D, Jarowski C I, Wang C Y, Halper J, Broxmeyer H E 1977 Proceedings of the National Academy of Science, USA, 74: 4012–4016

Wortmann R L, Mitchell B S, Edwards N L, Fox I H 1979 Proceedings of the National Academy of Science, USA 76: 2434–2437

Wu A M, Gallo R C 1977 In: Hoffbrand A V, Brain M C, Hirsh J (eds) Recent advances in haematology, 2nd edn. Churchill Livingstone, Edinburgh, p 289–324

Zola H, McNamara P, Thomas M, Smart I J, Bradley J 1981 British Journal of Haematology (in press)

11. Cytogenetic studies in hematologic disorders

Janet D Rowley

INTRODUCTION

Our understanding of the pattern of chromosome changes in the affected cells of patients with various hematologic disorders has expanded enormously in the past 10 years since the introduction of new staining techniques that allow the precise identification of every human chromosome. Some diseases, such as chronic myelogenous leukemia (CML) have been extensively studied and, therefore, a great deal of information is available regarding the chromosome abnormalities that occur both in the chronic and acute phases. Other disorders, such as the lymphoproliferative disorders, have been less adequately studied and many of the associations that I will discuss in this chapter are tentative at best. Even in a well studied disease such as CML, the introduction of new techniques requires that additional patients be studied using multiple techniques to be able to correlate chromosome changes with the new parameters. Thus, a number of laboratories have studied terminal deoxynucleotidyl transferase (TdT) or cell surface markers in the blast crisis of CML but there are few reports in which these analyses have been correlated with chromosome changes in the same sample. There are even fewer data correlating chromosome changes and cell surface markers in patients with acute lymphoblastic leukemia. Since both of these are areas in which substantial progress will be made in the next years, the preliminary correlations described here may have to be modified, possibly substantially, as the result of additional evidence.

The study of chromosome abnormalities in leukemia serves two functions; one of these is to assist in more accurate diagnosis, and therefore in the more rational choice of the most appropriate treatment for a particular patient. The other function is to provide clues as to the particular chromosome sites which are abnormal so that, in the future, we can understand the alterations in the regulation of genes that are located at these affected sites. This chapter will provide a general overview of the evidence regarding particular patterns of chromosome change in various hematologic disorders. The primary data that support these conclusions are presented in a number of current reviews of these diseases (Mitelman & Levan, 1978; Sandberg, 1980; Rowley, 1980c); moreover, an issue of Clinics in Haematology was recently devoted to cytogenetics in hematology (Vol. 11, No. 1, February 1980).

METHODS

An analysis of chromosomal patterns, to be relevant to a malignant disease, must be based on a study of the karyotype of the tumor cells themselves. In the case of leukemia, the specimen is usually a bone marrow aspirate that is processed immediately or cultured for a short time (Testa & Rowley, 1980b). In patients with a white blood cell count higher than $15.5 \times 10^9/l$, with about 10 per cent immature myeloid cells, a sample of peripheral blood can be cultured for 24 or 48 hours without adding phytohemagglutinin (PHA). The karyotype of the dividing cells will be similar to that obtained from the bone marrow. It is more difficult to obtain chromosomes from lymph nodes or spleen; however, careful attention to the details of tissue culture can provide mitotic cells in about 70 per cent of the samples in our laboratory. Lymph node cells are usually processed directly or are cultured for only 24 to 48 hours before chromosome preparations are made.

When an abnormal karyotype is found in a tumor, it is important to analyze cells from normal tissues, such as skin fibroblasts or peripheral blood lymphocytes stimulated to divide with PHA. In most instances, cells from these unaffected tissues will have a normal karyotype. The chromosome abnormalities observed in the tumor cells thus represent somatic mutations in an otherwise normal individual.

Chromosomes obtained from bone marrow cells, particularly from patients with leukemia, frequently are very fuzzy, and the bands may be indistinct. In patients with complex chromosome changes, multiple staining techniques are required for correct identification of the chromosomes involved in the rearrangements, and for more accurate definition of the chromosome bands affected by the breaks. In my laboratory, we are able to obtain a precise identification of the chromosome abnormalities in more than 90 per cent of leukemic patients and in about 70 per cent of lymphoma patients. Unused material can be stored in fixative in the freezer; usable quinacrine-fluorescent bands can be obtained from such material even after 12 years.

The observation of at least two 'pseudodiploid' or hyperdiploid cells or three hypodiploid cells, each showing the same abnormality, is considered evidence for the presence of an abnormal clone; patients with such clones are classified as abnormal. Patients whose cells show no alterations, or in whom the alterations involve different chromosomes in different cells, are considered to be normal. Isolated changes may be due to technical artifacts or to random mitotic errors. In malignancies with a very low mitotic index, however, a single abnormal cell may be the only malignant cell undergoing mitosis.

In the following discussion, the chromosomes are identified according to the Paris Nomenclature (1971), and the karyotypes are expressed as recommended under this system. The total chromosome number is indicated first, followed by the sex chromosomes, and then by the gains, losses, or rearrangements of the autosomes. A plus (+) sign or minus (−) sign before a number indicates a gain or loss, respectively, of a whole chromosome; a + or − after a number indicates a gain or loss of part of a chromosome. The letters 'p' and 'q' refer to the short and long arms of the chromosome, respectively; 'i' and 'r' stand for 'isochromosome' (i.e. chromosome with both arms the same) and 'ring chromosome'. 'Mar' is marker, 'del' is deletion, 'ins' is insertion, and 'inv' is inversion. Translocations are identified by 't' followed by the chromosomes involved in the first set of brackets; the chromosome bands in which the breaks occurred are indicated in the second brackets. Uncertainty about the chromosome or band involved is signified by '?'.

MYELOPROLIFERATIVE DISORDERS

Ph'-positive myelogenous leukemia

Cytogenetic studies on patients with chronic myelogenous leukemia (CML) have been the keystone for karyotype analysis of other human malignancies. New discoveries that have resulted from examination of CML have subsequently been confirmed in other hematologic malignancies, and in many solid tumors as well.

Chromosome studies of chronic myelogenous leukemia prior to banding
Nowell & Hungerford (1960) reported the first consistent chromosome abnormality in human cancer; they observed an unusually small G-group chromosome, which appeared to have lost about one-half of its long arm, in leukemic cells from patients with CML. Whether the deleted portion was missing from the cell or was translocated to another chromosome could not be answered at that time, because it was impossible to identify each human chromosome precisely with the techniques then available. Furthermore, the identity of this chromosome as either a No 21 or No 22 could not be established. Despite this uncertainty, the Ph' chromosome was a very useful marker in the study of CML.

Bone marrow cells from approximately 85 per cent of patients who have clinically typical CML are Ph'+; the other 15 per cent of patients usually have a normal karyotype (Ph'−). Chromosomes obtained from PHA-stimulated lymphocytes of patients with Ph'+ CML are normal.

A perplexing observation, still not explained, was that patients with Ph'+ CML had a much better prognosis than those with Ph'− CML (42- vs 15-month survival), and that patients with a Ph' chromosome and additional chromosome abnormalities did not have a substantially poorer survival than those who had only a Ph' chromosome. However, a change in the karyotype was a grave prognostic sign; the median survival after such a change was about 2 months.

Chromosome studies of CML with banding chronic phase of CML
Chromosome banding techniques were first used in the cytogenetic study of leukemia for identification of the Ph' chromosome as a deletion of No 22 (22q−). Since quinacrine fluorescence revealed that the chromosome present in triplicate in Down's syndrome was No 21, the abnormalities in Down's syndrome and CML were shown to affect different pairs of chromosomes.

The question of the origin of the Ph' (22q−) chromosome was answered when Rowley (1973a) reported that the Ph' chromosome results from a translocation rather than a deletion. Additional dully fluorescing chromsomal material was observed at the end of the long arm of one No 9 (9q+) and was approximately equal in length to that missing from the Ph' chromosome; it had staining characteristics similar to those of the distal portion of the long arm of No 22 (Fig. 11.1). It was proposed, therefore, that the abnormality of CML was an apparently balanced reciprocal translocation (9; 22) (q34; q11). Other studies with fluorescent markers or chromosome polymorphisms have shown that, in a particular patient, the same No 9 or No 22 is involved in each cell.

Karyotypes of 802 Ph'+ patients with CML have been examined with banding techniques by a number of investigators, and the 9;22 translocation has been identified in 739 (92 per cent) (Rowley, 1980a). It is now recognized that, in addition to the typical t(9;22), variant translocations may occur (Mitelman & Levan, 1978; Sandberg, 1980). These appear to be of two kinds; one is a simple translocation involving No 22 and some chromosome other than No 9, which has been seen in 29

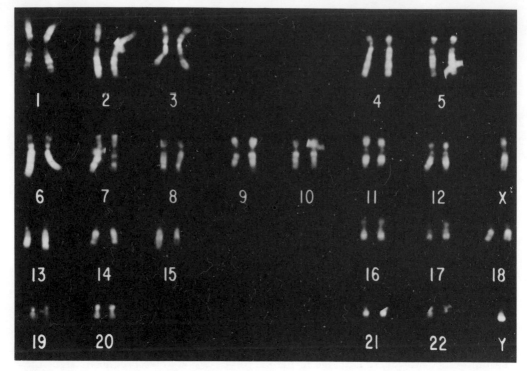

Fig. 11.1   Karyotype of a metaphase cell from a bone marrow aspirate obtained from an untreated male patient with CML. The chromosomes were stained with quinacrine mustard, and photographed with ultraviolet fluorescence. In addition to the Ph' (22q−) chromosome, the No 9 on the right (9q+) has an additional pale band that is not present on the normal No 9.

patients. The other is a complex translocation involving three or more different chromosomes; except in two cases, two of the chromosomes involved were found to be No. 9 and No 22. This type of translocation has been observed in 31 patients. Three patients have been reported who are said not to have had a translocation. The great specificy of the translocation involving Nos 9 and 22 remains an enigma. The survival curves for patients with variant translocations appeared to be the same as those for patients with the standard t(9;22).

Acute phase of CML
When patients with CML enter the terminal acute phase, about 20 per cent appear to retain the 46,Ph'+ cell line unchanged, whereas other chromosome abnormalities are superimposed on the Ph'+ cell line in 80 per cent of patients (Rowley, 1980a). In a number of cases, the change in the karyotype preceded the clinical signs of blast crisis by 2 to 4 months. In general, if patients have a clone of Ph'+ cells with a unique marker during the chronic phase, this clone will be the one involved in the transformation.

Bone marrow chromosomes from 242 patients with Ph'+ CML, who were in the acute phase, have been analyzed with banding techniques (Rowley, 1980a). Forty showed no change in their karyotype, whereas 202 had additional chromosome abnormalities. The most common changes frequently occur in combination to produce modal numbers of 47 to 52 (Table 11.1). The following gains or structural rearrangements of particular chromosomes were observed in 202 patients who had relatively complete analyses: gain of No 8 (95) gain of an isochromosome No 17q (74); gain of No 19 (38), and gain of Ph' (78).

Table 11.1 Modal chromosome number in aneuploid patients with leukemia whose cells have been studied with banding

Type of leukemia	Number of patients	Modal chromosome number										
		<44	44	45	46	47	48	49	50	51	52	>53
Ph'+ CML in acute phase	197	0	1	9	56[a]	60	27	12	11	8	5	8
ANLL	191	7	6	43	63[b]	58	4	2	1	2	1	4
ALL	54	2	0	2	17[b]	3	2	4	3	4	4	13

[a] Cells have the Ph' chromosome and other new abnormalities.
[b] All patients are pseudodiploid.

Since virtually all patients who are studied in the acute phase of CML have been treated, usually with busulphan, it is impossible to determine whether this therapy affects the pattern of abnormalities described earlier. Evidence has been presented recently that aggressive chemotherapy in the chronic phase may alter the pattern of chromosome abnormalities seen in the acute phase (Alimena et al, 1979).

Ph'-positive acute leukemia

Our interpretation of the biologic significance of the Philadelphia chromosome has been modified over the course of the last nine years, as our clinical experience with this marker has widened. Patients with acute myeloblastic leukemia (AML) in whom the Ph' chromosome was present were classified as cases of CML in blast transformation. This notion, which was broadened to include the cases that appeared to be acute lymphoblastic leukemia (ALL) at diagnosis, was generally accepted until about 1977. More recently, however, the tendency has been to refer to patients who have no prior history suggestive of CML as having Ph'-positive leukemia (Rowley, 1980a). It is becoming increasingly evident that the observed interrelations of Ph'+ leukemias are complex indeed, and that the distinctions between some categories are difficult to make. Moreover, although the Ph' chromosome is used as the marker that defines these leukemias, the cytogenetic studies on patients have often been woefully inadequate. Chromosome banding is an essential requirement not only for establishing whether the 'Ph'' is a 22q− rather than a 21q− chromosome, but also because there is some evidence that variant translocations may occur more often in the Ph'+ acute leukemias. Moreover, most of these patients become chromosomally normal in remission; cytogenetic studies on patients in remission are thus essential.

Some patients who are first seen with what appears to be acute leukemia and a Ph' chromosome have a high percentage of lymphoblasts, others have a high percentage of myeloblasts, and still others have a mixture of myeloblasts and lymphoblasts. In some instances, cells from the last group have been analyzed for cell surface markers. More recently, levels of TdT have been determined in patients with CML in blast crisis and in patients with Ph'+ acute leukemia. It is important to determine whether there is any correlation between the karyotype and TdT levels in patients who have elevated blast cell counts. The data available for 21 patients (Rowley, 1980a) suggest that CML patients with a lymphoid blast crisis and elevated TdT levels tend to remain only Ph'+ (5 of 5 patients), whereas patients with a myeloid blast crisis may have low or high levels of TdT and tend to show chromosome changes commonly associated with CML blast crisis (4 of 6 patients). Clearly, more patients will have to be examined so that we can determine whether these are consistent differences.

Levels of TdT were elevated in 7 of 8 patients with Ph'+ acute leukemia, regardless of whether the blasts were predominantly or only partially of lymphoid origin (Rowley, 1980a). Two patients remained only t(9;22), whereas other, apparently variable abnormalities occurred in six. Patients with mixed lymphoid and myeloid blasts seemed to have a mosaic karyotype with some cells having 46,Ph'+, and with a variable percentage having other abnormalities. Seven of the 8 patients were studied in remission, and all had a normal karyotype. Lymphoid cells in 5 of the 8 were of the null-cell type. Four of the 8 patients achieved a complete remission on treatment with vincristine and prednisone, and 3 had no response to a variety of drug combinations.

Acute nonlymphocytic leukemia (ANLL)

The use of chromosome banding techniques has markedly increased our understanding of the types and frequency of chromosome abnormalities in ANLL. Extra,

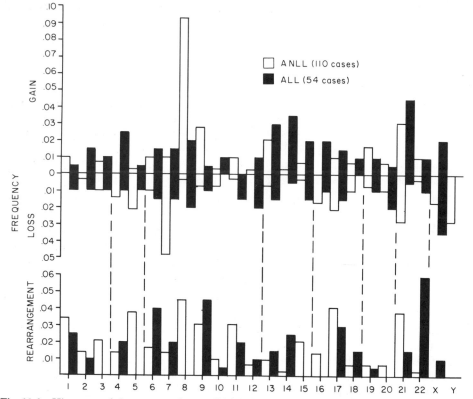

Fig. 11.2 Histogram of chromosome abnormalities (gain, losses, and rearrangements) in 110 cases of ANLL and in 54 cases of ALL, excluding documented cases of secondary karyotypic evolution. The frequency of each abnormality is calculated as a proportion of all abnormalities. (Reproduced from Cimino et al, 1979.)

missing, or rearranged chromosomes previously described on the basis of morphology alone can now be identified precisely in terms of the particular chromosomes or chromosome bands involved.

We and others have also shown that the karyotype pattern of the leukemic cells is correlated with survival. Patients with a normal karyotype have a significantly longer median survival (10 months) than do patients with an abnormal karyotype (4 months) (Golomb et al, 1978; First Workshop, 1978).

Approximately 50 per cent of the patients studied with banding have detectable karyotypic changes; these abnormalities are present prior to therapy and usually disappear when the patient enters remission. The same aberrations reappear in relapse, sometimes showing evidence of further karyotypic change superimposed on the original abnormal clone (Sandberg, 1980; Mitelman & Levan, 1978; Testa & Rowley, 1980a).

Although the karyotypes of patients with ANLL may be variable, examination of the chromosome changes seen in 191 chromosomally abnormal patients are available for analysis (Testa & Rowley, 1980a). The modal numbers for the changes are listed in Table 11.1. The non-random distribution of chromosome losses and gains is particularly evident in patients with 45 to 47 chromosomes (Fig. 11.2). A gain of No 8, the most common abnormality in ANLL, was seen in 48 cases, and loss of one No 7, the next most frequent change, was seen in 22 patients. Gains or losses of some chromosomes occurred only in patients with more complex karyotypes; they are likely to represent secondary changes occurring in clonal evolution, rather than primary events.

The 8;21 translocation in AML

Two structural rearrangements seen in ANLL appear to have special significance. The more common of these was first recognized by Kamada et al (1968) as most likely representing a translocation between a C- and a D-group chromosome. A high incidence of this aberration also was noted by other investigators. The precise nature of the abnormality was resolved by Rowley (1973b), who used the Q-banding technique to determine that it is a balanced translocation between Nos 8 and 21 [t(8;21)(q22;q22)] (Fig. 11.3). Chromosomes 8 and 21 can also participate in three-way rearrangements similar to those involving Nos 9 and 22 in CML. The 8;21 translocation is frequently associated with loss of a sex chromosome; 32 per cent of the males with the 8;21 translocation are $-Y$, and 36 per cent of the females are missing an X (Second Workshop, 1980). This association is especially noteworthy since sex chromosome abnormalities are otherwise rarely seen in ANLL.

The frequency with which this translocation occurs varies from one laboratory to another, but it probably amounts to about 8 per cent of all cases of AML. It appears to be restricted to patients with AML (M2 in FAB classification). These patients also have a much longer median survival than do patients with other chromosome abnormalities (Sandberg, 1980; Second Workshop, 1980). Data on survival of 48 patients with t(8;21) were reviewed at the Second Workshop (1980); the median survival of the whole group was 11.5 months.

The 15/17 translocation and acute promyelocytic leukemia (APL)

Another significant structural rearrangement is that observed in APL. The FAB

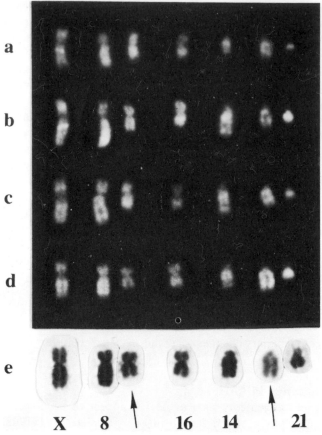

Fig. 11.3 Partial karyotype of four cells from a female patient with an 8;21 translocation and a missing X chromosome. (Rows a-d) Chromosomes stained with quinacrine mustard and photographed with ultraviolet fluorescence; (Row e) Standard Giemsa stain of chromosomes in row d. The 8q− chromosome (↑) is broken in band q22 and it it resembles a No 16; the 21q+ chromosome (↑) is broken in band q22 and it resembles a No 14.

cooperative study group recently (1980) recognized that not all patients have coarse granules in promyelocytes and has thus added a category called the M3 variant. The variant category was identified largely on the basis of the clinical features and a specific chromosome abnormality, namely, a translocation involving the long arms of Nos 15 and 17 [t(15;17)(q25;q22)] (Rowley et al, 1977). We have now studied a total of 7 patients with APL; each had the t(15;17). The breakpoint in No 15 appears to be distal to band q24, and in No 17 it appears to be in q22 (Second Workshop, 1980) (Fig. 11.4). The translocation was present in about 40 per cent of patients with APL; it was not seen in patients with other types of acute leukemia (Second Workshop, 1980). Eighty patients with APL were reviewed at the Second Workshop (1980). Forty patients had a normal karyotype, 33 had the t(15;17) alone or with other abnormalities, and 7 had other types of chromosome changes. Two patients with complex translocations involving Nos 15 and 17 and either No 2 or No 3 have recently been described (Bernstein et al, 1980). Therefore, the same pattern of variation of a specific translocation involves t(15;17) as well as t(9;22) and t(8;21).

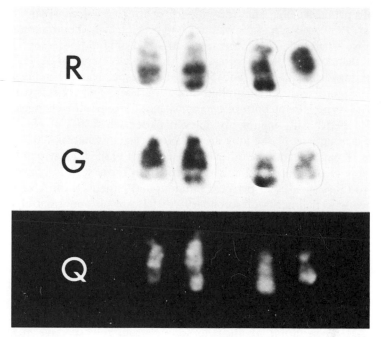

Fig. 11.4   Partial karyotype of chromosome pairs No 15 and No 17 from two patients with APL. The translocation chromosome is on the right in each pair. (Top row) R-banding with acridine orange from patient with the M3 variant form of APL. (Middle row) Modified trypsin G-banding of a cell from the same patient as in top row. (Bottom row) Q-banding of cell from another patient with the M3 variant form of APL.

It is important to make a correct early diagnosis because the initial therapy, which includes the use of heparin for control of bleeding, is associated with a significant improvement in survival. Whereas the correct diagnosis should not be difficult in typical cases, the M3 variant, in which granules may be lacking or reduced in number, may cause confusion. Every one of our M3 variant patients also had the typical translocation.

There is a curiously uneven and as yet unexplained frequency in the geographic distribution of this chromosome abnormality. It is seen in 100 per cent of our patients in Chicago, in about 70 per cent of patients seen in Belgium, and has not been identified in a single patient in Sweden.

Secondary acute leukemia

The occurrence of ANLL in patients who have been treated for other diseases is being recognized with increasing frequency. It has been observed in patients treated for Hodgkin's disease, non-Hodgkin's lymphoma, and other solid tumors, as well as non-malignant diseases. The fact that virtually every one of these patients has a clone of chromosomally abnormal cells in the bone marrow is not well known, nor is the fact that the chromosome changes observed are non-random. In addition, these data are particularly relevant to the identification of patients with ANLL de novo who may have been exposed to potentially mutagenic agents.

We studied the karyotype of 27 patients who developed ANLL either after treatment of a primary malignancy (26 patients) or after a renal transplant (one patient) (Rowley et al, 1980). Fifteen of the patients had previously had both radiotherapy and chemotherapy, 8 had only chemotherapy, and 4 had only radiotherapy. The median times from diagnosis of initial disease to the development of ANLL for these treatment groups were 61, 59, and 59 months, respectively. Nineteen of the 27 patients had a clone with a hypodiploid modal number. Twenty-six patients had an abnormal karyotype; one or both of two consistent chromosome changes were noted in 23 of 26 patients with aneuploidy. Eleven patients had loss of No 5, and three others were lacking part of the long arm of No 5 (5q−), whereas No 7 was missing from cells of 18 patients and one other had loss of part of the long arm of No 7 (7q−). Although these changes are distinctly different from those seen in lymphomas, they are similar to those seen in 25 per cent of aneuploid patients with ANLL de novo.

The cytogenetic hallmarks of secondary ANLL are an abnormal clone of cells, usually with a hypodiploid modal number, that is associated with the non-random loss of chromosomes 5 and/or 7. Our observations regarding the non-random abnormalities of Nos 5 and 7 are germane to the question whether the leukemic cells of patients with ANLL de novo contain specific karyotypic changes that allow one to distinguish between patients who have and those who have not been exposed to an environmental mutagen. Although this question cannot be answered at present, several lines of evidence suggest that the answer may be positive. The first of these comes from studies of ANLL in children, and the second from retrospective studies of the correlation of the karyotype with occupational exposure.

Three series describing ANLL de novo in 49 children have recently been published (Benedict et al, 1979; Hagemeijer et al, 1979; Morse et al, 1979). Not one of the 30 aneuploid patients had an abnormal clone with a hypodiploid modal number. Moreover, not one of the abnormal clones was missing a No 5, and only one was missing a No 7 and this was from a child who was also +8. Five patients had deletions involving 7q, but only two had a deletion at 7q22, which is the abnormality seen in adult ANLL de novo and in secondary ANLL.

Two studies reported by Mitelman and his colleagues in Sweden and in Rome provide some additional relevant information. The first study was a retrospective analysis of 56 patients who had ANLL and whose karyotypes and occupations were known. Twenty-three had a history suggesting an occupational exposure to chemical solvents, insecticides, or petroleum products, whereas 33 had no such known exposure (Mitelman et al, 1978). Only 24.2 per cent of patients in the non-exposed group had clonal aberrations, compared with 82.6 per cent in the exposed group. There was a distinctly non-random pattern of abnormalities in the exposed group, with 84.2 per cent of these patients having at least one of four changes, namely, −5, −7, +8, or +21. Only two patients in the non-exposed group had any of these aberrations.

These observations have been confirmed in a collaborative study consisting of more patients in the Swedish series combined with patients studied in Rome (Mitelman et al, 1979b). Thus of 156 patients with ANLL, 76 per cent of exposed patients and 32 per cent of non-exposed patients had a chromosomally abnormal clone of cells. When the exposed population was divided into those with an exposure to chemical solvents and pesticides, versus those with an exposure to petroleum products, 94 per cent (32 of 34) of the former patients were abnormal compared with 25 per cent (3 of 12) of the latter group.

Refractory anemia and preleukemia

It has been recognized for thirty years that some patients with unexplained cytopenias may develop acute leukemia. These patients may or may not have an increased frequency of blasts in the bone marrow. Data on 244 such patients were analyzed at the Second Workshop (1980). As in ANLL, about 50 per cent of patients had a normal karyotype. The types of chromosome changes were very similar to those seen in ANLL. Fifty-two patients had progressed to overt ANLL at the time of the Workshop. Some clear differences emerge between those patients who had and those who did not have a normal karyotype. Only 34 of 118 patients (29 per cent) with a normal karyotype were dead, roughly one-half of these having developed ANLL, whereas 66 of 111 patients (60 per cent) with autosomal abnormalities were dead, about one-half of them of ANLL. None of the 7 patients with loss of a sex chromosome developed acute leukemia. Thus, the data indicate that the presence of a chromosome abnormality in patients with cytopenias is a sign of a poor prognosis.

Polycythemia Vera (PV)

Early cytogenetic studies in PV before the advent of chromosomal banding techniques had revealed clonal abnormalities in a small percentage of them. Two abnormalities that were frequently reported were trisomy C and partial deletion of an F group chromosome (Lawler et al, 1970). Since a partially deleted F group chromosome had rarely been reported in other diseases, several investigators suggested that this abnormality had some degree of association with PV.

The incidence of clonal chromosome abnormalities in PV varies with the stage of the disease. Thus, fewer than 15 per cent of patients have abnormalities prior to myelosuppressive therapy, whereas the incidence is 35 to 40 per cent in initial samples from treated patients (Testa, 1980). Some PV patients develop leukemia late in their disease course; more than 80 per cent have abnormal karyotypes at this time. Gains of chromosomes are usually seen in abnormal clones from untreated PV patients, and therefore the modal number is generally hyperdiploid. Structural rearrangements are more frequent in clones from treated patients, which are typically pseudodiploid.

In 47 patients studied with banding techniques, gain of chromosomes, usually Nos 8 and/or 9 was most common (Testa, 1980). Clonal loss of a chromosome is an infrequent finding in PV. The two chromosomes most frequently rearranged were Nos 1 (10 patients) and 20 (14 patients). Nine of the 10 rearrangements of No. 1 resulted in trisomy of all or part of the long arm; trisomy of 1q, particularly bands 1q25 to 32, can be a common finding in various hematologic disorders (Rowley, 1977).

Most of the rearrangements seen in PV were found in treated patients. For example, 11 of the 14 patients with a rearranged No 20 had been treated, usually with ^{32}P, prior to their initial cytogenetic analysis. The deletion can also be found in patients treated with chemical agents, or in those who had a phlebotomy only. It has been suggested that the 20q− chromosome might have some diagnostic value in PV. However, a deleted F group chromosome has also been associated with idiopathic acquired refractory sideroblastic anemia and other myeloproliferative disorders.

Essential thrombocytosis (ET)

This myeloproliferative disorder is closely related to PV; although the majority of patients have a normal bone marrow karyotype, various abnormalities have recently been described in a few cases.

Deletion of the long arm of No 21 (21q−), was first described in Italy by Zaccaria (1978) in 6 of 7 patients, frequently in a small percentage (10–30) of cells. The abnormal cells are reduced in number after therapy. More recently, Van Den Berghe et al (1979b) described three patients with a 21q− chromosome among 18 patients with ET; a translocation involving 11q[t(11;21)(q25;q11)] was seen in all three. Whether there was a translocation in the earlier cases has not been established. The frequency of the 21q− chromosome is still unknown; it has not been observed in the cases reviewed by the PV Study Group.

LYMPHOPROLIFERATIVE DISORDERS

Two major problems with chromosome analysis in some of the lymphoproliferative disorders (LPD) are the small number of dividing cells and the difficulty of distinguishing the origin of these dividing cells. This is particularly difficult in chronic lymphatic leukemia (CLL), in which most of the mitotic cells described in studies before 1979 were derived from the non-malignant lymphocyte population.

Malignant lymphoma

Chromosome abnormalities in malignant lymphomas have been reported since 1962. Many of these studies were completed prior to banding; they have been reviewed recently by Mark (1977) and will not be referred to here. The studies revealed that the majority of patients with lymphomas had an abnormal karyotype, with no clear evidence of a consistent chromosome change in the same type of tumor obtained from different individuals. They also showed that the modal chromosome number in the non-Hodgkin lymphomas was near-diploid in the majority of cases, and that it was polyploid in more than one-half of the cases of Hodgkin disease. The proportion of karyotypically normal cells appeared to be higher in Hodgkin disease, suggesting that the normal host cell reaction might be increased in Hodgkin disease over that in other lymphomas.

Surprisingly few lymphomas have been studied with banding. The modal chromosome number seen in some lymphomas is summarized in Table 11.2. The results have confirmed the previous observations of a complex karyotype with many structural rearrangements (Mark et al, 1979; Rowley & Fukuhara, 1980). Some recurring types of chromosome change have been discerned.

Hodgkin's disease

Data are available for only 14 cases of Hodgkin's disease (HD); they are too few to provide useful information regarding chromosome patterns. Nine patients had modal numbers of 46 to 48, three were near-triploid, and two had modal numbers of 83 to 102. This agrees with the data obtained prior to banding that cells from HD frequently were in the triploid–tetraploid range. Reeves's (1973) patients had 10 to 25 per cent of lymph node cells or spleen cells with a normal karyotype; histopathologically, these cases were said to be of the mixed-cell type. The percentage of normal metaphases tends to be lower in patients with lymphocyte depletion than in those with mixed-cell HD. We have also noted that the frequency of normal metaphases is higher in patients with lymphocytic predominance HD.

Six patients clearly had a 14q+ marker. In all, the material appeared to be added at 14q32. The donor chromosome was identified in three patients and was 1q, 6q, or 10q. Chromosome studies show that the abnormal cells are clonal in origin. Many patients have a mosaic population of cells, with some near-diploid cells combined with triploid or tetraploid cells. The use of marker chromosomes clearly shows that the diploid cells are the precursors for the polyploid Reed-Sternberg cells.

Burkitt's lymphoma

Burkitt's lymphoma is an excellent example of a disease in which continued study of samples has revealed a complexity in the karyotype which was not suspected on the basis of the initial reports. Fresh tumor tissue obtained from six patients with African Burkitt's lymphoma was studied with quinacrine banding by Manolov and Manolova (1972). They reported on the presence of an extra band at the end of the long arm of one chromosome No 14 (14q+) in 5 of the 6 tumors, and in 5 of 6 cell lines established from tumors from other patients. Zech et al (1976) reported that the material at the end of No 14 represented a translocation from the end of No 8 [t(8;14)(q24;q32)] in 8 of the 10 African Burkitt's tumors in which it could be scored; two other tumors had the 14q+ chromosome, but the fluorescence was inadequate and involvement of No 8 could not be determined (Table 11.3). Kaiser-McCaw et al (1977) observed the t(8;14) in cell lines from two American Burkitt's lymphomas that had cultured for only 4 to 6 weeks; one of these was EBV-negative. Similar results were observed in a larger series of 18 patients with American Burkitt's lymphoma reported by Douglass et al (1980); 15 of the 18 patients had either a t(8, 14) or a 14q+ chromosome. Recently, Manolova et al (1979) determined that the break in No 8 is in the proximal pale portion of band 8q24, and in No 14, is in the distal part of 14q32 in all five cell lines studied. They concluded that the origin of the markers involves a reciprocal translocation of the terminal segments of 8q and 14q.

The heterogeneity of the translocation in Burkitt's lymphoma has only recently been recognized. There are now several patients with non-African Burkitt's lymphoma whose cells show a translocation involving the short arm of No 2 and the long arm of No 8 [t(2;8) (p12;q24)] (Van Den Berghe et al, 1979a; Miyoshi et al, 1979). Tumor cells from several other patients have a different variant translocation involving the long arms of No 8 and No 22 [t(8;22)(q24;q11)] (Berger et al, 1979b). Thus the consistent change in the t(8;14), t(2;8), and t(8;22) is the involvement of band 8q24. The frequency of the variant translocations is unknown, but may be about 10–30 per cent of Burkitt's lymphomas. Some patients with variant translocations have been EB virus positive and others have been negative. The data are too preliminary to determine whether there are important differences in the biological behavior of the Burkitt's cells with translocations other than t(8;14).

Poorly differentiated lymphocytic lymphoma (PDL)

Partial or complete data on the chromosome analysis are available for 38 patients with PDL. Some of the cases were described as PDL, whereas others were called lymphosarcoma, which may also include patients who had moderately- (MDL) or well-differentiated lymphoma (WDL) (Rowley & Fukuhara, 1980). Among the 38 patients, cytogenetic analysis was performed on a clearly involved specimen (lymph nodes or effusion) in 27; peripheral blood was studied in the remainder (Table 11.2). With one exception, a chromosomally abnormal clone was obtained from specimens that contained malignant cells, i.e. lymph nodes or effusions. In more than one-half of the lymph nodes, 12 to 50 per cent of the cells had a normal karyotype. A chromosomally abnormal clone was also seen in all except two peripheral blood specimens.

Patients with PDL often have very few dividing cells in their lymph nodes, and the banding pattern in many is somewhat indistinct. Complete karyotypes were available for only some of the 35 chromosomally abnormal patients, and the changes appeared to be somewhat variable; some changes, however, occurred more often than others, the predominant one, the 14q+ chromosome was identified in 24 of the 35 patients in whom chromosomally abnormal cells were found. Some other abnormality of No 14 was seen in three other patients. The identity of the donor chromosome is summarized in Table 11.3. Structural rearrangements of 11q and 18q were usually associated with translocation to No 14. The long and short arms of No 1 were involved in rearrangements 9 times. Some abnormality of No 1 was noted in 5 of our 9 patients with a 14q+ marker; abnormalities of No 1 were described in eight other patients, three of whom had a 14q+ chromosome, another of whom could have had a Dq+ marker, and two of whom were 14+. Abnormalities of the long arm usually were associated with trisomy for 1q. Six patients with an extra No 7 also had a 14q+ marker. No other abnormalities showed a consistent association.

Diffuse histiocytic lymphoma (DHL)

Chromosome analyses with the use of banding have been performed on 32 patients with DHL (Rowley & Fukuhara, 1980). In most cases, the analysis was done on involved lymph nodes or tissue from extra-nodal sites, although cells from pleural or ascitic fluid or circulating cells in the leukemic phase were also used. Every patient had a chromosomally abnormal clone of cells; in a few patients, two different, but related clones were observed. In many cases, the karyotypic pattern showed a remarkable consistency among the mitotic cells from any one individual. Where the data were provided, only a few normal cells were observed; many patients had no dividing normal cells in the samples that were analyzed.

Table 11.2 Modal chromosome number in patients with chronic leukemia and lymphoma[a]

Type of disorder	Number of patients	Modal chromosome number						
		<45	45	46	47	48	49–53	>70
Histiocytic	32	0	7	4	10	3	3	5
Poorly differentiated lymphocytic	35	3	2	9	10	4	4	3
T-cell dyscrasias	18	3	3	5	5	1	1	0

[a] Modification of table in Rowley & Fukuhara (1980)

As was noted prior to banding, the modal chromosome number tended to be near-diploid (Table 11.2). The chromosome pattern in some patients was extremely complex, with 15 or more structurally rearranged chromosomes per cell (Fig. 11.5). Under these circumstances, correct identification of all the breaks and rearrangements becomes very difficult. Some valid conclusions can nevertheless be reached at this time, based on data from 28 patients in whom the analysis was sufficiently complete to give fairly adequate information. Not a single patient had a gain of a No 1; gains of Nos 6, 14, or the Y chromosome also were not observed. Although all chromosomes were involved in structural rearrangements, deletions, inversions, and rings, there was a great difference in the frequency with which individual chromosomes were affected. The single most common abnormality was a translocation to the end of the long arm of No 14, usually to band 14q32; this occurred in 15 patients. The donor chromosome involved in the translocation was identified in all 15 cases (Table 11.3).

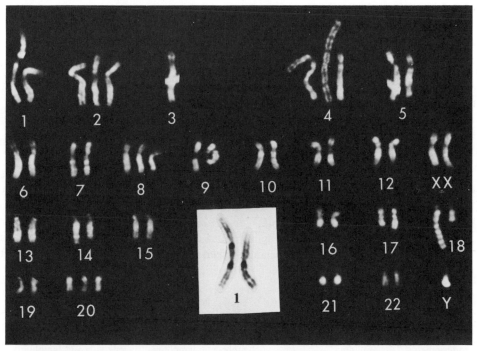

Fig. 11.5 Q-banding karyotype of a cell from the peripheral blood of a 59-year-old male patient in the leukemic phase of diffuse histiocytic lymphoma (the tumor was composed of large non-cleaved cells); the patient's leukemic cells were IgMk. This cell has 50 chromosomes, with additional Nos 2, 4, 8, 20, and an X, and with a missing No 3. Chromosome No 1 is involved in a complex rearrangement which includes duplication of all of the long arm. The first two No 4 chromosomes have a series of repeating bands of unknown origin at the end of the short arm (4p+). The end of the first 18q (18q+) also has a series of repeating bands. The first No 14 has an extra band which appears to be a translocation from the end of the third No 8 [t(8;14)(q24;q32)]. C-banding of No 1 (inset) shows that the 1q+ marker represents a duplication of all of 1q. (Reproduced from Fukuhara et al, 1978, Blood 52: 989.)

The identification of cell surface markers provides important information about the immunologic function of lymphoid tumor cells. Data are available on cell surface marker studies of tumor tissue obtained directly from only three patients with DHL. Two of our patients who were in the leukemic phase had monoclonal surface immunoglobulins (SIg) [IgM kappa].

Table 11.3 Frequency of 14q+ marker chromosome in lymphoid disorders[a]

Type of disorder	Number of patients			Donor chromosome						
	Total[b]	Abnormal	With 14q+	1q	8q	11q	14q	18q	Other	Unknown
Burkitt	43	43	35		25					10
Histiocytic	28	28	15	2	2	2	2	0	6	1
Poorly differentiated lymphocytic	28	27	24	0	2	8[c,d]	2	6[c,d]	0	7
T-cell	18	18	9	0	0	1	4	1	3	0

[a] Modified from Rowley & Fukuhara (1980).
[b] Number of patients on whom a reasonably complete analysis was done.
[c] Identification uncertain in two cases.
[d] One patient had two 14q+ chromosomes.

T-cell dyscrasias

It is frequently impossible to distinguish T-cell from B-cell malignancies without specific immunologic studies. However, some specific histologic types are closely associated with one or the other of these cells of origin — for example, Burkitt lymphoma and poorly differentiated lymphocytic lymphoma with B-cell origin and mycosis fungoides and Sézary syndrome with T-cell origin. The patients included here have been shown with the use of immunologic markers to have T-cell abnormalities.

Chromosomes from fewer than 20 patients with malignancies of T-cell origin have been analyzed with banding. Results on 15 patients have been reported, in addition to three of my unreported cases (Rowley & Fukuhara, 1980) (Table 11.2). Although this does not provide an adequate sample, very interesting differences can be noted in T-cell disorders, compared to the lymphomas that have been discussed thus far (Tables 11.3, 11.4). Some of the variability seen in this group may be related to the well-recognized heterogeneity of the T-cell malignances.

Table 11.4 Chromosomes commonly affected in chronic leukemia and lymphoma[a]

Type of chromosome change	Diffuse histiocytic lymphoma[b] (28 patients)	Number of chromosomes Poorly differentiated lymphocytic lymphoma (28 patients)	Chronic T-cell leukemia and lymphoma (18 patients)
Gain	7, 8	3, 7	Infrequent
Loss	6, 15, 13	11	13, 17, 20, 22
Break in short arm	1, 3, 6, 8	1	1, 9
Break in long arm	1, 14, 3, 9	14, 11, 18, 8	14, 2, 9, 13, 18

[a] Reproduced from Rowley & Fukuhara (1980).
[b] Listed in order of descending frequency.

Gains and losses of chromosomes are not a particularly prominent feature of these disorders. Five structural rearrangements, however, merit special attention; in addition to the 14q+ abnormality, translocations and deletions most often involve the long arm of Nos 2, 9, 13, and 18, in that order. Nine of the 18 patients with T-cell malignancies had a structural rearrangement of No. 14 leading to a 14q+ chromosome

(Table 11.3). In four cases, a tandem translocation was found; the break point occurred in q11-13 in one No 14 and in q32 in the other No 14 [t(14;14)(q11-13; q32)] One patient had one normal No 14 as well as the translocation (Rowley, unpublished). Three of the patients had ataxia-telangiectasia (AT) and had the 14q+ translocation in the stable phase of AT. In each patient, this chromosomally marked clone was the one involved in the leukemic transformation to CLL (2 patients) or atypical subacute lymphocytic leukemia. Two of the patients included here would fall within the recently described category of adult T-cell leukemia (Uchiyama et al, 1977); a 14q+ marker has been seen in these patients. Among the other structural rearrangements noted, those affecting No 2 are noteworthy, since this chromosome is rarely involved in abnormalities in myeloid disorders or in other non-Hodgkin lymphomas.

Ataxia-telangiectasia (AT)
It has been recognized for some time that patients with AT frequently have a small clone of PHA-stimulated lymphocytes that show consistent chromosome rearrangements. This clone may represent as few as 1 per cent of cells when the patients are first seen; but it expands and may subsequently become the major clone. With the development of banding, it was possible to show that, in most patients, the rearrangement was the result of a tandem translocation involving both No 14 chromosomes. One No 14 broke near the centromere, usually in band 14q12 or 13, and the rest of the long arm was translocated to the other No 14 at q32. The break point in the 'donor' No 14 may be somewhat variable; it did not always occur in 14q12. There was variability in the recipient chromosomes as well; the findings were summarized by Kaiser-McCaw et al (1975). Because these abnormalities are seen in PHA-stimulated lymphocytes, it is assumed that the T cell is the one affected.

Multiple myeloma
Reports on banding studies are available for relatively few patients with multiple myeloma (MM) or plasma cell leukemia (PCL) (Rowley, 1980c). Bone marrow cells from many of these patients have appeared to have a normal karyotype. This may be related to the very low mitotic index of the myeloma cells, so that the only cells in division are normal myeloid elements. In patients with abnormalities, the modal number tends to be hyperdiploid (47–55). The presence of a 14q+ marker chromosome has been reported in cells from 6 patients with MM and 2 patients with PCL. Many of these patients had other complex rearrangements as well; usually patients with a 14+ chromosome also had abnormalities of 1q. Gains of other chromosomes, particularly Nos 3, 5, 7, 9, and 11, occur together or in various combinations.

Chronic lymphocytic leukemia (CLL)
In the past, chromosome studies of patients with CLL have revealed mainly normal karyotypes. It is generally agreed that this result reflects the absence of dividing malignant cells. The early studies used primarily PHA, which is a T-cell mitogen; more recently, a variety of mitogens have been used with an emphasis on those that stimulate B-cells, such as lipopolysaccharide and Epstein Barr (EB) virus (Autio et al, 1979; Gahrton et al, 1979, 1980). This is appropriate since the majority (90 per cent) of CLL cells are of B-cell origin. These more recent studies have revealed a variety of chromosome abnormalities, two of which stand out. One of these is an abnormality of

No 14 in which material from some other chromosome is translocated to the end of No 14 producing a 14q+ chromosome similar to that described for the lymphomas. At least 3 patients with CLL have been identified whose cells have a 14q+ chromosome (Finan et al, 1978; Gahrton et al, 1979). More recently, Autio et al (1979) and Gahrton et al (1980) have identified 5 patients whose cells have an extra No 12 when they were stimulated with B-cell mitogens. This will be a very productive area for further research.

Acute lymphoblastic leukemia (ALL)

Chromosome abnormalities have been observed in about one-half of the patients with ALL (Mitelman & Levan, 1978; Sandberg, 1980; Rowley, 1980b). Even when banding techniques are used, about 50 per cent of patients appear to have a normal karyotype. It has long been recognized that aneuploid patients with ALL have higher modal chromosome numbers than do patients with ANLL (Sandberg, 1980) (Table 11.1). Considerably fewer data are available on the types and frequency of chromosome changes in ALL than in ANLL.

Only two unselected series of patients with ALL, each studied with banding, have been reported; Oshimura et al (1977) in 31 patients and Cimino et al (1979) in 16 patients. There have been a number of other reports on one or a few patients, all selected for some unusual cytogenetic abnormalities, most frequently the presence of a Ph' chromosome (see earlier). The small number of patients and the complexity of the karyotypes make the identification of non-random patterns in ALL difficult. At least one karyotypic abnormality however, seems to be consistently associated with one type of ALL. It seems reasonable to assume that other associations will become apparent in the future.

Fifty-three patients with ALL whose karyotypes were abnormal have been reported (Rowley, 1980b). The most frequent single change was a gain of one No 21; the second a gain of one No 14, and third a gain of one No 13 (Fig. 11.2). The only chromosome lost with any frequency was one X chromosome. Abnormalities of the Y chromosome have not been described. The most common deletion is that involving the long arm of No 6; the break point in 6q appears to be somewhat variable, involving the region from 6q11 to 6q25. As can be seen in Figure 11.2, the chromosome changes in ALL differ from those seen in ANLL. These differences probably reflect the action of different genes that provide a proliferative advantage in myeloid as compared with lymphoid disorders.

Patients with B-cell ALL constitute about 4 per cent of those with ALL. With one exception, every B-ALL patient identified had an abnormality of No 14 (14q+). The exceptional case, reported by Berger et al (1979b), had a t(8;22)(q24;q11). It should be noted that the break in No 8 is similar to that noted in the typical Burkitt t(8;14) as well as in the t(2;8) variant. The donor chromosome involved with No 14 was identified in 12 cases; it was 11q in the patient of Roth et al (1979) and 8q in the 10 cases of Berger et al (1979a) and the case of Mitelman et al (1979a). Some of the cases of Berger et al (1979a) and one patient of Slater et al (1979) had a Burkitt-type solid tumor as well as leukemic phase, which indicates that at least some B-ALLs may represent the leukemic phase of Burkitt lymphoma. The precise relationship of these two manifestations of malignant B cells is unclear at present. Karyotypic analysis will be useful in clarifying this relationship. Other abnormalities in addition to the 14q+

chromosome have been trisomy for part or all of the long arm of No 6, an additional No 7 and rearrangements of 1q and 13q. Cells from two patients were examined for EB virus and were found to be negative (Mitelman et al, 1979a). In one patient, the cells had a characteristically low level of adenosine deaminase (Roth et al, 1979).

We have recently studied a patient with pre-B ALL whose cells had a t(8;14) as well as other abnormalities (Rowley, unpublished). This provides further evidence for the close association of the 8;14 translocation and B-cell malignancies.

CONCLUSIONS

The primary focus in this chapter has been on the identification of non-random chromosome changes in various myeloproliferative and lymphoproliferative disorders. Although the data available for these disorders are quite variable both with regard to the number of patients studied and the quality of banding, patterns of chromosome changes can be discerned that differ among the various groups. Wherever possible, these patterns have been related to structural and functional characteristics of these cells as determined by others, as well as to the clinical correlations of particular chromosome changes. In the future, these correlations must be extended to relate specific chromosome aberrations, particularly translocations and deletions, to alterations of the function of genes located at these sites.

ACKNOWLEDGMENTS

This work was supported in part by Grants CA-16910, CA-19266, CA-23954, and CA-25568 from the National Cancer Institute, Department of Health, Education and Welfare, and by the University of Chicago Cancer Research Foundation. The Franklin McLean Memorial Research Institute was operated by the University of Chicago for the US Department of Energy under Contract No EY-76-C-02-0069.

REFERENCES

Alimena G, Brandt L, Dallapiccola B, Mitelman F, Nilsson P G 1979 Cancer Genetics and Cytogenetics 1: 79–85
Autio K, Turunen O, Penttilä O, Erämaa E, de la Chapelle A, Schröder J 1979 Cancer Genetics and Cytogenetics 1: 147–155
Benedict W F, Lange M, Greene J, Derencsenyi A, Alfi O S 1979 Blood 54: 818–823
Berger R, Bernheim A, Brouet J-C, Daniel M T, Flandrin G 1979a British Journal of Haematology 43: 87–90
Berger R, Bernheim A, Weh H-J, Flandrin G, Daniel M T, Brouet J-C, Colbert N 1979b Human Genetics 53: 111–112
Bernstein R, Mendelow B, Pinto M R, Morcom G, Bezwoda W 1980 British Journal of Haematology 46: 311–314
Cimino M C, Rowley J D, Kinnealey A, Variakojis D, Golomb H M 1979 Cancer Research 29: 227–238
Douglass E C, Magrath I T, Lee E C, Whang-Peng J 1980 Blood 55: 148–155
First International Workshop on Chromosomes in Leukaemia 1978 British Journal of Haematology 39: 311–316
French-American-British (FAB) Co-operative Group Bennett J M, Catovsky D, Daniel M T, Flandrin G, Galton D A G, Gralnick H R, Sultan C 1980 Annals of Internal Medicine 92: 261
Gahrton G, Robèrt K-H, Friberg K, Zech L, Bird A G 1980 Lancet i: 146–147
Gahrton G, Zech L, Robèrt K-H, Bird A G 1979 New England Journal of Medicine 301: 438
Golomb H M, Vardiman J W, Rowley J D, Testa J R, Mintz U 1978 New England Journal of Medicine 299: 613–619

Hagemeijer A, Van Zanen G E, Smit E M E, Hahlen K 1979 Pediatric Research 13: 1247–1254
Kaiser-McCaw B, Epstein A L, Kaplan H S, Hecht F 1977 International Journal of Cancer 19: 482–486
Kaiser-McCaw B, Hecht F, Harnden D G, Teplitz R L 1975 Proceedings of the National Academy of
    Science, USA 72: 2071–2075
Kamada N, Okada K, Ito T, Nakatsui T, Uchino H 1968 Lancet i: 364
Lawler S D, Millard R E, Kay H E M 1970 European Journal of Cancer 6: 223–233
Manolov G, Manolova Y 1972 Nature 237: 33–34
Manolova Y, Manolov G, Kieler J, Levan A, Klein G 1979 Hereditas 90: 5–10
Mark J 1977 Advances in Cancer Research 24: 165–222
Mark J, Dahlenfors R, Ekedahl C 1979 Cancer Genetics and Cytogenetics 1: 39–56
Mitelman F, Anvret-Andersson M, Brandt L, Catovsky D, Klein G, Manolov G, Manolova Y,
    Mark-Vendel E, Nilsson P G 1979a International Journal of Cancer 24: 27–33
Mitelman F, Brandt L, Nilsson P G 1978 Blood 52: 1229–1237
Mitelman F, Levan G 1978 Hereditas 89: 207–232
Mitelman F, Nilsson P G, Brandt L, Alimena G, Montuoro A, Dallapiccola B 1979b Lancet ii: 1195–1196
Miyoshi I, Hiraki S, Kimura I, Miyamoto K, Sato J 1979 Experientia 35: 742
Morse H, Hays T, Peakman D, Rose B, Robinson A 1979 Cancer 44: 164–170
Nowell P C, Hungerford D A 1960 Science 132: 1197
Oshimura M, Freeman A I, Sandberg A A 1977 Cancer 40: 1161–1172
Paris Conference 1971 1972 In: Birth Defects, Original Article Series, Vol 8, No 7. The National
    Foundation — March of Dimes, New York
Reeves B R 1973 Humangenetik 20: 231–250
Roth D G, Cimino M C, Variakojis D, Golomb H M, Rowley J D 1979 Blood 53: 235–243
Rowley J D 1973a Nature (London) 243: 290–293
Rowley J D 1973b Annales de Génétique 16: 109–112
Rowley J D 1977 Proceedings of the National Academy of Science, USA, 74: 5729–5733
Rowley J D 1980a Clinics in Haematology 9: 55–86
Rowley J D 1980b Cancer Genetics and Cytogenetics 1: 263–271
Rowley J D 1980c In: Zucker-Franklin D, Greave M F, Grossi C E, Marmont A M (eds) Biology and
    Pathology of Blood Cells. Edi Ermes, Milan, Italy (in press)
Rowley J D, Fukuhara S 1980 Seminars in Oncology 7: 255–266
Rowley J D, Golomb H M, Vardiman J W 1980 Submitted for publication
Rowley J D, Golomb H M, Vardiman J, Fukuhara S, Dougherty C, Potter D 1977 International Journal of
    Cancer 20: 869–872
Sandberg A A 1980 Chronomsomes in Human Cancer and Leukemia. Elsevier North-Holland, New York
Second International Workshop on Chromosomes in Leukemia 1980 Cancer Genetics and Cytogenetics
    2: 89–113
Slater R M, Philip P, Badsberg E, Behrendt H, Hansen N F, van Heerde P 1979 International Journal of
    Cancer 23: 639–647
Testa J R 1980 Cancer Genetics and Cytogenetics 1: 207–215
Testa J R, Rowley J D 1980a Cancer Genetics and Cytogenetics 1: 239–247
Testa J R, Rowley J D 1980b In: Catovsky D (ed) The Leukemic Cell. Churchill Livingston, Edinburgh
    p184–202
Uchiyama T, Yodoi J, Sagawa K, Takatsuki K, Uchino H 1977 Blood 50: 481–492
Van Den Berghe H, Parloir C, Gosseye S, Englebienne V, Cornu G, Sokal G 1979a Cancer Genetics and
    Cytogenetics 1: 9–14
Van Den Berghe H, Petit P, Broeckaert-Van Orshoven A, Louwagie A, De Baere H, Verwilghen R 1979b
    Cancer Genetics and Cytogenetics 1: 63–68
Zech L, Haglund U, Nilsson K, Klein G 1976 International Journal of Cancer 17: 47–56

12. Platelets, the vessel wall and antiplatelet drugs

C N Chesterman   A S Gallus   D G Penington

INTRODUCTION

The blood circulation is an efficient system of fluid conduction; one of its outstanding properties is a highly developed mechanism for stemming the flow of blood from an injured vessel. The efficiency of the circulation depends upon a complicated relationship between blood vessel components and flowing blood, not only with respect to functions such as fluid and solute passage to surrounding tissues but also with haemostatic components. The main requirements are a luminal surface which differs substantially in its thrombogenic properties from tissue immediately surrounding. In this way the signals to activate platelets and coagulation are retained external to the lumen and the sensitivity of the system to this signal can be very great. This sensitivity relates not only to the degree but to the rapidity of response. Platelets responding to an endothelial breach and adhering to subendothelial tissue are estimated to react within a few milliseconds (Born, 1977).

The important contribution of platelets to end-stage artery occlusion in patients with pre-existing atherosclerosis is well known, but recent evidence suggests that platelets may also contribute to the pathogenesis of atherosclerosis itself. This broader prospective has further stimulated interest in platelet-vessel wall interactions, and in their modifications by antiplatelet drugs.

PLATELETS

A detailed description of platelet morphology and function is inappropriate for this review; the subject will be briefly outlined with emphasis on aspects which relate to platelet-blood vessel interaction. Platelets circulate in a disc-shaped form 2 to 5 μm in diameter, maintaining a non-reactive surface to both endothelium and other platelets.

Membrane functions

The functional component of platelets which maintains their integrity while retaining requisite sensitivity to environmental changes is the *peripheral zone*. The peripheral zone has been divided into three areas: the outer plasmatic atmosphere, the glycocalyx and the inner platelet membrane (Jamieson & Smith, 1976).

The 'outer plasmatic atmosphere' contains a number of coagulation factors although these are loosely bound and may be removed by washing (Ardlie & Han, 1974). This zone is ill-defined compared to comparatively well-characterised receptors for specific coagulation factors on the platelet membrane (see below).

The glycocalyx is 20 to 50 nm in thickness and rich in glycoproteins several of which are unique to platelets. Surface labelling techniques (Phillips, 1980) have enabled the identification and subsequent partial characterisation of these proteins. The carbohydrate containing portions of these molecules are almost certainly oriented to the outer surface of the platelet membrane, and some of the glycoproteins are transmembrane (Phillips & Agin, 1974) possibly related to post-receptor signals.

Glycolipids and phospholipids are arranged in bilayers around the glycoproteins, sphingomyelin on the outer aspect of the membrane and phosphatidylcholine and phosphatidylethanolamine being on both membrane surfaces (Schick et al, 1976). The sites of phospholipids and specific phospholipases involved in the release of arachidonic acid for prostaglandin synthesis are not defined.

The functions of several membrane glycoproteins have been clarified. Convincing evidence is available for the following:

Thrombin receptor. Davey & Luscher (1967) proposed that thrombin hydrolyses a protein on the surface of platelets. More recent studies support this conclusion and have identified glycoprotein V as the 'sensitive' protein (see Phillips, 1980). Membrane binding of thrombin, however, is not altered by active-site inhibition of thrombin. Other studies have characterised a separate receptor. It has been reported that the platelet has about 500 high affinity sites (K_d 0.2 nM) and 50 000 low affinity sites (K_d 30 nM) for thrombin. The receptors appear to be a component of the glycocalyx (Tollefsen et al, 1974). Membrane glycoprotein I has been reported to be functionally and immunologically identical to *glycocalicin* (Jamieson et al, 1980) and the probable thrombin receptor. Bernard-Soulier platelets aggregate slowly with thrombin and their number of thrombin binding sites is reduced in proportion to the reduction of glycoprotein I (glycocalicin) (Jamieson et al, 1980).

Ristocetin — Factor VIII von Willebrand Factor receptor. This receptor, reduced in patients with Bernard-Soulier syndrome, has been identified also as glycoprotein I.

Platelet-platelet receptor. Many membrane changes take place following stimulation to platelet aggregation and release. Among earlier proposals was the formation of an intramolecular bridge between actin and myosin molecules (Booyse & Rafelson, 1972). Supporting evidence has not been forthcoming. Von Willebrand Factor is a possible candidate for this function by virtue of its large molecular radius and repetitive subunit structure (Coller & Gralnick, 1977). The most compelling data supports the notion that fibrinogen has a major role in this process. Membrane receptors for fibrinogen become available after stimulation by ADP and adrenaline, well demonstrated by radiolabelled fibrinogen studies (Marguerie et al, 1979) and confirmed by platelet agglutination by fibrinogen coupled to polymer particles (Pfueller & Firkin, 1978; Coller, 1980). Thrombasthenic platelets lack receptors on the basis of the above techniques (Peerschke et al, 1980; Coller, 1980) and this absence is associated with the classical defect in aggregation (and adhesion) in this disorder. This leads to the conclusion that either or both of glycoproteins IIb and IIIa which are absent in thrombasthenia may normally function as fibrinogen receptors.

Collagen receptor. Collagen is the basement membrane component responsible for platelet adherence, release and aggregation which are dependent on its quarternary structure (Jaffe, 1976). Adhesion is enhanced by Ca^{2+}, fibrinogen and Von

Willebrand Factor. Glycoproteins of the platelet glycocalyx are involved, in particular glycoprotein I (glycocalicin) as Von Willebrand's and Bernard-Soulier diseases are associated with defective platelet adhesion. It has been suggested that fibronectin (cold insoluble globulin), released by platelets (Zucker et al, 1979) and which binds collagen may be involved in platelet to collagen binding (Plow et al, 1979) although evidence to the contrary has been put forward (Santore & Cunningham, 1979).

Other receptors. Other receptors on platelet membrane have been more or less characterised and include those for adrenaline, ADP, serotonin, vasopressin, insulin and Factor Xa. It is clear that platelets play a significant role in prothrombin generation via the binding of Factor Xa to the platelet surface and such binding is dependent on Factor V activation (Kane et al, 1980).

Platelet granules

The electron dense granules contain ADP and serotonin both of which are of importance in platelet aggregation and probably in blood vessel tone. *α-granule* content is released simultaneously with ADP and serotonin. Fibrinogen, platelet factor 4 (PF4), β-thromboglobulin (β TG) and platelet derived growth factor (PDGF) are important α-granule components (Kaplan et al, 1979) although other platelet factors may also derive from these granules including coagulation factors V, VIII and XIII, fibronectin and antiplasmins. Both PF4 and PDGF have been identified in megakaryocytes and are probably synthesised there.

Antiheparin activity derived from platelets was described in 1948 by Conley and coworkers. A number of platelet proteins have heparin binding properties (Budzinski et al, 1979) but the major antiheparin activity resides in PF4, a protein with a subunit molecular weight (MW) of 7767 existing as a non-covalent bonded tetramer and which is released bound to a chondroitin sulphate complex of MW 350 000. In plasma it appears at least partially dissociated and exists in a number of smaller forms (Doyle et al, unpublished). It is rapidly cleared from the circulation (Dawes et al, 1978). Functions assigned to PF4 have been paracoagulation of fibrin monomer and more recently anticollagenase activity (Hiti-Harper et al, 1978).

β-thromboglobulin (Moore et al, 1975) is structurally closely related to PF4 (Begg et al, 1978), is a weaker heparin binder and is released unassociated with glyco-saminoglycan (GAG). Originally thought to be a 'structural' protein it has recently been shown to partially inhibit endothelial prostacyclin production (see p. 259).

Platelet derived growth-factor is a potent mitogen which is required for the proliferation in culture of a number of connective tissue cells (Ross et al, 1978). These include fibroblasts, glial cells and vascular smooth muscle. Recent evidence suggests that this protein has an approximate MW of 33 to 35 000 (Heldin, 1980; Chesterman et al, 1979) but is structurally dissimilar to PF4 and BTG (Heldin, 1980; Antoniades et al, 1979). It is heat stable but its activity is destroyed by trypsin and by reduction to two chains of MW 17 000 and 14 000; PDGF exists in platelets at concentrations orders of magnitude lower than PF_4 and β TG.

Exposure of fibroblasts or smooth muscle cells in culture to PDGF for as little as 60 minutes commits the cells to synthesise DNA. Other plasma factors are required to enable the cells to undergo cell proliferation; somatamedin C may be one such essential component (Stiles et al, 1979). Fluid endocytosis, lactic acid production, glucose uptake and other cellular events are stimulated by PDGF (Ross et al, 1978).

A number of other platelet released proteins and activities may have relevance to the vessel wall. Lysosomal enzymes common to other cells are released by platelets but additionally small amounts of neutral protease, elastase-like enzyme, collagenase and also heparitinase are present.

Prostaglandin metabolism (Fig. 12.1)

Release and aggregation of platelets is mediated by intracellular Ca^{2+} flux associated with a reduction in cyclic AMP levels in the cytosol. Prostaglandin intermediates produced as a result of excitation by thrombin and collagen are probably in large part responsible for this chain of events. It is important to note that platelet function is not totally dependent on prostaglandins as complete pharmacologic blockage of their synthesis, congenital absence of enzymes and modification of substrate fatty acids result in only minor haemostatic defects. Further, in vitro aggregation can be achieved by increasing the dose of 'release' agents. Prostaglandin metabolism remains an important basic modulator of platelet function. Platelet prostaglandin pathways have been thoroughly reviewed in recent years (Burch & Majerus, 1979; Moncada & Vane, 1979).

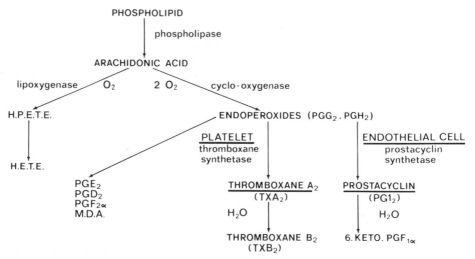

Fig. 12.1 A diagrammatic scheme of prostaglandin metabolism in the platelet and the vascular endothelial cell.

Membrane phospholipid, in particular phosphatidylinositol and possibly phosphatidylcholine comprise the substrate for phospholipases resulting in production of arachidonic acid. This release represents the major control mechanism in prostaglandin metabolism. It was postulated that phospholipase A was the enzyme responsible but recent work suggests reactions involving phospholipase C specific for phosphatidylinositol and a diacylglycerol lipase which acts on the diglyceride liberated by the phospholipase (Bell & Majerus, 1980). Two potential pathways for arachidonic acid metabolism exist. Ordinarily the minor pathway is by the action of lipoxygenase which brings about the conversion of arachidonic acid to 12-hydroperoxyeicosatetra-enoic acid (HPETE) with subsequent reduction to (12-hydroxyeicosatetraenoic acid (HETE). HETE is chemotactic for neutrophil and eosinophil leukocytes (Goetz et al, 1977).

The major pathway of arachidonic acid metabolism depends on cyclo-oxygenase, which produces cyclic endoperoxides, PGG_2 and PGH_2. Subsequent reactions result in their conversion to thromboxane A_2 (TXA_2). While the cyclic endoperoxides are active aggregating substances, TXA_2 is the most powerful but is also transient with a half-life of 30 seconds in aqueous medium and about 5 minutes in plasma. The stable end product thromboxane B_2 (TXB_2) is readily measured by radioimmunoassay.

Alternative metabolic pathways are responsible for the production of small amounts of PGE_2, PGD_2 and PGF_2 which have possible effects on inflammatory response.

Vascular effects of reduced platelet numbers or function

Haemostasis is compromised by thrombocytopenia or by platelet dysfunction. In the absence of complicating factors the skin bleeding time correlates well with the circulating platelet count. A role for platelets in endothelial 'integrity' has support from a number of studies. In rabbits, induced thrombocytopenia results in the development of endothelial fenestration and thinning (Kitchens & Weiss, 1975). These changes correlate with increases in vascular permeability and are restored by the return of normal platelet numbers. In an organ perfusion system it has been documented that platelets are important for vascular integrity (Gimbrone et al, 1969). Platelets have been reported to enhance growth (Saba & Mason, 1975) and migration (Maca et al, 1979) of cultured endothelial cells. Platelet lysate on the other hand did not effect DNA synthesis or migration of cultured endothelial cells (Thorgeirsson & Robertson, 1978).

THE VESSEL WALL

Components of the vessel wall

The endothelial cell

The lumen of the vessel is lined by a continuous monolayer of endothelial cells and this respresents the most important vascular component. Endothelial cells are elongated, with their long axis lying in the direction of blood flow. Their dimensions are 25 to 50 μm long by 10 to 15 μm wide (Cotran, 1965) and they overlap to a minor degree. Two forms of junctions between endothelial cells are described, tight and gap junctions. Tight junctions are more common in arteries but both types occur throughout the circulation with the exception of capillaries where gap junctions are absent. Presumably the form of junctions are critical for limiting transendothelial exchange of substances other than water and small molecules.

Endothelial cells have certain clear functions, perhaps the most obvious being a mechanical barrier with a facility for selective diffusion and transport. Tissue culture of endothelial cells (Fig. 12.2) has enabled the definition of a number of other potential functions. The interpretation of these capabilities, which are for the most part metabolic, is open to question because of the artificial nature of the systems employed. They remain, however, a starting point in delineating cell function and

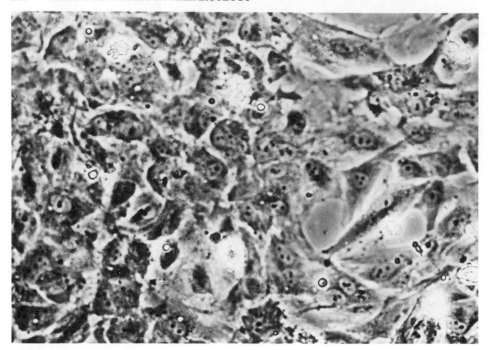

Fig. 12.2   Human umbilical vein endothelial cells form a monolayer in culture. The cells to the left have reached confluence while those on the right show the appearance of single cells spread on the surface of the culture dish (Phase contrast ×175).

in many instances culture characteristics parallel those suggested using other experimental techniques.

Endothelial cells contain the usual apparatus of eukaryotic cells. Microfilaments and microtubules (Weibel-Palade bodies) may participate in contractility and cell movement. This latter is of importance in the migration and spreading of endothelial cells following vascular injury and in neovascularisation of growing tissue. A rather specific structural component is a perinuclear arrangement of intermediate (10 nm) filaments (Blose & Chacko, 1976) which probably plays a role in orienting the spindle during mitosis. It also may help position other intracellular organelles.

PROTEIN SYNTHESIS

Endothelial cells display a high protein synthetic activity. Angiotensin converting enzyme, responsible for the cleavage of angiotensin I to produce angiotensin II, has been recognised as a useful and specific marker for endothelial cells in culture (Caldwell et al, 1976). Factor VIII related antigen is present in platelets, synthesised in megakaryocytes but also localised in vascular endothelial cells by immunohistological methods (Bloom et al, 1973) and demonstrable in cultured endothelial cells (Jaffe et al, 1973). Von Willebrand factor associated with Factor VIII related antigen is also produced by endothelial cells in culture (Jaffe et al, 1974) but procoagulant activity has not been detected.

Plasminogen activator has been identified with the vascular endothelium since the fibrinolysis autographs studied by Todd in 1958. Synthesis and release of plasminogen activator by cultured vascular endothelium from several species has since been demonstrated (Loskutoff & Edgington, 1977; Levin & Loskutoff, 1979). The simultaneous release of an inhibitor of this enzyme by endothelial cells suggests a complex regulation of fibrinolysis. Changes in culture conditions and the stage of cell growth cycle result in substantial variation in synthesis and release of plasminogen activator (Loskutoff & Levin, 1980); such observations underscore the pitfalls inherent in tissue culture experiments.

Antithrombin III (ATIII) has been identified in cultured endothelial cells by immunofluorescent studies (Chan & Chan, 1979). Further proteins pertinent to blood coagulation in endothelial cells are tissue factor activity (Maynard et al, 1977) and Hageman Factor activator activity which has been demonstrated in disrupted rabbit venous endothelium (Wiggins et al, 1980). Last but not least, endothelial cells synthesise basement membrane components (see below).

PROSTAGLANDIN METABOLISM (FIG. 12.1)
Vane and coworkers (1976) reported a potent vasodilator with a marked ability to inhibit platelet aggregation which was produced by aortic microsomes from the cyclic endoperoxide PGH_2. They later identified this substance as prostacyclin (PGI_2). Prostacyclin is synthesised by all cells of the vessel wall, endothelial cells producing the most and media and adventitia the least. PGI_2 is probably synthesised from arachidonic acid rather than extracellular cyclic endoperoxides (Needlemam et al, 1978). PGI_2 production is stimulated by thrombin, Ca^{++} ionophore (Weksler et al, 1978), angiotensin II (Dusting & Mullins, 1980), and inhibited by low density lipoprotein (Nørdoy et al, 1978) and platelet β-thromboglobulin (see p. 255). PGI_2 production may be altered by a number of drugs (see p. 268).

OTHER METABOLIC CAPABILITIES
Endothelial cells in culture metabolise exogenous nucleotides, adenosine triphosphate (ATP) and diphosphate (ADP), with the production of adenosine monophosphate and adenosine (Dosne et al, 1978). Recently, more detailed studies suggest the presence of a nucleoside diphosphate kinase with the conversion of excess ADP to ATP (Pearson et al, 1980). Exogenous serotonin is similarly taken up and metabolised by endothelial cells (Shepro et al, 1975).

Basement membrane and intercellular matrix
The basement membrane underlying the endothelial layer contains three important components: structural collagen fibres, a filtering system of proteoglycans and the cell-binding proteins, laminen (Timpl et al, 1979) and fibronectin (cold insoluble globulin). The endothelium is probably responsible for the synthesis of these substances while smooth muscle cells in the media of arteries are responsible for similar components in the media and internal elastic lamina. Elastin is important in both the internal elastic lamina and the media. Other glycoproteins throughout the vessel wall are thought to be organised into microfibrils and presumably play a supporting role.

Smooth muscle cells
The cellular component of the mammalian blood vessel media is solely the smooth

muscle cell while the adventitia also contains fibroblasts. The role of smooth muscle is predominantly twofold; the synthesis of the vessel supporting matrix and the ability to contract. As with endothelium, cell and tissue culture techniques have aided the investigation of these functions and factors which influence them.

SYNTHESIS

Smooth muscle cells form Type III collagen, to a lesser extent Type I collagen and elastin as the protein components of the media and internal elastic lamina. Chondroitin sulphate and dermatin sulphate are the major glycosaminoglycans (GAG) synthesised by smooth muscle cells as demonstrated by uptake of labelled precursors (Wight & Ross, 1975).

After birth the number of smooth muscle layers does not increase, medial thickening being due to connective tissue production (Gerrity & Clift, 1975). In the 8th to 16th weeks in the life of the rat, elastin increases from 6 per cent to 35 per cent and collagen from 8 per cent to 26 per cent in dry weight of the media. In the adult synthesis of extracellular matrix occurs only very slowly (Kao et al, 1961).

CONTRACTILITY

Contraction is the other major function of vascular smooth muscle both in response to the autonomic nervous system and to a number of locally released substances. The ultrastructural characteristics of smooth muscle myofilaments are well defined (Chamley-Campbell et al, 1979). Endothelial cell modulation of smooth muscle tone by the production of angiotensin converting enzyme, adenine nucleotides, and prostacyclin suggest a complex control system. In addition the substances released from platelets discussed below, are likely to result in smooth muscle contraction, particularly thromboxane A_2 and serotonin.

PROLIFERATION

Following wounding there is loss of differentiation in some of the smooth muscle cells with subsequent appearance of mitoses and cell division (Poole et al, 1971). This loss of differentiation includes reduction in myofilaments and the appearance of large numbers of synthetic organelles such as microsomes and rough endoplasmic reticulum and is seen to occur in smooth muscle cells over a 5–7 day period in cell culture (Chamley-Campbell et al, 1979).

Proliferation, migration and synthesis of smooth muscle cells are influenced by a number of plasma components which probably include insulin, somatomedins and lipoproteins as well as locally produced prostaglandins. An essential requirement for proliferation in culture is derived from platelets (see p. 255).

The non-thrombogenic property of the vessel wall

It has been noted that the non-thrombogenic property of the vessel wall resides in the endothelial cell. A number of factors have been identified as important for this function (Table 12.1). The negative surface charge, formerly regarded as significant in repelling similarly charged platelets may not be so critical. Desialation and subsequent loss of charge does not result in increased thrombogenicity in in vitro experiments (Danon & Skutelsky, 1976).

Adenine nucleotide metabolism by endothelial cells and in particular ADPase activity in reducing local ADP concentrations is potentially important in reducing platelet aggregation following adherence and release. Uptake of released serotonin by endothelium might have a similar function. Other enzymes likely to contribute to the inhibition of thrombus function are plasminogen activator and angiotensin converting enzyme. Local activation of plasminogen to plasmin may appear important following thrombosis rather than in its prevention; however the case for fibrinogen as a major component in platelet-platelet interaction suggests a primary role for fibrinolysis or fibrinogenolysis in endothelial defence against platelet aggregation.

Table 12.1 Non-thrombogenic properties of the vascular endothelium

Glycocalyx functions
   negative charge
   heparin binding (interaction with antithrombin III)
   ?α2 macroglobulin binding.
Metabolism of platelet released aggregating substances.
   ADPase
   serotonin uptake.
Proteinases
   plasminogen activator
   angiotensin converting enzyme
Antithrombin III release
Prostacyclin production
   antiplatelet activity locally
   vasodilation.

An interesting feedback from the endothelial angiotensin converting enzyme has recently been proposed. Angiotensin II produced by this enzyme may result in a burst of endothelial prostacyclin production (Dusting & Mullins, 1980).

Antithrombin III, heparin, heparan sulphate and other sulphated GAG are molecules closely related to endothelial cells with potential antithrombotic effects. A specific heparin-binding site has been reported on cultured endothelial cells (Glimelius et al, 1979). Heparin thus located can bind ATIII, possibly released by the endothelial cell itself. 'Activated' ATIII is then available at the endothelial surface. Heparan sulphate on the endothelial membrane may be capable of a similar relationship with ATIII (Busch et al, 1980).

Recent work has focused on PGI$_2$ production as the major endothelial inhibitor of platelets. PGI$_2$ binds to a specific platelet receptor and activates adenylate cyclase thus raising the cyclic AMP level in platelets (Best et al, 1977). As might be expected, the subsequent inhibition of ADP and thrombin-induced aggregation is paralleled by inhibition of mobilisation of membrane fibrinogen receptors (Hawiger et al, 1980). In vitro adherence and aggregation of platelets to exposed subendothelium is readily inhibited by PGI$_2$. Similarly, perfusion of PGI$_2$ in extracorporeal circulations significantly reduces platelet loss onto the artificial surface (see p. 271).

Vein wall biopsy in diabetic patients and atherosclerotic vessels have been reported to show reduced prostacyclin production. However a patient with congenital cyclo-oxygenase deficiency and no apparent endothelial prostacyclin production has not suffered thrombotic disease (Pareti et al, 1980). To confuse matters a less-well documented patient is reported to suffer from extensive atherosclerosis suggesting that PGI_2 production may help prevent the development of vascular disease (Rak & Boda, 1980).

The proposal (Moncada et al, 1978) that PGI_2 may circulate as an anticoagulant has been challenged (Haslam & McClenaghan, 1979). It is most likely that the prime role of PGI_2 is as a local modulator of platelet function, acting in the immediate vicinity of the vessel wall.

Thrombogenicity of the vessel wall

While the net effect of the intact endothelium is to inhibit platelets and coagulation, certain components have the potential for the opposite effect. Tissue factor and a Hageman factor activator have been described in disrupted endothelial cells (see above). In addition the factor VIII/VWF produced by endothelial cells and localised at this site has haemostatic effects. Thus endothelial disruption in vivo may contribute positively to thrombosis.

Endothelial loss or dysfunction

Endothelial dysfunction or damage is associated with loss of the protective barrier and exposure of subendothelial collagen fibrils. The adherence of platelets is well demonstrated (Fig. 12.3) with several methods of producing endothelial desquamation, for example, balloon catheter trauma and air injection (Fishman et al, 1975). In vitro models of de-endothelialised vascular strips have been used to study many

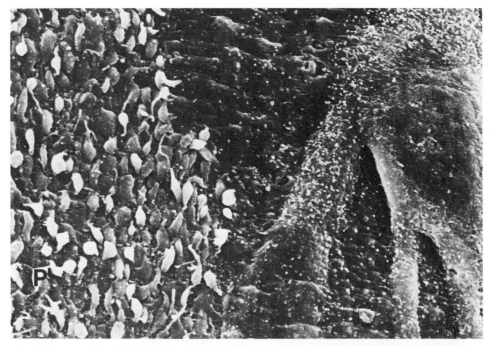

Fig. 12.3   Scanning electron micrograph of rat carotid artery following endothelial injury. Large numbers of platelets (P) are attached to the denuded surface (on the left). Regenerating endothelium is spreading across the denuded surface from above; the bulge on the right contains an endothelial cell nucleus; the endothelial surface shows multiple small microvilli ×2800. (Courtesy of Professor G. B. Ryan)

aspects of platelet/vessel wall interaction, in particular for pharmacological purposes (Baumgartner, 1979).

In vivo endothelial loss is related to several events. Shear stress particularly at vessel junctions where turbulence occurs is a continuing process (Barnhart & Baechler, 1978), with increased endothelial cell turnover. Immune complexes may result in endothelial cell damage. Leukocyte adherence to vascular endothelium is a manifestation of the inflammatory response. This phenomenon is thought to be mediated by activation of complement and in particular C5a. Stimulated granulocytes release lysosomal enzymes and thus induce vascular permeability by disrupting endothelial cell integrity (Craddock et al, 1979).

Viruses and bacteria may also cause endothelial desquamation possibly through the above mechanism although endotoxin may directly damage endothelium. It has also been proposed that elevated lipid levels may have direct toxic effects on endothelium.

Endothelial damage has been experimentally produced by toxic agents, for example homocystine (see p. 267). Investigation of the deleterious effects of cigarette smoking have shown that both carbon monoxide concentrations (Thomsen, 1974) and tobacco proteins may result in endothelial damage.

HYPERACTIVITY OF PLATELETS AND HYPERCOAGULABILITY

Vessel wall changes are likely to contribute the major stimulus for platelet adherence. The degree of reactivity of platelets to subendothelium may be influenced by factors unrelated to the vessel wall. The concept of hypercoagulability and platelet hyperactivity has a long history. Many laboratory correlates with clinical vascular disorders have been made (for review see Hirsh, 1977). In particular, evidence for platelet reactivity has been sought and found in atherosclerosis (see p. 267). In almost all instances such hyperactivity may be the result of vessel wall changes but nevertheless it may contribute to further atherosclerotic change or to consequent thromboembolic phenomena.

It is clear that there are factors, for example lipid levels and composition which can influence platelet behaviour independently. Platelets from patients with familial hypercholesterolaemia are abnormally sensitive to aggregating agents (Carvalho et al, 1974) and the acquisition of cholesterol by platelets is associated with increased sensitivity (Shattil et al, 1975). In vitro 'cholesterol-enriched' platelets released more labelled arachidonic acid and produced more TXB_2 than did control platelets in recent experiments (Stuart et al, 1980). A saturated fat diet in healthy subjects resulted in mildly elevated plasma PF4, increased platelet aggregates and increased heparin-neutralising ability of plasma when compared to a polyunsaturated fat diet (Jakubowski et al, unpublished).

In contrast, dietary differences have been identified which result in a reduction in platelet reactivity. The Eskimo population of Greenland has served as a model for this seemingly unique situation (Dyerberg et al, 1979). Their diet is largely animal fat (seal, fish, etc.) but the phospholipid content is rich in linolenic acid rather than linoleic acid. Increased eicosapentaenoic acid is released by membrane phospholipases; in platelets, the resulting prostaglandin intermediates formed, the trienoic series (in particular TXA3), are not aggregatory. Endothelial trienoic series prostaglandins (PGI_3) retain antiplatelet-aggregation activity.

Eskimos have mildly prolonged bleeding times, reduced reactivity to laboratory aggregating agents and notably a low incidence of ischaemic heart disease. In a further study, mackerel feeding to volunteers resulted in increased eicosapentaenoic acid in platelet phospholipid and to a reduction in platelet reactivity and TXB_2 production when exposed to collagen (Siess et al, 1980).

MOLECULAR EFFECTS OF PLATELET SECRETION ON THE VESSEL WALL

The adhesion of platelets to subendothelium may be followed by various sequelae (Table 12.2). Isolated platelets may shear off the surface. Frequently, however, adherence is followed by release and aggregation of further platelets. Apart from the release products and the exposure of binding sites involved in 'plasma' coagulation reactions, other components of the release reaction may have a direct effect on the vessel wall. Of potential importance are TXA_2, serotonin and other amines causing smooth muscle contraction. β-TG may result in local inhibition in endothelial prostacyclin production. Studies using cultured bovine aortic endothelial cells have demonstrated a reduction in prostacyclin activity following incubation with β-thromboglobulin at concentrations likely to be produced locally by thrombosis (Hope et al, 1979).

Table 12.2   Platelet release products and vessel walls

Products contributing to platelet aggregation and fibrin formation.
  Thromboxane A_2, serotonin, PF_3, coagulation factors I, V, VIII, XIII ? others.
  surface for coagulation
  inhibitors of plasminogen activator and plasmin
  antiheparin — PF4
Effects on vessel wall
  serotonin and thromboxane A_2 — vasoconstriction
  collagenase, elastase-proteolysis of basement membrane and supporting medium
  chemotaxis and permeability
  ? prostaglandin products
  β-thromboglobulin — ? reduction in endothelial prostacyclin.
  platelet derived growth factor — repair, smooth muscle and fibroblast proliferation
  intimal fibromuscular proliferation — atherosclerosis.

Furthermore, PF4 with its high affinity for GAG may bind heparin and haparan sulphate molecules on surrounding endothelium. Evidence for such a proposal is derived from the demonstration of ^{125}I-labelled PF4 binding to cultured endothelial cells (Busch et al, 1980). Bound PF4 is displaced by heparin. The intravenous injection of heparin in man causes an immediate but transient rise in plasma PF4 concentration (Dawes et al, 1978). A simultaneous rise in β TG levels does not occur, making it unlikely that the phenomenon is due to platelet release and suggesting displacement from the endothelial surface. PF4-bound to endothelial GAG may interfere with the ATIII interactions.

Heparinitase released from platelets may also result in degradation of heparin and heparan sulphate. Other enzymes, in particular the neutral proteases collagenase and elastase might reach local concentrations high enough to disrupt subendothelial basement membrane and the internal elastic lamina. Antiplasmin and an inhibitor to plasminogen activator relased in small quantities by platelets are directly antagonistic to the fibrinolytic component of endothelial defence. Other platelet activities including neutrophil chemotaxis by prostaglandin intermediates and effects on permeability may contribute to the inflammatory response following tissue damage. The release of PDGF is presently believed to promote repair processes although prolonged or repeated exposure of subendothelial components to PGDF may result in the initiation of atherosclerotic lesions (see below).

PATHOLOGICAL AND CLINICAL SEQUELAE OF ENDOTHELIAL LOSS AND PLATELET ADHERENCE

Minor events involving platelets and vessel wall must take place constantly. Presumably the degree of endothelial loss and possibly the 'hyperactivity' of platelets in certain conditions may tip the scale to produce pathological and clinical conditions which are platelet related.

Development of thrombi and thromboembolic disease
The initiation of thrombosis whether in the arterial circulation on the basis of atherosclerotic lesions, on prosthetic devices or in venous valves is almost certainly due to platelet adherence, aggregation and subsequent fibrin formation. The proportion of platelets to fibrin, red cells and granulocytes differs according to the vessel wall and conditions of flow. Similarly, embolic particles may be derived from either small platelet aggregates or from large fibrin and blood cell masses typical of pulmonary emboli.

Haemolytic-uraemic syndrome (HUS) and thrombotic thrombocytopenic purpura (TTP)
Two conditions in which the underlying pathophysiology involves the vessel wall and the platelet are HUS and TTP. Often regarded as variants of disseminated intravascular coagulation in the past, most reports suggest a minor coagulation component despite gross thrombocytopenia. The basic defect remains undefined but recent work has indicated mechanisms which may be responsible for mediating some of the abnormalities.

Kwaan and colleagues have observed that the vessel wall affected by the lesions of TTP are devoid of plasminogen activator activity (Kwaan, 1979) in contrast to both unaffected vessels in the same patient and thrombosed vessels in patients with DIC. They suggest that this defect may be causal.

The introduction of exchange transfusion and then therapeutic plasmapheresis in TTP (Bukowski et al, 1976) and more recently in HUS was originally based on the removal of putative immune complexes or immunoglobulin although the evidence for an immune mechanism in these diseases is not convincing. The subsequent observation that the infusion of plasma alone was equally effective, at least in some cases, led to the hypothesis of a missing inhibitor to platelet aggregation (Byrnes & Khurana, 1977). Such an inhibitor was partially characterised (Lian et al, 1979). Further case studies have provided evidence for reduced PGI$_2$ production in HUS and TTP in relapse. These observations have led to the proposal that a deficient plasma factor normally stimulates PGI_2 synthesis or release. Such a deficiency has been reported in a patient with HUS and two of her children (Remuzzi et al, 1980) also providing a possible explanation of the familial predisposition to the disease.

It is likely that these disorders represent a final common pathway of several pathogenetic factors and these suggested mechanisms may only apply in a proportion of cases.

Erythermalgia

Erythermalgia is an uncommon clinical entity consisting of redness, warmth and burning pain in the fingers or toes (Babb et al, 1964). It may be associated with myeloproliferative diseases and with disorders likely to result in abnormal vessels, for example diabetes mellitus, rheumatoid arthritis and SLE although more than half are idiopathic. Pathologically small platelet thrombi may occur in dermal blood vessels (Redding, 1977). In addition the discomfort is easily controlled by small doses of acetyl salicylic acid (aspirin). The symptoms were found to be associated with increased plasma levels of TXB_2 and β-TG in a case we have recently studied. During the three day period of relief afforded by 75 mg of aspirin the plasma levels of TXB_2 were unmeasurable and β-TG concentration was reduced significantly (unpublished observations). These clinical and laboratory findings suggest that this syndrome is mediated by platelet release although the exact nature of the production of symptoms is obscure.

Platelets and coronary spasm

Evidence has recently accumulated to suggest that platelets may play a more complex role in the production of ischaemic symptoms than previously believed. Platelet aggregates may initiate thrombus formation, or distal embolism of platelet aggregates may produce myocardial ischaemia. In addition coronary spasm either superimposed on atherosclerotic vessels or in comparatively normal vessels has recently been recognised as a definite occurrence, a cause of variant angina (Maseri et al, 1978) severe arrhythmia and acute myocardial infarction (Johnson & Detwiler, 1977). It is possible that platelet and vessel wall interactions may account for coronary spasm.

An increase in circulating catecholamines during exercise could cause increased sensitivity of platelets and the local release of TXA_2 at the site of an atherosclerotic plaque could result in vasoconstriction of major coronary vessels. Both an increase in plasma PF4 levels (Green et al, 1980) and TXB_2 in peripheral blood during exercise stress (Kuzuya et al, 1980), has been reported. PF4 levels showed some correlation with the production of angina and ECG abnormalities.

Experiments with anaesthetised animals have shown that intermittent thrombotic occlusions at coronary artery stenosis result in myocardial ischaemia which can be prevented by aspirin (Folts et al, 1976). Similar preservation of the myocardium after coronary artery ligation was afforded by a TXA_2 analogue which inhibits the production and the action of TXA_2 (Schrör et al, 1980). Antiplatelet agents may reduce the incidence of arrhythmias or ST depression on ECG in patients with ischaemic heart disease (see below). Such effects may be related to reduction in thrombotic occlusions but also may result from reduction in vasospasm caused by platelet release.

Atherosclerosis

Finally, platelets may play a causal role in the development of atherosclerosis. A traditional although not widely held theory to explain atherogenesis is the organisation and subsequent accretion of lipid into intravascular thrombi. While this mechanism may account for some lesions of atherosclerosis, a recent hypothesis has proposed a different role for platelets. This theory has support from experimental observations, animal models for atherosclerosis and isolated clinical studies.

The initial lesion of atherosclerosis has been characterised by three phenomena (1) intimal smooth muscle proliferation, (2) formation of a matrix of collagen, glycosaminoglycan and elastin; and (3) the deposition of lipid which is both intracellular and extracellular.

The adherence to subendothelium by platelets following endothelial desquamation and dysfunction has already been reviewed. The release of enzymes and other active components, in particular PDGF has been described. Ross and colleagues (for review see Harker & Ross, 1979) have proposed that the platelet response to endothelial injury and the action of PDGF is responsible for the initial migration of smooth muscle cells from the media to the intima and their subsequent proliferation. Lipid deposition may be either a subsequent or concomitant event and may itself result in endothelial disruption and smooth muscle proliferation.

Apart from in vitro experiments with cultured vascular smooth muscle cells a number of animal models suggest a requirement for platelets in the development of atheroma. Proliferative lesions in the vessels of rats are prevented by heparin administration (Clowes & Karnowski, 1977). Heparin may prevent platelet release but also might bind platelet proteins, particularly PDGF, which has similar heparin affinity to β-TG (Chesterman et al, 1979; Rucinski et al, 1979). Harker & Ross (1978) have studied 15 baboons made homocystinaemic by continuous intravenous infusion of homocysteine. Denudation of vascular endothelium was observed and a platelet response detected by increased consumption of ^{51}Cr-labelled platelets proportional to the endothelial loss. Severely affected animals developed eccentric fibromusculoelastic lesions within 3 months. Simultaneous administration of dipyridamole or sulphinpyrazone prevented the platelet consumption and development of intimal lesions.

Mechanical disruption of vascular endothelium in rabbits fed cholesterol-rich diets results in early atheromatous lesions which are preventable by rendering the animals thrombocytopenic during the period of damage. Aspirin administration reduced diet-induced coronary artery atherosclerosis in cynomolgus monkeys (Pick et al, 1979). Phenylbutazone and flufenamic acid but not aspirin were effective in reducing diet-induced atheroma in rabbits (Bailey et al, 1979). Swine with Von Willebrand's disease studied by Fuster et al (1978) are resistant to arteriosclerosis formation induced by cholesterol feeding.

In humans, platelet abnormalities have been described in many disorders associated with either the development of vascular disease or the presence of atherosclerosis. In the first category the evidence for platelet hyperreactivity has been reviewed (p. 263). In patients with established atheroma the results of platelet survival measurements have been controversial. Several authors have described subgroups of patients with coronary artery disease (CAD) who have shortened platelet survival. Patients with shortened platelet survival have fared less well following coronary artery grafting procedures (Steele et al, 1976) while the abnormality has been corrected by coronary grafting or by antiplatelet drugs in others (Ritchie & Harker, 1977). In one group of CAD patients shortened platelet survival was associated with increased plasma concentrations of PF4 and β TG suggesting a continuous tendency for in vivo platelet release (Doyle et al, 1980). Other authors have found groups of patients with stable CAD to have normal platelet survival (Salem et al, 1980).

Whether platelet activation is due to platelet hypersensitivity or to normal platelet interaction with grossly disordered vessel surfaces is not clear and it remains to be proven that the abnormalities described are responsible for adverse effects either short or long term.

PHARMACOLOGY OF DRUGS AFFECTING PLATELET AND ENDOTHELIAL FUNCTION

Aspirin and dipyridamole are perhaps the best known examples of a heterogeneous group of drugs which can inhibit platelet adhesion, aggregation, or release by altering platelet metabolism. These 'antiplatelet' drugs have surprisingly little effect on normal haemostasis, and there has been much recent interest in their potential value as antithrombotic agents. Among them, aspirin, dipyridamole, sulphinpyrazone, hydroxychloroquine and clofibrate have been the most widely evaluated in man. The newer generation of more specific antiplatelet drugs largely awaits clinical trial.

Effects of antiplatelet drugs on platelet metabolism and function, and their appropriate dose

Aspirin
This blocks platelet prostaglandin synthesis by inhibiting cyclo-oxygenase (Fig. 12.1). Enzyme inhibition is irreversible, due to active site acetylation, and, because platelets cannot generate new cyclo-oxygenase, the effect lasts throughout their life-span. There is therefore little or no platelet prostaglandin synthesis for 24 hours after an oral dose of 325 to 600 mg aspirin in man, followed by a gradual return to normal over 8 to 10 days as affected platelets are replaced. Even a dose as small as 80 mg has a substantial effect (Ali et al, 1980; Burch & Majerus, 1979). Aspirin treatment has been shown to prevent prostaglandin synthesis by rat megakaryocytes (Demer, Budin & Shaikh, 1980) but it is not known if this occurs in man.

Some platelet responses appear to be largely independent of prostaglandin synthesis and are unaffected by aspirin; these include platelet adhesion to collagen, and primary platelet aggregation by ADP, adrenaline and thrombin. On the other hand, aspirin reduces platelet aggregation by dilute collagen suspensions, and prevents the release reaction and secondary aggregation after exposure of citrated platelet rich plasma to adrenaline or ADP (Jobin, 1978; Packham & Mustard, 1977; Weiss, Aledort & Kochwa, 1968). Aspirin also prolongs the skin bleeding time, and reduces platelet retention in the bleeding time wound (Schwartz, Leis & Johnson, 1979). However, despite the obvious platelet function defect, aspirin does not prevent platelet adhesion or aggregation when flowing native blood is exposed to aortic subendothelium ex vivo (Baumgartner, 1979; Cazenave et al, 1978), and does not prevent increased platelet consumption in baboons with arteriovenous cannulae (over a dose range of 10 to 330 μmol or 2 to 60 mg/Kg/day) or in patients with prosthetic heart valves or arterial thrombosis (in the relatively high dose of 4 gm/day) (Harker & Slichter, 1972; Harker, Hanson & Kirkman, 1979).

The most appropriate antiplatelet dose of aspirin has become a question of some controversy. Aspirin can inactivate vascular as well as platelet cyclo-oxygenase, to block vascular prostacyclin production, a potentially adverse effect if prostacyclin production is indeed an important endothelial defence mechanism. However, cell culture experiments show that human endothelial cell cyclo-oxygenase is relatively insensitive to aspirin, and that the aspirin effect is transient due to continuing enzyme synthesis (Burch et al, 1978; Jaffe & Weksler, 1979), suggesting that aspirin should be given in small and infrequent doses which inhibit platelet cyclo-oxygenase but spare endothelial prostacyclin production. Dose-effect studies in human volunteers support this concept; in one report 3.5 mg/Kg aspirin was found to have a maximal effect on platelet aggregation and prostaglandin synthesis lasting for 24 hours, but only a small and transient effect on prostacyclin synthesis, which was totally suppressed by increasing the dose to 8 mg/Kg (Masotti et al, 1979). Most clinical trials of aspirin have used larger doses, usually 500 to 1500 mg/day often given in 2 to 4 divided doses. Whether smaller doses given once a day will be equally or more effective in practice remains to be determined.

Other non-steroidal anti-inflammatory drugs
Indomethacin, ibuprofen, naproxen, etc. also inhibit cyclo-oxygenase (Flower, 1974), but their effect in vivo is concentration dependent and reversible. Thus the aspirin-like platelet function defect is mild and transient after a single dose, though continued treatment sustains the antiplatelet effect, at least with indomethacin (Cockbill, Heptinstall & Taylor, 1979; Rane et al, 1978).

Sulphinpyrazone can be shown to inhibit platelet prostaglandin production (Ali & McDonald, 1977), and to reduce platelet aggregation by dilute solutions of adrenaline or collagen in vitro (Wiley et al, 1979), without affecting endothelial cell prostacyclin production (Gordon & Pearson, 1978). It also protects cultured human endothelial cells from injury by homocysteine in vitro and reduces in vivo endothelial injury by chronic homocysteine infusion in baboons (see p. 267). The drug may marginally prolong the bleeding time (Weston et al, 1977). Platelet survival studies suggest that the most appropriate antiplatelet dose is 200 mg given four times a day (Weily & Genton, 1970) which is consistent with the pharmacokinetics of sulphinpyrazone (Lecaillon et al, 1979).

Dipyridamole. High concentrations of dipyridamole inhibit platelet adhesion to collagen, platelet aggregation by collagen, ADP, and thrombin, and the platelet release reaction in vitro (Packham & Mustard, 1977). By contrast, the platelet function defect demonstrable in patients taking the drug is mild (Rajah et al, 1977). As dipyridamole is a phosphodiesterase inhibitor, its antiplatelet effect was initially attributed to increased platelet cyclic AMP levels. More recently, the drug has been shown to potentiate cyclic AMP elevation caused by prostacyclin and other adenylate cyclase stimulators (Best et al, 1979), and it has been suggested that the drug may act partly by potentiating the effects of endogenous, circulating prostacyclin (Moncada & Korbut, 1978). Dipyridamole may also stimulate endothelial prostacyclin synthesis

(Blass et al, 1980). Platelet survival studies suggest that the appropriate antiplatelet dose is 100 mg four times daily, or once a day when dipyridamole is given together with 1.2 gm of aspirin (Harker & Slichter, 1972).

Hydroxychloroquine inhibits platelet aggregation by ADP and collagen, as well as platelet release caused by low concentrations of collagen or thrombin; its effect on platelet prostaglandin metabolism is not known (Packham & Mustard, 1977).

Clofibrate inhibits collagen-induced aggregation and the second phase of ADP-induced aggregation (Packham & Mustard, 1977). It also reduces the increased platelet aggregability found in type IIa hyperlipoproteinaemia, perhaps by increasing membrane fluidity and so increasing the responsiveness of membrane-bound adenylate cyclase (Colman, 1978). Like all antiplatelet drugs, clofibrate has many pharmacologic actions. Hence any effect of clofibrate treatment on arterial thrombosis could equally be due to its cholesterol-lowering effect, which may itself reduce platelet reactivity (Stuart et al, 1980), or to its effect on fibrinogen levels and blood viscosity.

Promising new drugs like *ticlopidine*, which can reduce platelet aggregation by ADP and collagen for 4 to 8 days, apparently by increasing the responsiveness of adenylate cyclase to stimulators like PGE_1 (Ashida & Abiko, 1979; David et al, 1979; O'Brien et al, 1978) and *Bay g6575* which has been reported to stimulate prostacyclin release from blood vessels and to potentiate the antiplatelet effect of dipyridamole in man (Vermylen, Chamone & Verstraete, 1979), still await clinical evaluation. Prostacyclin and prostaglandin analogues with specific inhibitory effects on TXA_2 production have been studied in animals and clinical studies are underway in some areas.

Clinical trial of antiplatelet drugs

Regardless of the effect of potentially useful antiplatelet drugs on platelet function in vitro or ex vivo, their final evaluation depends on clinical trial. Further, as the antiplatelet drugs form a diverse group of substances with differing effects on platelet function, and as the thrombogenic stimulus differs in various thrombotic disorders, it is hardly surprising that every potential clinical application of each antiplatelet drug or drug combination has had to be tested separately, and that these drugs have not proved to be equally or universally effective.

The interpretation of clinical trial results has its own well-known problems. Trials of antiplatelet drugs have ranged in complexity from observations on the effects of treatment in single patients to large multicentre studies. Very few have met all or even most of the methodologic criteria for an ideal evaluation proposed by Gifford & Feinstein (1969) and elaborated by Genton et al (1975); many reportedly negative studies have involved too few patients to exclude even a large drug effect (see Freiman et al, 1978). Thus, the certainty with which a drug effect has been demonstrated or excluded has varied greatly in different studies.

In a number of clinical studies beneficial effects of antiplatelet drugs have been demonstrated in males with a notable absence of effect in females. At least one animal experiment has supported this strange sex difference (Kelton et al, 1978) but inadequate data is available to be sure that it is a true phenomenon.

Foreign surfaces exposed to flowing blood
Systemic embolism remains a substantial hazard after *prosthetic heart valve replacement*

despite improved valve design and adequate oral anticoagulant treatment (Murphy & Kloster, 1979). Adding dipyridamole to warfarin reduced the incidence of embolism from 14 per cent to 1 per cent in a one year study of 163 patients with early model ball valves (Sullivan, Harker & Gorlin, 1971) and from 11 per cent to 2 per cent in a more recent two year study of 117 patients by Rajah et al (1979). Aspirin has a similar effect; 500 mg per day reduced the embolism rate over two years from 18 per cent to 5 per cent in patients with Starr-Edwards valves treated with acenocoumarol (Altman et al, 1976), while Dale et al (1977) found that 500 mg bid reduced the incidence of embolism in anticoagulant treated patients with aortic ball valves from 9.3 to 1.8 episodes per 100 patient years. All of these studies were randomised, and two were double-blind (Dale et al, 1977; Sullivan, Harker & Gorlin, 1971). In the aspirin study of Dale et al (1977) the drug appeared to cause a five-fold excess of gastrointestinal bleeding; whether a smaller dose would be safer and remain effective is not known. It is important to note that antiplatelet drugs alone appear to be relatively ineffective in these patients.

Both sulphinpyrazone and aspirin have been shown to prevent shunt thrombosis in patients with *silastic arteriovenous shunts* for chronic haemodialysis. In double-blind, randomised trials the incidence of shunt thrombosis was reduced from 0.64 to 0.21 per patients month by 200 mg sulphinpyrazone tid (Kaegi et al, 1975), and from 0.46 to 0.16 per patient month by 160 mg aspirin per day (Harter et al, 1979); both statistically significant results. These are important trials because their end point was quite unequivocal, i.e. the removal of thrombus from a shunt. In addition, the study by Harter et al (1979) confirms for the first time that a very small daily dose of aspirin can be clinically effective.

Thrombus formation in *haemodialysis machines* can be reduced by aspirin (Lindsay et al, 1972; Stewart, Farrell & Dixon, 1975) and sulphinpyrazone (Woods et al, 1979), while dipyridamole may reduce platelet consumption during *cardiopulmonary bypass* (Nuutinen et al, 1977). However, the drug effects are relatively small and clinical application awaits the pharmaceutical development of more powerful agents like prostacyclin, which can prevent thrombocytopenia and preserve platelet function as demonstrated during extracorporeal membrane oxygenation in sheep and haemodialysis in greyhounds (Coppe et al, 1979; Longmore et al, 1979; Woods et al, 1978).

Artery surgery

Antiplatelet drugs have been evaluated in four settings: artery catheterisation, arteriovenous fistula formation, surgery for peripheral vascular diseases, and aorto-coronary bypass grafting.

Pretreatment with aspirin had no demonstrable effect on the incidence of partial or complete pulse loss after arteriography in two small randomised studies (Freed, Rosenthal & Fyler, 1974; Hynes et al, 1973), and its effect on the likelihood of cerebral embolism after coronary arteriography in a large, unrandomised study was equivocal (Storstein, Nitter-Hauge & Enge, 1977). On the other hand, Bedford & Ashford (1979) found that 600 mg aspirin given on the night before radial artery cannulation reduced the risk of subsequent artery occlusion detected with Doppler examination from 39 per cent to 13 per cent, the drug effect being most marked when the cannula occupied more than 30 per cent of the vessel lumen.

In a double-blind study of patients with a newly-fashioned arteriovenous fistula for haemodialysis, the incidence of early fistule thrombosis was reduced from 23 per cent to 4 per cent by 1 gm aspirin given every other day (Andrassy et al, 1974).

Another double-blind study, by Zekert et al (1975), suggests that aspirin may improve the early outcome of reconstructive artery surgery. Treatment with 1.5 gm/ day for 14 days after iliac or femoral artery bypass grafting was associated with a strong, but statistically not significant, trend towards a reduced early graft occlusion rate (from 30 per cent to 7 per cent), although in this study the incidence of graft occlusion among control patients seems surprisingly high. The drug had no apparent benefit after endarterectomy.

Ehresmann, Alemany & Loew (1977) also report evidence of long-term benefit after reconstructive artery surgery. Aspirin (1.5 gm/d) or a placebo was given to 428 patients; after one year, the incidence of artery occlusion was 22 per cent in control patients and 11 per cent in those treated with aspirin, a highly significant difference which was most evident when there was a suboptimal postoperative haemodynamic result. Sulphinpyrazone treatment, on the other hand, had no effect on the long-term results of peripheral artery surgery in a four year double-blind study of 169 patients (Blakely & Pogoriler, 1977; Rodvien & Salzman, 1978).

The theoretically attractive combination of aspirin with dipyridamole has been shown to prevent neointimal hyperplasia and graft occlusion during the first four months after placing a 'Dacron' or 'Gore-Tex' femoral artery graft in dogs (Oblath et al, 1978), but has not yet been tested after peripheral artery surgery in man.

Attempts have also been made to prevent aortocoronary bypass graft closure with antiplatelet drugs. Sulphinpyrazone (800 mg/d) apparently reduced the incidence of graft closure two weeks after surgery from 9.1 per cent to 3.8 per cent in one randomised study of 182 patients (Baur, van Tassel & Gobel, 1979), but neither 325 mg aspirin plus 75 mg dipyridamole given three times a day nor warfarin influenced the proportion of grafts which had closed by six months after surgery in another study of 50 patients (Pantely et al, 1979). Clearly, more information is needed about both short and long term effects of antiplatelet drug treatment in this situation.

Lastly, infusion of PGE_1 or prostacyclin has been reported to give long-term relief from rest pain in some patients with advanced peripheral artery disease (Carlson & Olsson, 1976; Szczeklik et al, 1979). The mechanism is not known, but is unlikely to be vasodilation, which leads to 'stealing' of blood from ischaemic tissue (Nielsen, Holstein & Nielsen, 1977).

Myocardial infarction
Despite over a decade of clinical trials, there is still more controversy than consensus about the role of antiplatelet drug treatment in patients with ischaemic heart disease.

The proposition that regular aspirin use may prevent myocardial infarction was supported by two consecutive surveys of hospital inpatients, which found that patients interviewed after myocardial infarction were one-fifth to one-half as likely to have regularly taken aspirin in the previous three months as in-patients with other disorders (Boston Collaborative Drug Surveillance Group, 1974; Jick & Miettinen, 1976). In addition, aspirin treatment in 125 men with rheumatoid arthritis followed for an average of 10 years at the Mayo Clinic was associated with a 30–50 per cent decrease in the incidence of myocardial infarction, sudden unexpected death, angina pectoris, and stroke when compared with that expected for their community. However, these trends were not statistically significant and were not seen in 378 women (Linos et al, 1978).

A comparison of aspirin use among 568 men who had died of coronary artery disease with that in living, age-matched, neighbourhood controls found no significant differences (Henneken et al, 1978), while a five year follow up of over one million people taking part in a cancer risk factor study found no correlation between frequent or occasional aspirin use at the start of the survey and subsequent death from coronary artery disease (Hammond & Garfinkel, 1975).

No prospective study of primary prevention has been reported with aspirin, but several have evaluated clofibrate, a particularly attractive drug for this purpose because it has effects on cholesterol and fibrinogen levels as well as platelet function.

The results of a large double-blind trial in 15 000 subjects recently completed in three countries under the auspices of the WHO argue strongly against the general use of clofibrate for primary prophylaxis. After five years of treatment, 1.6 gm clofibrate per day had lowered the serum cholesterol level in apparently healthy hypercholester-olemic men by an average of 9 per cent, but had no effect on mortality from ischaemic heart disease, while a statistically significant 26 per cent decrease in the incidence of non-fatal infarction was offset by a statistically significant excess of non-cardiac deaths (possibly coincidental) and a doubling of the cholecystectomy rate (Report from the Committee of Principal Investigators, 1978).

Two earlier and much smaller trials had suggested that clofibrate treatment may benefit patients with angina pectoris (Group of Physicians of The Newcastle Upon Tyne Region, 1971; Research Committee of the Scottish Society of Physicians, 1971). Clofibrate treatment for 3½ years was associated with a marked and statistically significant decrease in the likelihood of a first infarction, and a strong trend towards reduced cardiovascular mortality among 94 patients with angina in the Newcastle Study, while smaller trends in favour of clofibrate treatment were not statistically significant in the Scottish Study. In the absence of further trials the case for clofibrate in angina pectoris remains unproven.

Uncertainty also surrounds the role of antiplatelet drug treatment after myocardial infarction.

Aspirin has been evaluated in six double-blind randomised trials, most of which show suggestive, but statistically not significant trends towards reduced mortality and less reinfarctions in aspirin-treated patients.

Elwood et al (1974) found a trend towards reduced mortality which reached 34 per cent after two years, in their study of 1239 men treated with 300 mg aspirin per day or placebo for 2 to 30 months, starting an average of 10 weeks after infarction. Subgroup analysis suggested that any benefit from aspirin was limited to those patients starting treatment within six weeks of infarction, so a further trial of aspirin treatment starting during the initial hospital admission was begun. This second study found a 12.3 per cent mortality after one year in aspirin-treated patients, compared with 14.8 per cent in the placebo group. There was also a stronger trend towards reduced cardiovascular mortality and a significant 34 per cent decrease in non-fatal reinfarctions (Elwood & Sweetman, 1979).

Another, smaller trial compared results of treatment with 1.5 gm of aspirin per day, phenprocoumon, or a placebo, starting 30 to 42 days after myocardial infarction in 946 patients (Breddin et al, 1979). After two years, aspirin treatment was associated with a slightly lower mortality (8.5 per cent compared with 10.4 per cent in placebo patients and 14.1 per cent in patients given phenprocoumon), and a 42 per cent reduction in the 'coronary death rate' (from 7.1 per cent in placebo patients to 4.1 per cent) which was, however, not statistically significant.

Aspirin treatment starting late after infarction was evaluated in three other trials. In a study conducted by The Coronary Drug Project Research Group (1976), 1529 men who had taken part in previous CDP trials (and 75 per cent of whom had survived their most recent infarct by over five years) were given 972 mg aspirin or a placebo daily for an average of 22 months. Aspirin treated patients showed a 30 per cent decrease in mortality, as well as small reductions in the likelihood of sudden death and fatal or non-fatal reinfarction, none of which were statistically significant.

Similar trends were shown in the recent Persantine-Aspirin Reinfarction Study (PARIS), where 2026 patients received either 324 mg aspirin or 324 mg aspirin plus 75 mg dipyridamole three times daily (two study groups of 810 patients each) or a placebo (406 patients) for an average of 41 months, starting 2 to 60 months after their most recent myocardial infarct. Compared with the placebo group, patients given aspirin or aspirin plus dipyridamole had a lower mortality (by 18 per cent and 16 per cent), less coronary deaths (by 21 per cent and 24 per cent), and less non-fatal myocardial infarcts (by 30 per cent and 20 per cent), but none of these differences was statistically significant. Retrospective subgroup analysis showed the apparent treatment effect to be largely restricted to the small number of patients entering the study within six months of their qualifying infarct. In these patients, aspirin treatment was associated with a 51 per cent reduction and combined treatment with a 44 per cent reduction of mortality (The Persantine-Aspirin Reinfarction Study Research Group, 1980).

On the other hand, aspirin treatment was associated with excess mortality in the Aspirin Myocardial Infarction Study Research Group (1980) trial, where 0.5 mg aspirin or a placebo was given twice daily to 4524 patients, starting an average of 25 months after the most recent infarct. In this study, mortality after an average 38 months follow-up was 10.8 per cent in aspirin-treated patients and 9.7 per cent in the placebo group, while a small decrease of the non-fatal reinfarction rate from 8.1 per cent in controls to 6.3 per cent during aspirin treatment was not statistically significant.

Clearly these studies do not rule out the possibility of some benefit from aspirin treatment especially when started soon after infarction, although such benefit is likely to be small, as the inconclusive early treatment trial of Elwood & Sweetman (1979) was designed to detect a 25 per cent reduction of annual mortality with a probability below 0.05. Indeed, it has been claimed that aspirin can be shown to cause a 17 per cent decrease in mortality, a highly significant reduction of cardiovascular mortality, and a 21 per cent decrease in the likelihood of reinfarction when the results of these trials are grouped, regardless of their differing patient entry criteria and end point analyses (Editorial, 1980). Again the issue awaits further study.

A great deal of controversy has predictably surrounded the somewhat unexpected results of a recent trial of sulphinpyrazone after myocardial infarction. Labelled a 'rcinfarction' trial, this large multicentre study found that sulphinpyrazone had no effect on the reinfarction rate, but dramatically reduced the number of sudden deaths during the first seven months of treatment (The Anturane Reinfarction Trial Research Group, 1978; 1980). 1558 patients were given 200 mg sulphinpyrazone or a placebo four times daily, starting 25 to 35 days after infarction. An initial analysis after an average of 8.4 months follow-up showed sulphinpyrazone treatment to be associated with an annual mortality of 5.1 per cent and a 2.7 per cent likelihood of sudden death, compared with 9.5 per cent and 6.4 per cent in placebo patients. After an average of 16 months, sulphinpyrazone had apparently reduced cardiac mortality by 32 per cent (p = 0.058), and the risk of sudden death by 43 per cent (p = 0.041) in 'analysable' patients. This effect had developed fully by seven months after infarction, when sulphinpyrazone treatment was associated with a 51 per cent decrease in cardiac mortality, and a 74 per cent reduction in the number of sudden deaths; the survival curves in the two patient groups ran parallel after this time, indicating no further treatment benefit. At no time was the risk of reinfarction reduced.

That sulphinpyrazone should prevent sudden death without preventing reinfarction seems a paradox. It has been speculated that the drug has a previously undetected anti-arrhythmic effect, or prevents the release of vasoconstrictor materials by platelets, which may contribute to coronary artery spasm.

The trial was criticised because of its patient selection criteria, and the results cannot be extrapolated to patients with heart failure, cardiomegaly, untreated hypertension, or previous cardiac surgery, who were excluded from the study. Trial design and data analysis have also been extensively discussed, as have some discrepancies between the preliminary and final reports (e.g. Mitchell, 1980). Some criticisms were invalidated by the final analysis which showed that the effect of sulphinpyrazone on sudden deaths remained when 'unanalysable' events and patients who failed to complete the trial were included. However, a recent review of much of the original ART data by the American FDA has questioned whether allocations to the 'sudden death' category were consistently correct. Hence, a final opinion must await further analysis of other sulphinpyrazone trials like the Italian multicentre study begun in 1976 (Polli & Cortellaro, 1979).

Results of the long term clofibrate treatment after myocardial infarction have been disappointing. Further, there was no change in total or cardiovascular mortality in a trial of clofibrate plus nicotinic acid after myocardial infarction reported by Carlson et al (1977), although there was a statistically significant 50 per cent reduction in the risk of non-fatal reinfarction.

Dipyridamole had no effect on mortality or morbidity after myocardial infarction in a small study of 103 patients (Gent et al, 1968). Combined treatment with dipyridamole plus aspirin had little or no advantage over treatment with aspirin alone in the recent PARIS study (The Persantine-Aspirin Reinfarction Study Research Group, 1980).

Cerebral ischaemia

The aim of treatment in patients with *transient cerebral ischaemia* is to prevent stroke as well as further transient ischaemic attacks. In these patients stroke is most likely to develop within the first three months after presentation, may occur in up to 15 per cent of patients during the first year, and then has an incidence of 5 to 6 per cent per annum (Barnett, 1979; Millikan & McDowell, 1978). Case reports and small clinical trials have long suggested that aspirin, sulphinpyrazone, and dipyridamole may arrest transient ischaemic attacks in some patients. There is no evidence that aspirin treatment also reduces the high risk of stroke in men with these symptoms.

The Canadian Cooperative Study Group (1978) compared the effects of 325 mg aspirin qid and 200 mg sulphinpyrazone qid, given alone or together, and placebo, in a double-blind study of 585 patients with 'threatened stroke', defined as ischaemic episodes in the carotid or vertebral artery territory which resolved partly or completely within 24 hours. Eighty per cent of patients had more than one attack in the three months before they entered the study. After an average follow up of 26 months, the aspirin treated patients showed a 19 per cent reduction in the risk of stroke, death, or further transient ischaemic episodes (p < 0.05), and a 31 per cent decrease in the risk of stroke or death (p < 0.05). Subgroup analysis showed the apparent aspirin effect to be limited to men, in whom the likelihood of stroke or death was reduced by a dramatic 49 per cent (from 27.2 per cent to 14.5 per cent). There was no apparent benefit from sulphinpyrazone.

Aspirin also reduced the incidence of cerebral ischaemic attacks in a smaller multicentre trial with a shorter follow-up period reported by Fields et al (1977). Here, 178 patients with transient carotid territory ischaemia were given 650 mg aspirin twice daily or a placebo; after six months, 90 per cent of aspirin-treated patients and 74 per cent of the placebo group had less ischaemic attacks than before (p < 0.05) and there was a trend towards fewer strokes and a lower mortality in the aspirin group. There was a similar trend in a separate aspirin study of 125 patients who had carotid artery surgery before randomisation (Fields et al, 1978).

The case for aspirin must be seen in the context of other presently acceptable therapeutic approaches. Oral anticoagulants are the first choice in women, and should certainly be considered in men if aspirin fails. Indeed, Olsson et al (1980) concluded that coumadin may be superior to twice daily treatment with 0.5 gm aspirin plus 75 mg dipyridamole in men and women with threatened stroke. In their randomised study of patients with transient ischaemic attacks (TIA) or reversible ischaemic neurologic deficit (RIND), eight of 68 patients treated with coumadin, and 22 of 67 patients taking aspirin/dipyridamole developed further TIA, RIND, or stroke during two years (p < 0.05). However, bleeding complications were more frequent and serious during oral anticoagulant treatment. Failure of aspirin treatment in patients responding to oral anticoagulants was also reported by Jestico, Harrison & Marshall (1978).

The relative effectiveness of drug treatment and surgery is not known. In expert hands and with proper case-selection, mortality and morbidity after carotid endarterectomy can be low, but the complication rate is probably unacceptable outside specialised centres (Millikan & McDowell, 1978).

There is little evidence supporting antiplatelet drug treatment after a completed stroke, as randomised studies have not shown benefit from treatment with dipyridamole (Atcheson, Danta & Hutchinson, 1969), clofibrate (Atcheson & Hutchinson, 1972; Veterans Administration Cooperative Study Group, 1973) or sulphinpyrazone (Blakely, 1979).

Venous thrombosis

The use of antiplatelet drugs to prevent venous thrombosis has been evaluated in patients having elective abdominal surgery, total hip replacement or knee replacement, and after hip fracture. Results in orthopaedic surgery will be considered separately because this carries a particularly high risk of postoperative thrombosis which is relatively resistant to prophylaxis.

A consideration of the diagnostic methods used is particularly important for the correct interpretation of these trials. For instance, aspirin was found to reduce the incidence of *clinically* detectable venous thrombosis and pulmonary embolism after surgery (Loew et al, 1974), but may only have suppressed symptoms and signs through its anti-inflammatory and analgesic effects without preventing subclinical thromboembolism. Clinical diagnosis is also notoriously nonspecific for this disorder. Fibrinogen leg scanning is a much more reliable end point after general surgery, but not after hip surgery where the high incidence of isolated femoral vein thrombosis at the level of the operation site makes venography the preferred diagnostic test for prophylactic studies.

For practical reasons, most trials have examined the effects of drugs on the incidence of venous thrombosis rather than that of pulmonary embolism. A drug effect on the development of leg vein thrombosis probably implies a similar effect on pulmonary embolism, but some drugs (such as the oral anticoagulants, and perhaps dextran) can prevent embolism without preventing venous thrombosis.

Fibrinogen leg scanning studies in *general surgery* have shown that aspirin (1 to 1.3 gm/day) and sulphinpyrazone (400 mg bid) have little or no effect on the incidence of postoperative thrombosis (Gruber et al, 1977; Report of the Steering Committee, 1972), although there appears to be synergism between aspirin and low dose heparin prophylaxis at the cost of some increase in wound bleeding (Loew et al, 1977; Vinazzer et al, 1980). Positive results have been reported with the combination of aspirin and dipyridamole (Encke, Stock & Dumke, 1976; Plante et al, 1979; Renney, O'Sullivan & Burke, 1976), which appeared to be equally effective with low-dose heparin prophylaxis in one small study (Plante et al, 1979), and with hydroxychloroquine (Carter & Eban, 1974). However, experience with these drugs is still limited, and there have been no large-scale studies of their effect on the incidence of pulmonary embolism, as there have been with low-dose heparin, dextran, and the oral anticoagulants.

Harris et al (1977) found that aspirin reduces the high incidence of venous thrombosis after *elective total hip replacement* in men, but not in women. In their double-blind study of 95 patients who had venography 7 to 10 days after surgery, 0.5 gm aspirin twice daily reduced the incidence of venous thrombosis from 56 per cent to 17 per cent in men, but had no effect on the 35 per cent thrombosis rate in women. This result needs independent confirmation, not least because there was an 80 per cent thrombosis rate in a consecutive series of 30 aspirin treated patients studied by Stamatakis et al (1978) with venography 14 to 16 days after total hip replacement, while leg scan studies of patients after hip replacement by Shondorf, Hey & Lasch (1978) found postoperative aspirin to be ineffective in doses between 0.45 gm per 48 hours, and 1.8 gm per day.

Another result which needs independent confirmation is that of a double-blind study of 240 patients after hip fracture, by Zekert et al (1974). Here, all patients who died had an autopsy, which showed major pulmonary embolism in one of 120 patients treated with 0.5 gm aspirin thrice daily (t.i.d.) and in eight of 120 controls (p < 0.05).

Lastly, there is a report by McKenna et al (1980) who found that 1.3 gm of aspirin t.i.d., but not 325 mg t.i.d., significantly reduced the incidence of venous thrombosis in a small randomised study of 46 patients who had total knee replacement.

Oxyphenbutazone may be effective after total hip replacement (Tillberg, 1976), but controlled studies with dipyridamole, dipyridamole plus aspirin, flubiprofen, sulphinpyrazone, and hydroxychloroquine in orthopaedic patients have generally shown little or no effect on the incidence of postoperative venous thromboembolism.

Antiplatelet drugs have no place in the acute treatment of established venous thromboembolism, but there is suggestive evidence that the addition of sulphinpyrazone may prevent further recurrence in the small group of patients whose venous thromboembolism recurs despite continuing anticoagulant treatment (Steele et al, 1973).

Microvascular disorders

Aspirin is dramatically effective in the uncommon syndrome of erythermalgia (see p. 266). The use of aspirin and high doses of dipyridamole in patients with TTP or HUS is based on case reports which have described remission in some patients treated with these drugs, usually in conjunction with very complex therapeutic protocols. Currently, they should be used together with plasmapheresis and plasma infusion (Myers et al, 1980; Remuzzi et al, 1978).

Side effects

Bleeding complications of antiplatelet drug treatment are generally mild or non-existent. Aspirin damages gastric mucosa, and most chronically treated patients have minor, subclinical gastrointestinal bleeding, although the risk of major bleeding is small. There is evidence that the incidence of gastric lesions is lowest with enteric coated aspirin (Silvoso et al, 1979). Aspirin also increases the risk of minor wound bleeding after surgery (Loew et al, 1974), but this is not a problem with the other drugs.

Patients treated with oral anticoagulants are a special case; combined treatment with aspirin and the oral anticoagulants is particularly likely to be complicated by significant gastrointestinal bleeding (Dale et al, 1977), while both sulphinpyrazone and clofibrate have caused bleeding by prolonging the prothrombin time (Gallus & Birkett, 1980; O'Reilly, Sahud & Robinson, 1972).

CONCLUSION

The prospect of major advances in the management of patients with vascular disorders by the use of drugs with effects on platelet-vessel wall interaction appears very promising. Further developments in this area can be anticipated with confidence but painstaking and costly clinical trials will be essential in every instance before the place of any new compound or combination of drugs in clinical practice can be established, regardless of effects on platelets or endothelial cells in vitro or of effects on other models in the laboratory which have been developed with the aim of reproducing conditions similar to those in the body. Nonetheless, the growing understanding of the relationship between the endothelial cell and other elements of the vessel wall on the one hand, and platelets, the coagulation and fibrinolytic systems on the other augers well for steady progress in this important field.

REFERENCES

Acheson J, Danta G, Hutchinson E C 1969 British Medical Journal 1: 614–615
Acheson J, Hutchinson E C 1972 Atherosclerosis 15: 177–183
Ali M, McDonald J W D 1977 Journal of Laboratory and Clinical Medicine 89: 868–875
Ali M, McDonald J W D, Thiessen J J, Coates P E 1980 Stroke 11: 9–13
Altman R, Boullon F, Rouvier J, Raca R, de la Fuenta L, Favaloro R 1976 Journal of Thoracic and Cardiovascular Surgery 72: 127–129
Andrassy K, Malluche H, Bornefeld H, Comberg M, Ritz E, Jesdinsky H, Mohring K 1974 Klinische Wochenschrift 52: 348–349
Antoniades H N, Scher C D, Stiles C D 1979 Proceedings of the National Academy of Science USA 76: 1809–1813
Ardlie N G, Han P 1974 British Journal of Haematology 26: 331–356
Ashida S-I, Abiko Y 1979 Thrombosis and Haemostasis 41: 436–449
Aspirin Myocardial Infarction Study Research Group 1980 Journal of the American Medical Association 243: 661–669
Babb R R, Alarcon-Segovia D, Faibairn J F II 1964 Circulation 29: 136–141
Bailey J M, Makheja A N, Butler J, Salata K 1979 Atherosclerosis 32: 195–203
Barnett H J M 1979 Medical Clinics of North America 63: 649–679
Barnhart M I, Baechler C A 1978 Seminars in Hemostasis and Thrombosis 5: 50–86
Baumgartner H R 1979 Hemostasis 8: 340–352
Baur H R, Van Tassel R A, Gobel F L 1979 Circulation 60: II, 105
Bedford R F, Ashford T P 1979 Anesthesiology 51: 176–178
Begg G S, Pepper D S, Chesterman C N, Morgan F J 1978 Biochemistry 17: 1739–1744
Bell R L, Majerus P W 1980 The Journal of Biological Chemistry 255: 1790–1792
Best L C, Martin T J, Russell R G G, Preston F E 1977 Nature 267: 850–852
Best L C, McGuire M B, Jones P B B, Holland T K, Martin T J, Preston F E, Segal D S, Russell R G G 1979 Thrombosis Research 16: 367–379
Blakely J A, Pogoriler G 1977 Thrombosis and Haemostasis 38: 238
Blakely J A 1979 Thrombosis and Haemostasis 42: 161
Blass K E, Block H U, Förster W, Pönicke K 1980 British Journal of Pharmacology 68: 71–73
Bloom A L, Giddings J C, Wilks C J 1973 Nature New Biology 241: 217–219
Blose S H, Chacko S 1976 Journal of Cell Biology 70: 459–466
Booyse F M, Rafelson Jr M E 1972 Annals of New York Academy of Sciences 201: 37–60
Born G V R 1977 British Medical Bulletin 33: 193–197
Boston Collaborative Drug Surveillance Group 1974 British Medical Journal 1: 440–443
Breddin K, Loew D, Lechner K, Uberla K, Walter E 1979 Thrombosis and Haemostasis 41: 225–236
Bukowski R M, Hewlett J S, Harris J W, Hoffman G C, Battle J D Jr, Silverblatt E, Yang I V 1976 Seminars in Hematology 13: 219–232
Burch J W, Baenziger N L, Stanford N, Majerus P W 1978 Proceedings of the National Academy of Sciences of USA 75: 5181–5184
Burch J W, Majerus P W 1979 Seminars in Haematology 16: 196–207
Busch C, Dawes J, Pepper D S, Wasteson A 1980 Thrombosis Research 19: 129–138
Byrnes J J, Khurana M 1977 The New England Journal of Medicine 297: 1386–1389
Caldwell P R B, Seegal B, Hsu K, Das M, Soffer R L 1976 Science 191: 1050–1051
Carlson L A, Olsson A G 1976 Lancet 2: 810
Carlson L A, Danielson M, Ekberg I, Klintemar B, Rosenhamer G 1977 Atherosclerosis 28: 81–86
Carter A E, Eban R 1974 British Medical Journal 3: 94–95
Carvalho A C A, Colman R W, Lees R S 1974 New England Journal of Medicine 290: 434–438
Cazenave J P, Kinlough-Rathbone R L, Packham M A, Mustard J F 1978 Thrombosis Research 13: 971–981
Chan V, Chan T-K 1979 Thrombosis Research 15: 209–214
Chamley-Campbell J, Campbell G R, Ross R 1979 Physiological Reviews 59: 1–61
Chesterman C N, Diggle T, Doyle D J, Culliver H, Morgan F J, Penington D G 1979 Australian and New Zealand Journal of Medicine 9: 604–605
Clowes A W, Karnowsky M J 1977 Nature 265: 625–626
Cockbill S R, Heptinstall S, Taylor P M 1979 British Journal of Pharmacology 67: 73–78
Coller B S 1980 Blood 55: 169–178

Coller B S, Gralnick H R 1977 Journal of Clinical Investigation 60: 302
Colman R W 1978 Thrombosis and Haemostasis 39: 284–293
Conley C L, Hartmann R C, Lalley J S 1948 Proceedings of the Society for Experimental Biology and
    Medicine 69: 284–287
Coppe D, Wonders T, Snider M, Salzman E W 1980 Proceedings of the Workshop on Prostacyclins.
    Augusta, Michigan. October 1978. Raven Press, New York (in press)
Cotran R S 1965 American Journal of Pathology 46: 589–620
Craddock P R, Hammerschmidt D E, Moldow C F, Yamada O, Jacob H S 1979 Seminars in Hematology
    15: 140–147
Dale J, Myhre E, Storstein O, Stormorken H, Efskind L 1977 American Heart Journal 94: 101–111
Danon D, Skutelsky E 1976 Annals of the New York Academy of Science 275: 47–63
Davey M F, Luscher E F 1967 Nature (London) 216: 857
David J L, Monfort F, Herion F, Raskinet R 1979 Thrombosis Research 14: 35–49
Dawes J, Smith R C, Pepper D S 1978 Thrombosis Research 12: 851–861
Demers L A, Budin R E, Shaikh B S 1980 Proceedings Society for Experimental Biology and Medicine
    163: 24–29
Dosne A M, Le Grand C, Bauvois B, Bodevin E, Caen J P 1978 Biochemical Biophysical Research
    Communications 85: 183–189
Doyle D J, Chesterman C N, Cade J F, McGready J R, Rennie G C, Morgan F J 1980 Blood 55: 82–84
Dusting G I, Mullins E 1980 Clinical and Experimental Pharmacology and Physiology 7: 545–550
Dyerberg J, Bang H O 1979 Lancet 2: 433–435
Editorial 1980 Lancet 1: 1172–1173
Elwood P C, Cochrane A L, Burr M L, Sweetnam P M, Williams G, Welsby E, Hughes S J, Renton R 1974
    British Medical Journal 1: 436–440
Elwood P C, Sweetnam P M 1979 Lancet 2: 1313–1315
Ehresmann V, Alemany J, Loew D 1977 Medizinische Welt 28: 1157–1162
Ëncke A, Stock C, Dumke H O 1976 Chirurg 47: 670–673
Fields W S, Lemak N A, Frankowski R F, Hardy R J 1977 Stroke 8: 301–316
Fields W S, Lemak N A, Frankowski R F, Hardy R J 1978 Stroke 9: 309–319
Fishman J A, Ryan G B, Karnovsky M J 1975 Laboratory Investigation 32: 339–351
Flower R J 1974 Pharmacologic Reviews 26: 33–67
Folts J D, Crowell E B, Rowe G G 1976 Circulation 54: 365–370
Freed M D, Rosenthal A, Fyler D 1974 American Heart Journal 87: 283–286
Freiman J A, Chalmers T C, Smith H, Kuebler R R 1978 New England Journal of Medicine 299: 690–694
Fuster V, Bowie E J W, Lewis J C, Fass D N, Owen C A Jr, Brown A L 1978 The Journal of Clinical
    Investigation 61: 722–730
Gallus A S 1979 Drugs 18: 439–477
Gallus A S, Birkett D 1980 Lancet 1: 535–536
Gent A E, Brook C G D, Foley T H, Miller T N 1968 British Medical Journal 4: 366–368
Genton E, Gent M, Hirsh J, Harker L A 1975 New England Journal of Medicine 293: 1174–1178;
    1236–1240; 1296–1300
Gerrity R G, Cliff W J 1975 Laboratory Investigation 32: 585–600
Gifford R H, Feinstein A R 1969 New England Journal of Medicine 280: 351–357
Gimbrone M A, Aster R H, Cotran R S, Corkery J, Jandl J H, Folkman J 1969 Nature 222: 33–36
Glimelius B, Busch C, Hook M 1978 Thrombosis Research 12: 773–782
Goetzl J, Woods J M, Gorman R R 1977 Journal of Clinical Investigation 59: 179–183
Gordon J L, Pearson J D 1978 British Journal of Pharmacology 64: 481–483
Group of Physicians of the Newcastle upon Tyne Region 1971 British Medical Journal 4: 767–775
Gruber V F, Buser P, Frick J, Loosli J, Matt E, Segesser D 1977 European Surgical Research 9: 303–310
Green L H, Seroppian E, Handin R I 1980 The New England Journal of Medicine 302: 193–197
Hammond E C, Garfinkel L 1975 British Medical Journal 2: 269–271
Harker L A, Slichter S J 1972 The New England Journal of Medicine 287: 999–1005
Harker L A. Hanson S R, Kirkman T R 1979 Journal of Clinical Investigation 64: 559–569
Harker L A, Ross R 1978 In: Abe T, Sherry S (Eds) A new approach to reduction in cardiac death. Hans
    Huber, pp 59–71
Harker L A, Ross R 1979 Seminars in Thrombosis and Hemostasis 5: 274–292
Harris W H, Salzman E W, Athanasoulis C A, Waltman A C, De Sanctis R W 1977 The New England
    Journal of Medicine 297: 1246–1249
Harter H R, Burch J W, Majerus P W, Stanford N, Delmez J A, Anderson C B, Warts C A 1979 The New
    England Journal of Medicine 301: 577–579
Haslam R J, McClenaghan M D 1979 Thrombosis and Haemostasis 42: 118 (Abst)
Hawiger J, Parkinson S, Timmons S 1980 Nature 283: 195–196

Heldin C-H 1980 Studies on growth factors for human cultured cells. Doctoral Thesis of University of Uppsala

Hennekens C H, Karlson L K, Rosner B 1978 Circulation 58: 35–38

Hirsh J 1977 Seminars in Hematology 14: 409–425

Hiti-Harper J, Wohl H, Harper E 1978 Science 199: 991-992

Hope W, Martin T J, Chesterman C N, Morgan F J 1979 Nature 282: 210–212

Hynes K M, Gan G T, Rutherford B D, Kazmier F J, Frye R L 1973 Circulation 47: 554–557

Jaffe R M 1976 In: Gordon J L (Ed) Platelets in biology and pathology. Elsevier/North Holland, Amsterdam, pp 261–292

Jaffe E A, Hoyer L W, Nachman R L 1973 Journal of Clinical Investigation 52: 2757–2764

Jaffe E A, Hoyer L W, Nachman R L 1974 Proceedings of the National Academy of Science USA 71: 1906–1909

Jaffe E A, Weksler B B 1979 Journal of Clinical Investigation 63: 532–535

Jakubowski J A, Ardlie N, Morgan F J, Chesterman C N (unpublished)

Jamieson G A, Okumura T, Hasatz M 1980 Thrombosis and Haemostasis 42: 1673–1778

Jamieson G A, Smith D F 1976 In: Gordon J L (Ed) Platelets in biology and pathology. Elsevier/North Holland, Amsterdam, pp 89–109

Jestico J, Harrison M J G & Marshall J 1978 British Medical Journal 1: 1188

Jick H, Miettinen O S 1976 British Medical Journal 1: 1057

Jobin F 1978 Seminars in Thrombosis and Hemostasis 4: 199–240

Johnson A D, Detwiler J H 1977 Circulation 55: 947–950

Kaegi A, Pineo G F, Shimizu A, Trivedi H, Hirsh J, Gent M 1975 Circulation 42: 497–499

Kao K-Y T, Hilker D M, McGavack T H 1961 Proceedings of the Society for Experimental Biology and Medicine 106: 335–338

Kand W H, Lindhout M J, Jackson C M, Majerus P W 1980 The Journal of Biological Chemistry 225: 1170–1174

Kaplan K L, Broekman M J, Chernoff A, Lesznik G R, Drillings M 1979 Blood 52: 604–618

Kelton J G, Hirsh J, Carter C J, Buchanan M R 1978 Blood 52: 1073–1076

Kernoff P B A, Willis A L, Stone K J, Davies J A, McNicol G P 1977 British Medical Journal 2: 1441–1444

Kitchens C S, Weiss L 1975 Blood 46: 567–578

Kuzuya T, Tada M, Inoue M, Kodama K, Takada H, Mishima M, Inui M, Abe H 1980 American Journal of Cardiology 45: 454 (Abst)

Kwaan H C 1979 Seminars in Thrombosis and Hemostasis 5: 184–198

Lecaillon J B, Souppart C, Schoeller J P, Humbert G, Massias P 1979 Clinical Pharmacological Therapeutics 26: 611–617

Levin E G, Loskutoff D J 1979 Thrombosis Research 15: 869–878

Lian E C Y, Harkness D R, Byrnes J J, Wallach H, Nunez R 1979 Blood 53: 333–338

Lindsay R M, Prentice C R M, Ferguson D, Burton J A, McNicol G P 1972 Lancet 2: 1287–1290

Linos A, Worthington J W, O'Fallon W, Fuster V, Whisnant J P, Kurland L T 1978 Mayo Clinic Proceedings 53: 581–586

Loew D, Wellmer H K, Baer V, Merguet H, Rumpf P, Petersen H, Bromig G, Persch W F, Marx F J, von Bary S M 1974 Deutsche Medizinische Wochenschrift 99: 565–572

Loew D, Brucke P, Simma W, Vinazzer H, Dienstl E, Boehme K 1977 Thrombosis Research 11: 81–86

Longmore D B, Bennett G, Gueirrara D, Smith M, Bunting S, Moncada S, Reed P, Read N G, Vane J R 1979 Lancet 1: 1002–1005

Loskutoff D J, Edgington T S 1977 Proceedings of the National Academy of Sciences USA 74: 3903–3907

Loskutoff D J, Levin E G 1980 In: Mann and Taylor (Eds) The regulation of coagulation. Elsevier North Holland Publishing Co. Amsterdam, pp 589–595

Maca R D, Fry G L, Hoak J C, Loh P T 1977 Thrombosis Research 11: 715–727

Marguerie G A, Plow E F, Edgington T S 1979 The Journal of Biological Chemistry 254: 5357–5363

Maseri A, Severi S, DeNes M, L'Abbate A, Chierchia S, Marzilli M, Ballestra A M, Parodi O, Biagini A, Distante A 1978 American Journal of Cardiology 42: 1019–1035

Masotti G, Galanti G, Poggesi L, Abbate R, Neri Serneri G G 1979 Lancet 2: 1213–1216

McKenna R, Galante J, Bachman F, Wallace D L, Kanshal S P, Meredith P 1980 British Medical Journal 1: 514–517

Maynard J R, Dryer B E, Stemerman M B, Pitlick F A 1977 Blood 50: 387–396

Millikan C H, McDowell F H 1978 Stroke 9: 299–308

Mitchell J R A 1980 British Medical Journal 1: 1128–1130

Moncada S, Higgs E A, Vane J R 1977 Lancet 1: 18–20

Moncada S, Korbut R 1978 Lancet 1: 1286–1289

Moncada S, Korbut R, Bunting S, Vane J R 1978 Nature 273: 767–768

Moncada S, Vane J R 1979 The New England Journal of Medicine 300: 1142–1147

Moore S, Pepper D S, Cash J D 1975 Biochemica Biophysica Acta 379: 360–369
Murphy E S, Kloster F E 1979 Modern Concepts of Cardiovascular Disease 48: 59–66
Myers T J, Wakem C F, Ball E D, Tremont S J 1980 Annals of Internal Medicine 92: 149–155
Nielsen P O, Holstein P, Nielsen S L 1977 Lancet 1: 192
Nordoy A, Svensson B, Wiebe D, Hoak J C 1978 Circulation Research 43: 527–534
Nuutinen L S, Pihlajaniemi R, Saarela E, Kärkölä P, Hollmen A 1977 Journal of Thoracic and
    Cardiovascular Surgery 74: 295–298
Oblath R W, Buckley F O, Green R M, Schwartz S I, De Weese J A 1978 Surgery 84: 37–43
O'Brien J R, Etherington M D, Shuttleworth R D 1978 Thrombosis Research 13: 245–254
Olsson J E, Brechter C, Bäcklund H, Krook H, Müller R, Nitelius E, Olsson O, Tornberg A 1980 Stroke
    11: 4–9
O'Reilly R A, Sahud M A, Robinson A J 1972 Thrombosis et Diathesis Haemorrhagica 27: 309–318
Packham M A, Mustard J F 1977 Blood 50: 555–573
Pantely G A, Goodnight S H, Rahimtoola S H, Harlan B J, De Mots H, Calvin L, Rösch J 1979 The New
    England Journal of Medicine 301: 962–966
Pareti F I, Mannucci P M, D'Angelo A, Smith J B, Sautebin L, Galli G 1980 Lancet i: 898–901
Pearson J D, Carleton J S, Gordon J L 1980 Biochemical Journal 190: 421–429
Peerschke E I, Zucker M B, Grant A A, Egan J J, Johnson M M 1980 Blood 55: 841–847
The Persantine-Aspirin Reinfarction Study Research Group (1980) Circulation 62: 449–461
Pfueller S L, Firkin B G 1978 Thrombosis Research 12: 979–990
Phillips D R 1980 Thrombosis and Haemostasis 42: 1638–1651
Phillips D R, Agin P P 1973 Series Haematologica 6: 292–310
Pick R, Chediak J, Glick G 1979 Journal of Clinical Investigation 63: 158–162
Plante J, Boneu B, Vaysse C, Barret A, Gonzi M, Bierme R 1979 Thrombosis Research 14: 399–403
Plow E F, Birdwell C, Ginsberg M H 1979 Journal of Clinical Investigation 63: 540–543
Polli E E, Cortellaro M 1979 In: Abe T, Sherry S (Eds) A new approach to reduction of cardiac death,
    Bern: Hans Huber, pp 73–77
Poole J C F, Cromwell S B, Benditt E P 1971 American Journal of Pathology 62: 391–414
Rajah S M, Crow M J, Penny A F, Ahmad R, Watson D A 1977 British Journal of Clinical Pharmacology
    4: 129–133
Rajah S M, Sreeharan N, Rao S, Watson D A 1979 Thrombosis and Haemostasis 42: 160
Rak and Boda 1980 Lancet 2: 44
Rane A, Oelz O, Frolich J C, Seyberth H W, Sweetman B J, Watson J J, Wilkinson G K, Oates J A 1978
    Clinical Pharmacology and Therapeutics 23: 658–668
Redding K G 1977 Archives of Dermatology 113: 468–471
Remuzzi G, Mecca G, Livio M, De Gaetano G, Donati M B, Pearson J D, Gordon J L 1980 Lancet 1: 656
Remuzzi G, Misiani R, Marchesi D, Livio M, Mecca G, de Gaetano G, Donati M B 1978 Lancet
    2: 871–873
Renney J T, O'Sullivan E F, Burke P F 1976 British Medical Journal 1: 992–994
Report from The Committee of Principal Investigators 1978 British Heart Journal 40: 1069–1118
Report of The Steering Committee of a Trial Sponsored by The Medical Research Council 1972 Lancet
    2: 441–444
Research Committee of the Scottish Society of Physicians 1971 British Medical Journal 4: 775–784
Ritchie J L, Harker L A 1977 The American Journal of Cardiology 39: 595–598
Rodvien R, Salzman E W 1978 Thrombosis and Haemostasis 39: 254–262
Ross R, Vogel A, Davies P, Raines E, Kariya B, Rivest M J, Gustafson C, Glomset J 1979 In: Sato G and
    Ross R (Eds) Hormones and cell culture (Book A) Cold Spring Harbour, pp 3–16
Rucinski B, Niewiarowski S, James P, Walz D A, Budzynski A Z 1979 Blood 53: 47–62
Saba S R, Mason R G 1975 Thrombosis Research 7: 807–812
Salem H H, Koutts J, Firkin B G 1980 Thrombosis Research 17: 707–711
Santoro S A, Cunningham L W 1979 Proceedings of the National Academy of Sciences USA 76: 2644–
    2648
Schick P K, Kurica K B, Chacko G K 1976 Journal of Clinical Investigation 57: 1221–1226
Schöndorf T H, Hey D, Lasch H G 1978 Klinische Wochenschrift 56: 1113–1118
Schrör K, Smith E F III, Bickerton M, Smith J B, Nicolaou K C, Magolda R, Lefer A M 1980 American
    Journal of Physiology 238: H87–H92
Schwartz B S, Leis L A, Johnson G J 1979 Journal of Laboratory and Clinical Medicine 94: 574–584
Shattil S J, Anaya-Galindo R, Bennett J, Colman R W, Cooper I 1975 Journal of Clinical Investigation
    55: 636–643
Shepro D, Bortbouta J C, Robblee L S, Carson M P, Belamarich F A 1975 Circulation Research
    36: 799–806
Siess W, Roth P, Scherer B, Kurzman I, Böhlig B, Weber P C 1980 Lancet 1: 441–444

Silvoso G R, Ivey K J, Butt J H, Lockhard O O, Holt S D, Sisk C, Baskin W N, Mackercher P A, Hewett J 1979 Annals of Internal Medicine 91: 517–520
Stamatakis J D, Kakkar V V, Lawrence D, Bentley P G, Nairn D, Ward V 1978 British Medical Journal 1: 1031
Steele P, Battock D, Pappas G, Genton E 1976 Circulation 53: 686–687
Steele P, Ellis J, Genton E 1978 American Journal of Medicine 64: 441–445
Stewart J H, Farrell P C, Dixon M 1975 Australian and New Zealand Journal of Medicine 5: 117–122
Stiles C E, Capone G T, Scher C T, Antoniades H N, Van Wyk J J, Pledger W J 1979 Proceedings of the National Academy of Sciences USA 76: 1279–1283
Storstein O, Nitter-Hauge S, Enge I 1977 Acta Radiologica (Diagnosis) 18: 555–560
Stuart M J, Gerrard J M, White J G 1980 The New England Journal of Medicine 302: 6–10
Sullivan J M, Harken D E, Gorlin R 1971 The New England Journal of Medicine, 284: 1391–1394
Szczeklik A, Nizankowski R, Skawinski S, Szczeklik J, Gluszko P, Gryglewski R J 1979 Lancet 1: 1111–1114
The Anturane Reinfarction Trial Research Group 1978 The New England Journal of Medicine 298: 289–295
The Anturane Reinfarction Trial Research Group 1980 The New England Journal of Medicine 302: 250–256
The Canadian Co-operative Study Group 1978 The New England Journal of Medicine 299: 53–59
The Coronary Drug Project Research Group 1975 Journal of the American Medical Association 231: 360–381
The Coronary Drug Project Research Group 1976 Journal of Chronic Diseases 29: 625–642
Thorgeirsson G, Robertson A L Jr 1978 Atherosclerosis 30: 67–78
Tillberg B 1976 British Medical Journal 1: 1256–1257
Timpl R, Rohde H, Robey P G, Rennard S I, Foidart J-M, Martin G R 1979 254: 9933–9937
Todd A S 1958 Nature 181: 495
Tollefsen D M, Feagler J R, Majerus P W 1974 Journal of Biological Chemistry 249: 2646–2651
Vermylen J, Chamone D A F, Verstraete M 1979 Lancet 2: 518–520
Veterans Administration Co-operative Study Group 1973 Stroke 4: 684–693
Vinazzer H, Loew D, Simma W, Brucke P 1980 Thrombosis Research 17: 177–184
Weily H S, Genton E 1970 Circulation 42: 967–972
Weiss H J, Aledort L M, Kochwa S 1968 Journal of Clinical Investigation 47: 2169–2180
Weksler B B, Ley C W, Jaffe E A 1978 Journal of Clinical Investigation 62: 923–930
Weston M J, Rubin M H, Langley P G, Westaby S, Williams R 1977 Thrombosis Research 10: 833–840
Wiggins R C, Loskutoff D J, Cochrane C G , Griffin J H, Edgington T S 1980 The Journal of Clinical Investigation 65: 197–206
Wight T N, Ross R 1975 Journal of Cell Biology 67: 675–686
Wiley J S, Chesterman C N, Morgan T J, Castaldi P A 1979 Thrombosis Research 14: 23–33
Woods H F, Ash G, Weston M J, Bunting S, Moncada S, Vane J R 1978 Lancet 2: 1075–1077
Woods J H, Ash G, Parsons V, Weston M J 1979 Clinical Nephrology 12: 122–126
Zekert F, Kohn P, Vormittag E, Poigenfurst J, Thien M 1974 Monatschrift der Unfallheilkunde 77: 97–110
Zekert F, Kohn P, Vormittag E, Piza F, Thien M 1975 In: Colfarit Symposium III, p 109–119, Köln: Bayer
Zucker M B, Mosesson M W, Broekman M J, Kaplan K L 1979 Blood 54: 8–12

13. Biochemistry of coagulation

M P Esnouf

INTRODUCTION

The cascade hypothesis of blood coagulation (Macfarlane, 1964) which proposed that all the clotting factors were zymogens undergoing sequential activation to enzymes, was an ideal base to set out from on a biochemical investigation of coagulation. Even today, 17 years on, many of the essential features embodied in this idea are still valid. The only exceptions to this hypothesis being factor V and possibly factor VIII, which act as high molecular weight cofactors for the activation of prothrombin and factor X respectively. The uncertainty in the behaviour of factor VIII is due to the fact that it is the only coagulation factor which has not been fully characterized.

A further advance in our understanding of coagulation was the concept of 'Self Damping'. This was formulated by Nemerson et al (1974) and was based on the observation that thrombin rapidly degraded prothrombin to prethrombin 1, which is only slowly activated by the physiological activators. The other product of the reaction, fragment 1, competes with prothrombin for the binding site in the prothrombinase complex, further reducing the rate of prothrombin conversion. Evidence is now accumulating that at other stages of coagulation there are control points which either stimulate (positive feedback) or inhibit (negative feedback) individual zymogen activations.

More recently, following the recognition of the function of vitamin K in the synthesis of the vitamin K dependent factors, it has been possible to define the role of calcium ions as an essential cofactor for coagulation. This work has also led to the discovery of at least three new vitamin K dependent plasma proteins, two of which at least appear to antagonize the clotting system.

There is also a growing awareness that the hitherto rigid distinctions between the intrinsic and extrinsic clotting systems may have no physiological significance, and the role of the contact activation of factor XII as a prime activator of the clotting cascade is being questioned. However, for the purpose of this brief review, coagulation will be considered along traditional lines.

CONTACT ACTIVATION OF FACTOR XI

Since the classical work of Lister, who in 1863 showed that blood exposed to glass coagulated more readily than when it remained enclosed in a blood-vessel, and the much later finding of Ratnoff & Colopy (1955) of a patient whose plasma did not readily clot on exposure to glass, led to the idea that there was a single plasma protein, *factor XII*, which became activated on contact with glass. However, the physiological role of factor XII was hard to assess, because patients with factor XII deficiency did not appear to bleed. One explanation for this was that deficiency was not absolute and

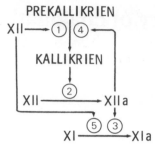

Fig. 13.1   Contact phase of coagulation. These reactions require High Molecular Weight Kininogen and a suitable surface.

the plasma contained sufficient factor XII to initiate coagulation. This view received some support from the work of Hathaway et al (1965) who suggested that an additional protein, Fletcher factor, potentiated the activation of factor XII by foreign surfaces. Fletcher factor has now been identified with *plasma prekallikrein* (Wuepper, 1972).

A third component of the contact phase was apparent from the work of Schiffman & Lee (1974). This was required for the rapid activation of factor XI. This factor, formerly called Fitzgerald factor and now identified as *High Molecular Weight Kininogen*, is also necessary for the activation of factor XII by the foreign surface.

The probable sequence of events following the contact of plasma with a foreign surface has been described by Heimark et al (1980) and is illustrated in Fig. 13.1. All the reactions shown in this figure take place in the presence of High Molecular Weight Kininogen and a foreign surface, such as Kaolin. The first reaction in the sequence is the conversion of prekallikrein to Kallikrein by factor XII. Heimark et al (1980) have shown that the initial rate of Kallikrein formation is the same if factor XII is replaced by factor XIIa (reaction 4). They suggest reaction 1 is a substrate induced catalysis of the conversion prekallikrein to Kallikrein which then cleaves the single chain factor XII to two chain factor XIIa.

Silverberg et al (1980), on the other hand, take the view that the initial reaction in coagulation is the autoactivation of factor XII in the presence of a foreign surface and does not require prekallikrein.

The formation of the two chain factor XIIa is followed by the rapid activation of factor XI (reaction 3). Heimark et al (1980) have further shown that single chain factor XII will also activate factor XI, in the presence of High Molecular Weight Kininogen, but at a rate four times slower than with factor XIIa (Reaction 5).

Factor XII is a single chain glycoprotein (mol wt 74 000) with little or no enzymic activity. On activation a two chain protein is formed with a heavy chain (mol wt 46 000) and a light chain (mol wt 28 000). The activation of the single chain prekallikrein (mol wt 82 000) is achieved by the cleavage of an internal peptide bond giving a two chain (mol wt 52 000 and 33 000) serine protease. The role of High Molecular Weight Kininogen in these reactions is to stimulate both the rate of Kallikrein formation and factor XI activation by a mechanism as yet unexplained. An interesting control aspect of these two reactions is that Kallikrein degrades High Molecular Weight Kininogen to Kinin (Han et al, 1978) and this is accompanied by the loss of stimulating activity.

The activation of *factor XI*, which is a glycoprotein (mol wt 124 000) composed of two nearly identical polypeptide chains, joined by disulphide bond(s), is by the cleavage of an internal peptide bond in both chains by factor XIIa or by factor XII to give a serine protease (Kurachi et al, 1980).

ACTIVATION OF FACTOR X

Intrinsic factor X activator

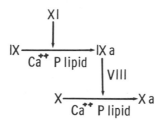

Fig. 13.2   Intrinsic activation of Factor X.

The activation of *factor IX* by factor XIa is a two step reaction requiring calcium ions (Fujikawa et al, 1974). In the first step, factor IX, which is a glycoprotein (mol wt 55 400) and composed of a single chain, is cleaved to give a light chain (mol wt 16 000) formed from the N-terminal region and a heavy chain (mol wt 38 000); both chains are joined by disulphide bond(s). In the next step a peptide (mol wt 9000) is removed from the N-terminal region of the heavy chain. This step is accompanied by the appearance of coagulant activity and a reactive serine residue which is located on the heavy chain. The light chain contains the vitamin K dependent calcium binding sites in the N-terminal region. Factor IXa has only slight activity on tripeptide nitroanilide substrates or arginine ester substrates. Factor IXa will slowly convert factor X to Xa in the presence of phospholipid and calcium ions but the rate of factor X activation is considerably increased in the presence of factor VIII.

Factor VIII is the only remaining coagulation factor to be purified and characterized. It seems likely that if factor VIII is a single entity with only coagulant activity, then the two other activities invariably associated with the coagulant activity, both in plasma or in many 'purified' preparations, must be the result of the formation of a stable complex between at least three proteins. In support of this, Hougie et al (1975) have shown that the different activities can be selectively inhibited by antibodies, and Ekert et al (1976) have observed patients in which the different activities are present in the complex in different proportions.

More recently, some success has been achieved in the separation of the factor VIII related activities by chromatography on antibody-sepharose columns (Holmberg & Ljung, 1978; Tuddenham et al, 1979). A disadvantage of this procedure is that the recovery of the different activities, especially of the coagulant activity, is low.

On the other hand, Switzer & McKee (1976) were unable to resolve coagulant activity from factor VIII-related antigen and platelet aggregating activity by gel filtration at high ionic strength. These authors conclude that the polypeptide chains carrying these activities were covalently joined by disulphide bonds.

It is apparent that greater success has been achieved in resolving the components of the factor VIII complex if the dissociation has been attempted immediately after cryoprecipitation, which is used as the initial step in the purification. If dissociation of the components is attempted after a more lengthy purification procedure, this is unsuccessful. It may be that reactive sulphydryl groups on the different polypeptide chains are brought together and oxidize to form interchain disulphide bonds. A recently published method for the purification of factor VIII (Vehar & Davie, 1980) uses glycine precipitation in the presence of sulphydryl reducing agents. These authors use chromatography on factor X-sepharose columns as a final step and obtain a purification of 320 000-fold, but the recovery of coagulant activity is only 1 per cent.

The purified protein consists of three polypeptide chains with molecular weights of approximately 85 000; 88 000; 93 000, which is consistent with an estimate of the apparent molecular weight of 250 000 to 300 000 for factor VIII based on gel filtration experiments. Vehar & Davie (1980) also showed that the long recognized activation of factor VIII by thrombin is associated with cleavage of one of the polypeptide chains. Incubation of the thrombin activated factor VIII with protein C (see later), which causes rapid inactivation of the coagulant activity, is accompanied by further proteolysis.

It has been generally supposed that factor VIII behaves as a high molecular weight cofactor for the activation of factor X by factor IXa, in the same way as factor V accelerates the conversion of prothrombin to thrombin. This is based on the fact that thrombin activated factor VIII does not have any direct action of factor X. However, this view may have to be reconsidered following the demonstration by Vehar & Davie (1980) that at least in the case of bovine factor VIII, the thrombin activated protein was inhibited by 30 mM diisopropyl fluorophosphate, suggesting that some aspect of its activity depended on a reactive serine residue. This observation has not yet been confirmed by others.

Extrinsic factor X activator

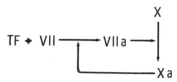

Fig. 13.3 Extrinsic activation of Factor X.

The active agent present in tissue, tissue factor, has been known for many years to be a lipoprotein complex; this when dissociated into its lipid and protein components loses coagulant activity, which is restored when the lipid and the protein are combined (Studer, 1946). The protein component has been isolated from a number of different tissues. The protein from bovine brain has been extensively purified and found to have a molecular weight of 45 000 (Nemerson et al, 1980). The wide distribution of this protein, especially in the plasma membranes of endothelial cells and in human atheromatous plaque (Zeldis et al, 1973) may indicate the importance of tissue factor in haemostasis and thrombosis.

Factor VII The exposure of plasma to tissue factor causes the activation of factor X however, this only occurs in the presence of factor VII. This is a single chain glycoprotein (mol wt 45 500), which requires vitamin K during its synthesis, and has been isolated from bovine plasma (Kisiel & Davie, 1975; Radcliffe & Nemerson, 1975). A unique feature of the native bovine protein is that it has an unusually reactive serine residue, as seen by its reaction with diisopropyl fluorophosphate. The human protein differs from the bovine protein in this respect and is quite inert with respect to this inhibitor (Davie et al, 1978). In spite of the reactivity of the bovine protein it has little action on its substrate, factor X, in the absence of tissue factor. The interaction of tissue factor and factor VII has been extensively investigated by Nemerson and his colleagues (Nemerson et al, 1980). They compared the kinetics of the activation of factor X by factor VII, phospholipid and calcium ions in the presence and absence of tissue factor and showed that in the presence of tissue factor the K_{cat} was enhanced 3000-fold and the K_m was decreased 10-fold. At plasma concentrations of factor X, tissue factor increases the rate of factor X activation 16 000-fold. Thus in plasma, when tissue factor is released by vascular injury, the rate of factor X activation is increased above a certain critical threshold.

As a result of the activation of factor X the reactivity of the factor VII is increased approximately 50-fold. Factor VII activity is also enhanced by thrombin and factor XIIa (Jackson & Nemerson, 1980). This is due to a proteolytic cleavage of an internal peptide bond giving a two chain protein (α VIIa) and is an example of positive feedback. On prolonged exposure to factor Xa, the coagulant activity of α factor VIIa is lost, and a three chain protein β factor VIIa is formed which still retains esterolytic activity. This phase is seen as negative feedback.

THE COMMON PATHWAY

Factor X

Bovine factor X is a two chain zymogen with a molecular weight of 55 000. The light chain (mol wt 16 500) contains in its N-terminal sequence the vitamin K dependent calcium binding region. The heavy chain (mol wt 39 300) possesses in addition to the reactive serine residue, two carbohydrate chains attached to Asn^{35} and Thr^{300}. The heavy and light chains are covalently joined by disulphide bond(s). The primary structures of both the light chain (Enfield et al, 1975) and the heavy chain (Titani et al, 1975) has been determined. Bovine factor X is eluted from ion-exchange columns as two separate components X_1 and X_2, X_2 behaving as if it was more acidic than X_1. This increased acidity of X_2 can be partially accounted for by the sulphation of Tyr^{18} (Morita & Jackson, 1979). The specific coagulant activity of factor X_2a is significantly higher than factor X_1a (Ong & Esnouf, 1979), and since the modified tyrosine residue is in the activation peptide, lost during the purification of factor Xa, this cannot account for the difference in coagulant activities of X_1a and X_2a. One possibility is that the γ-carboxy glutamic acid (Gla) content of X_1 and X_2 are different (Neal et al, 1976). However, because Gla is found at twelve positions in the amino acid sequence of both forms of factor X (Thøgersen et al, 1978) it may be that the occupancy of Gla at these positions is less than 100 per cent in the case of X_1a. This could account for both the difference in acidity and coagulant activity of the two forms of factor X. The esterase activities of the two forms of factor X are identical.

Human factor X (mol wt 58 900) differs from bovine factor X in that the heavy chain contains an additional 15–20 residues (Davie et al, 1979) and the specific activity is considerably lower (Kisiel & Hanahan, 1973).

The activation of factor X by either the extrinsic or intrinsic activator is achieved by the cleavage of the Arg^{51}-Ile^{52} bond. The same bond is also cleaved by the coagulant protein from Russell's Viper Venom or by insolubilized trypsin (Jesty et al, 1974).

The cleavage of this bond results in the loss of a fragment (mol wt 10 000) from the N-terminus of the heavy chain and the appearance of both esterolytic and coagulant activities.

The activation peptide also carries 80 per cent of the carbohydrate of factor X. This fact has been made use of by Silverberg et al (1977), who selectively tritiated the carbohydrate and were able to follow the activation of factor X by the release of radioactivity. This method is more sensitive than the conventional assay for factor Xa.

The first product of the activation of factor X [αXa] (mol wt 45 300) undergoes a second autolytic cleavage in the presence of calcium ions and phospholipid. In the reaction, the bond Arg^{290}–Gly^{291} is cleaved and a peptide (mol wt 2700) is lost from the C-terminus of the heavy chain. This peptide contains seventeen amino acids, of which five are proline, and the remainder of the carbohydrate. The formation of βXa (mol wt 42 600) is not accompanied by any change in the coagulant or enzymic activity. The physiological significance of this last step is not clear.

Conversion of prothrombin to thrombin

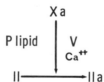

Fig. 13.4   The conversion of prothrombin.

The rapid conversion of prothrombin requires additional factors, namely, phospholipid, calcium ions and factor V.

Factor V accelerates the conversion of prothrombin by factor Xa some 20 000-fold. It has, however, no demonstrable activity on either Xa or prothrombin and would appear to act as a high molecular weight cofactor for the proteolysis of prothrombin.

The existence of factor V was first postulated by Nolf in 1908, who called it 'thrombogen', but only within the last two years have homogenous preparations of the bovine 'native' protein been described (Nesheim et al, 1979; Esmon, 1979). Factor V is a single chain polypeptide (mol wt 330 000) which also contains carbohydrate. Recently Dahlbäck (1980) has published a method for the isolation of factor V from human plasma and the protein has properties similar to the bovine protein.

Recent work by Bartlett et al (1980) suggests that factor V (mol wt 330 000) may in fact be derived from a precursor having a molecular weight of one million. The work of Esmon (1979) and Nesheim et al (1978) shows that the well known activation of factor V by thrombin is the result of limited proteolysis of the molecule. Although there are some differences in the interpretation of the fragmentation of the parent protein, both groups agree that the active peptide has a molecular weight of around 75 000. It is uncertain whether the active peptide is associated with any other part of the protein, since the electrophoretic separation of the intermediates was carried out under dissociating conditions.

Esmon (1979) favours the view that the formation of the 75 000 dalton component is sufficient to activate the factor V. Esmon & Jackson (1974) have shown that thrombin activated factor V binds both to prothrombin-Sepharose and prethrombin-1-Sepharose, while inactive factor V will not. Ong & Esnouf (unpublished observations) have further shown the activiated factor V binds to prothrombin fragment-2-Sepharose and that fragment 2 will elute factor V bound to prethrombin-1-Sepharose columns. The interaction between factor V and these prothrombin derivatives does not require calcium ions. In addition to the fragment 2 region of prothrombin, factor V also binds to columns of Xa-sepharose. This would suggest that during the activation of factor V the binding sites for both Xa and prothrombin are exposed. Prolonged incubation of factor V with thrombin or with protein C (see later) causes its inactivation.

Phospholipid. The acceleration of prothrombin conversion by factor V is only seen in the presence of phospholipid. An explanation for this is that in the presence of the phospholipid surface, two binding sites are available to the prothrombin. Nelsestuen (1980) comparing the rates of prothrombin conversion in the presence and absence of phospholipid shows that the apparent K_m value for the binding of prothrombin in presence of phospholipid is less than $1\,\mu M$, while in the absence of phospholipid then a K_m of $30\,\mu M$ was obtained. The affinity of factor Xa for platelet surfaces (Factor V) (Miletich et al, 1978) is several orders of magnitude greater than the affinity of Xa for phospholipid alone (Nelsestuen & Broderius, 1977). Thus factor V and phospholipid effectively increase the affinity of prothrombin for factor Xa. It is also possible that they may provide a more favourable arrangement of the substrate (prothrombin) with respect to the enzyme (factor Xa).

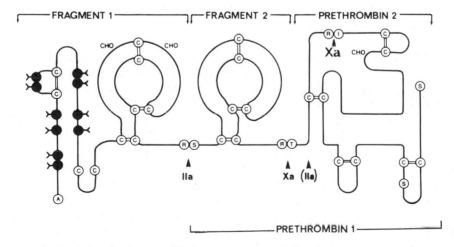

Fig. 13.5 A schematic diagram of prothrombin.
C = C disulphide bond: ꙮ γ carboxyglutamic acid (Gla).
CHO carbohydrate: Other letters are the single letter amino acid code.

Prothrombin is a single chain glycoprotein which has been isolated from both human and bovine plasma. The molecular weight of the protein from both species is close to 70 000. The primary and secondary structure of bovine prothrombin has been elucidated (Magnusson et al, 1975), and X-ray diffraction studies on crystals of bovine fragment 1 are in progress.

The conversion of prothrombin to thrombin is the result of the cleavage of the polypeptide chain (Fig. 13.5) by Xa at the point Arg^{274}–Thr^{275} $(R)(T)$ between fragment 2 and prethrombin 2. This is followed by proteolysis of the bond Arg^{323}–Ile^{324} $(R)(I)$ giving the A and B chains of thrombin. Thrombin cleaves prothrombin between fragment 1 and fragment 2 at Arg^{156}–Ser^{157} $(R)(S)$. Fragment 1 contains at its N-terminus the vitamin K dependent calcium binding region and two carbohydrate chains attached to Asn^{72} and Asn^{101}. These residues reside in the triple looped structure (Kringle), which shows considerable sequence homology with the equivalent structure in fragment 2, which suggests that there has been duplication of an ancestral gene. Fragment 2 contains the binding site for factor V.

The activation of prothrombin has been investigated by many laboratories and two paths have been identified. In the factor Xa mediated route, which can be demonstrated only in the presence of a thrombin inhibitor, prothrombin is cleaved at the two points indicated by the arrows (Fig. 13.5). If the thrombin is not inhibited then prothrombin is cleaved between fragments 1 and 2. The consequence of this is two-fold; firstly prethrombin 1, which does not possess the calcium binding region, is a poor substrate for the prothrombin activator complex; and secondly fragment 1 competes with prothrombin for the calcium binding site (Jesty & Esnouf, 1973).

In the case of human prothrombin, there is a second thrombin cleavage point, shown in brackets in Figure 13.5, removing thirteen residues from the N-terminus of the A chain of human thrombin (Lanchatin et al, 1975).

One paradox of the conversion of prothrombin to thrombin is the order of the bond cleavage. If prothrombin is cleaved first between fragment 1:2 and prethrombin 2, how is the bond between the A and B chains of thrombin split by Xa when prethrombin 2 like thrombin has no binding site for the prothrombinase complex? This problem was resolved by Esmon et al (1974), who showed that after the formation of prethrombin 2, the two halves of the original prothrombin molecule remained associated until the proteolysis of the bond between the A and B chains of thrombin. The finding that the rate of thrombin formation from a mixture of prethrombin 2 and fragment 1:2 is not less than that observed with intact prothrombin (Esmon et al, 1974) is consistent with this sequence of events.

Thrombin is the only serine protease originating from a vitamin K dependent protein which does not retain its calcium binding region. At present there is no obvious function of the 49 residue A chain for the catalytic activity of thrombin. It may be its only role is to facilitate the cleavage of prethrombin 2 by the prothrombinase complex. The B chain contains a serine active centre ($Ser^{528}(S)$) and exhibits considerable sequence homology with the pancreatic proteases, but differs from them in that it contains carbohydrate attached to Asn^{376}, and only three disulphide loops compared with four found in the pancreatic enzymes. Early attempts to gain information on the tertiary structure of thrombin by X-ray crystallography have been unsuccessful, but much can be inferred about its three-dimensional structure by comparison with chymotrypsin.

Thrombin has a considerably broader specificity than the other activated clotting factors; cleaving peptide bonds of the type Arg-X in a wide range of proteins, including itself. The autolysis of α thrombin first gives β thrombin in which the A chain is reduced to a 16 residue fragment attached to a shortened B chain at residue 74. β thrombin is further degraded to γ thrombin by an internal cleavage in the central disulphide loop (Kingdon et al, 1979). The transition from the α to β form of thrombin is accompanied by a 20-fold reduction in its activity towards fibrinogen, while γ thrombin has little activity on macromolecular substrates.

Thrombin in addition to its action on its natural substrate fibrinogen, activates both factor VIII, factor V, protein C and factor XIII by limited proteolysis and because of its specificity for arginyl bonds has been used to cleave a number of proteins for sequence studies.

Thrombin inhibitors

There are two important inhibitors of thrombin in plasma, α_2 macroglobulin and antithrombin III (heparin cofactor).

α_2 macroglobulin (mol wt 750 000) is present in plasma at a concentration of 2 to 4 μm. It binds the enzymes in an equimolar ratio, which involves proteolysis of the inhibitor by the enzyme. The thrombin-α_2 macroglobulin complexes retain slight coagulant activity whereas the activity against low molecular substrates is not severely decreased (Harpel & Rosenberg, 1976).

Antithrombin III (mol wt 65 000) is present in plasma in at least two-fold molar excess over the sum of all the clotting factors and is probably the most important inhibitor for regulating the activity of the activated factors with the possible exception of factor VII. Heparin has a dramatic effect in enhancing the rate at which the activated factors are inhibited, and appears to act catalytically in these reactions (Rosenberg et al, 1980). The inhibitor-enzyme complex is formed following the proteolysis of a fragment of Antithrombin III leading to formation of an acyl-enzyme complex. It should be remembered in assessing the importance of Antithrombin III as a physiological inhibitor that much of the experimental work has been carried out with heparin, which in the case of man is present in plasma in insignificant amounts. In this instance, other sulphated polysaccharides, e.g. dermatan sulphate must serve as catalytic agents.

Thrombin–fibrinogen interaction

The interaction of thrombin with fibrinogen to form fibrin monomer initiates the final phase of coagulation, which consists of the subsequent polymerization and steriliza-tion of the fibrin. Fibrinogen is a rod-shaped molecule which is a dimer composed of three non-identical chains $(\alpha_2\beta_2\gamma_2)$ with a molecular weight of 340 000. The α chains contain 610 amino acid residues, the β chain contains 410 residues as well as carbohydrate and the γ chain 411 residues and carbohydrate. The entire primary sequence of the molecule has now been completed (Doolittle et al, 1979). The two halves of the molecule are joined at the N-terminal region by disulphide bonds between pairs of α and γ chains (Blombäck & Blombäck, 1972). Fibrinogen also contains 4.5 per cent carbohydrate, but as yet no specific function has been ascribed to these residues.

The first stage of the conversion of fibrinogen to fibrin is the thrombin catalysed removal of the A peptide, an acidic peptide, from the N-terminus of the α chains. This allows the fibrin to form 'end to end' aggregates giving a thread-like polymer. Blombäck & Blombäck (1972) further suggest that the removal of the A peptide leads to a conformational change exposing the B peptide, situated at the N-terminus of the β chain, to proteolytic attack by thrombin. This is consistent with the fact that the B peptide is only released after a lag phase. The loss of the B peptide allows the side to side aggregation of the fibrin molecules, increasing the thickness of the fibrils. The fibrin polymer formed in this way is susceptible to the action of proteolytic enzymes present in the plasma and would readily dissolve.

Fibrin stabilization

In the final stage of coagulation the fibrin clot is rendered more resistant to enzymic degradation by the action of a plasma transaminase enzyme, factor XIII.

Factor XIII (mol wt 320 000) is composed of two A chains (mol wt 75 000) and two B chains (mol wt 88 000) (Schwartz et al, 1973) and circulates in plasma in an inactive form. Factor XIII is activated by a two-step reaction involving both thrombin and calcium ions (Chung et al, 1974). In the first stage a peptide (mol wt 4000) is removed from the N-terminus of the A chains, giving an inactive tetrameric intermediate. In the second stage, which requires calcium ions, the intermediate dissociates into an enzymically active chain composed of the modified A chains and an inactive dimer of B chains.

Activated factor XIII catalyses the formation of ε-(γ-glutamyl)-lysine isopeptide peptides, between specific glutamine and lysine residues located on different γ chains forming γ–γ dimers; there is a second slower reaction in which α chains are joined to give γ polymers (McKee et al, 1970). The fibrin clot cross-linked in this way is considerably more resistant to the action of plasmin.

THE ROLE OF VITAMIN K

Prothrombin, factors VII, IX and X have been recognized for many years to be dependent on Vitamin K at some stage for their synthesis. It was also thought that these four plasma proteins were unique in their dependence on Vitamin K. However, recent work has shown that there are at least three other plasma proteins which are vitamin K dependent in addition to other non-plasma proteins. All these proteins are characterized by the fact that they require calcium ions for their activity, or are associated with insoluble calcium salts such as phosphates or carbonate.

For the purpose of this review only the three plasma proteins will be considered because at least two of them (Protein C and Protein S) appear to inhibit the coagulation cascade.

The amino acid sequence of the first fourteen residues of the seven vitamin K dependent plasma proteins is similar (Table 13.1), and in the case of prothrombin and factor X the sequences are homologous for the first thirty-five residues, after which the sequences differ. The characteristic feature of the vitamin K dependent proteins is that they all contain a modified glutamic residue which has an extra carboxy-group attached to the γ-carbon. This carboxy-group is added at a post-translational vitamin K dependent step (see below).

Table 13.1 N-terminal sequence of bovine vitamin K dependent proteins

	1	2	3	4	5	6	7	8	9	10	11	12	13	14	
Prothrombin	Ala–	Asn–	Lys–	Gly–	Phe–	Leu–	Gla–	Gla–	Val–	Arg–	Lys–	Gly–	Asn–	Leu–	Magnusson et al (1975)
Factor X (LC)	Ala–	Asn–	Ser–	–	Phe–	Leu–	Gla–	Gla–	Val–	Lys–	Gln–	Gly–	Asn–	Leu–	Thøgersen et al (1979)
Factor IX	Tyr–	Asn–	Ser–	Gly–	Lys–	Leu–	Gla–	Gla–	Phe–	Val–	Arg–	Gly–	Asn–	Leu–	Katayama et (1979)
Factor VII	Ala–	Asn–	–	Gly–	Phe–	Leu–	?–	?–	Leu–	Leu–	Pro–	Gly–	Ser–	Leu–	Kisiel & Davie (1975)
Protein C (LC)	Ala–	Asn–	Ser–	–	Phe–	Leu–	Gla–	Gla–	Leu–	Arg–	Pro–	Gly–	Asn–	Val–	Stenflo (1976)
Protein S	Ala–	Asn–	Thr–	–	Leu–	Leu–	Gla–	Gla–	Thr–	Lys–	Lys–	Gly–	Asn–	Leu–	Stenflo & Jönsson (1979)
Protein Z	Ala–	Gly–	Ser–	Tyr–	Leu–	Leu–	Gla–	Gla–	Leu–	Phe–	Gla–	Gly–	X–	Leu–	Petersen et al (1980)

LC = Light chain
Gla = γ carboxyglutamic acid

Protein C (Stenflo, 1976) is a two-chain zymogen (mol wt 44 000) which is activated to a serine protease by thrombin, and in the active form inhibits both the binding of Xa to platelets and the conversion of prothrombin to thrombin. In each case activated Protein C acts by proteolysis of factor V (Stenflo & Dahlbäck, 1980), and Vehar & Davie (1980) have shown that factor VIII is inactivated in the same way. In addition, Comp & Esmon (1980) have found that activated Protein C apparently stimulates the release of vascular plasminogen activator by a mechanism not as yet understood. Thus Protein C not only inhibits the coagulation mechanism but also may stimulate fibrinolysis.

Stenflo & Jöhnsson (1979) have characterized a second vitamin K dependent plasma protein, *Protein S* (mol wt 57 100). This protein unlike Protein C does not appear to be activated to a serine protease. Recently Walker (1980) has some evidence to suggest that it may act as a cofactor for the inactivation of factor V by Protein C.

A third protein, *Protein Z*, described by Prowse & Esnouf (1977) and presently being sequenced by Magnusson and his colleagues (Petersen et al, 1980) has, as yet, no known function either as an antagonist or promoter of coagulation.

Calcium ions are required as a cofactor for the action of all the vitamin K dependent proteins and the mechanism by which calcium acts is a recent growing point of coagulation research. It has become clear that in the case of prothrombin and factor X, and presumably the other K dependent proteins, in the presence of calcium ions these proteins bind cooperatively at least three moles of calcium per mole of protein. This cooperative behaviour is interpreted as being due to conformational change taking place as the protein is 'switched' into a reactive form by calcium ions. Although, Jackson (1980) in a discussion of this, is inclined to the view that the results of metal ion binding experiments are better explained on the basis of ion induced self-association of the proteins. Whatever the nature of these changes it is clear that the γ-carboxyglutamic acid residues, particularly the Gla-Gla pairs, form the high affinity calcium binding sites in these proteins.

As mentioned above, γ-carboxyglutamic acid is formed by a vitamin K dependent reaction, and the inhibition of this reaction by oral anticoagulants results in the appearance in the plasma of non-carboxylated forms of these proteins with little or no biological activity. This is because the abnormal proteins are slowly converted to serine proteases (Esnouf & Prowse, 1977). The carboxylation of the specific glutamic acid residues in the N-terminal regions of these proteins occurs as a post translational event, and unlike other biological carboxylation reactions, there is no dependence on biotin or high energy phosphate. The only requirements are reduced vitamin K, molecular oxygen and carbon dioxide and an enzyme present in liver microsomes (Olson & Suttie, 1977). The mechanism by which the carbon is 'activated' and transferred to the γ-carbon is not fully understood. However, it is possible that the reduced vitamin reacts with molecular oxygen to form a peroxy intermediate (possibly a peroxy radical). Our present research suggests that this peroxy radical then reacts with carbon dioxide to form a peroxycarbonate adduct of the vitamin which decomposes to carboxylate the glutamic acid residues in the presence of the carboxylase, and the vitamin K is converted to the epoxide. Under physiological conditions the epoxide is converted back to the reduced vitamin (Suttie, 1980). It is the conversion of the vitamin K epoxide back to the vitamin that is inhibited by oral anticoagulants based on dicoumarol, thus creating an effective vitamin K deficiency and inhibiting the carboxylation reaction.

Since the activity of both the procoagulant and anticoagulant vitamin K dependent proteins are affected by oral anticoagulants it is worthwhile reassessing the theoretical aspects of this form of therapy.

CONCLUSIONS

The interaction of the clotting factors described in this brief review are summarized in

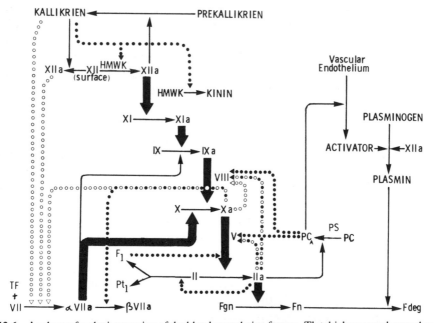

Fig. 13.6 A scheme for the interaction of the blood coagulation factors. The thick arrows denote the sequence of zymogen activations proposed in the cascade hypothesis. Open circles indicate positive feedback while closed circles represent negative feedback.

Figure 13.6. A comparison of this scheme with the original cascade hypothesis (Macfarlane, 1964) shows that while the basic concept of successive zymogen activation is still valid, the idea of the specific action of the activated factors has to be abandoned. The clotting cascade was seen as a biological amplifier; now it is apparent that the gain of the amplifier is modulated by several negative and positive feedback loops. The case of thrombin activating both factors VIII and V is an example of positive feedback, while the subsequent inactivation of these factors is negative feedback. Similarly, the destruction of prothrombin by thrombin giving rise to prethrombin 1, a poor substrate for the prothrombinase complex, and to fragment 1 which is a competitive inhibitor of prothrombin conversion, is also an example of negative feedback.

The activation of factor VII by Xa and Kallikrein, is of special interest since this implies that both the contact phase and the extrinsic clotting systems activate the tissue factor pathway. The importance of factor VII as a 'trigger' for coagulation is further emphasized by the fact that it is the only active factor which is virtually unaffected by antithrombin III, thus enhancing the sensitivity of plasma to low concentrations of tissue factor. Factor VII in addition to activating factor X will also activate factor IX (Østerud & Rapaport, 1977) and is a further example of the interconnection of the extrinsic and intrinsic clotting system. However, since the rate of activation of bovine factor IX by the bovine factor VII-tissue factor complex is about seven times slower than that seen for the direct activation of factor X (Jesty & Silverberg, 1980), it is difficult to assess the physiological importance of this pathway. It may be in human plasma that factor IX is activated more rapidly and provides a kinetically more advantageous route to thrombin formation than the direct activation of factor X.

The role of Proteins C and S in controlling the efficiency of the clotting cascade has not yet been fully assessed, but it is clear that they are able to buffer the system and render it less sensitive to vitamin K deficiency or to the action of oral anticoagulants.

There has always been some doubt about the role of the contact phase, particularly since patients with a recognized factor XII deficiency do not bleed. It may be that this phase is of greater significance for the production of Kinin and for plasmin activation than for initiating blood coagulation. Against this is the fact that patients with factor XI deficiency do show a tendency to bleed. The rate of factor XI activation by the contact phase is subject to both positive and negative feedback control. Positive feedback is seen in the activation of factor XII by Kallikrein, while the overall effect of this feedback loop is itself controlled by the rate of destruction of the High Molecular Weight Kininogen by Kallikrein. This is because the High Molecular Weight Kininogen is a necessary cofactor for the activation of factor XII, Prekallikrein and factor XI.

It is the evaluation of the physiological significance of these various pathways which will present the biochemist with perhaps the greatest challenge in research into blood coagulation.

REFERENCES

Bartlett S, Latson P, Hanahan D J 1980 Biochemistry 19: 273–277
Blombäck B, Blombäck M 1972 Annals of New York Academy of Sciences 202: 77–97
Chung S I, Lewis M S, Folk J E, 1974 The Journal of Biological Chemistry 249: 940–950

Comp P C, Esmon C T 1980 In: Mann, K G, Taylor F B Jr (eds) Regulation of coagulation. Elsevier: North Holland, New York, pp 583–587

Dahlbäck B 1980 The Journal of Clinical Investigation 66: 583–591

Davie E W, Fujikawa K, Kurachi K, Kisiel W 1978 Advances in Enzymology 48: 277–318

Doolittle R F, Watt K W K, Cottrell B A, Strong D D, Riley M 1979 Nature 280: 464–468

Ekert H, Ananthakrishan R, Muntz R H, Dowling S, D'Souza S 1976 Thrombosis and Haemostasis 36: 78 85

Enfield D L, Ericsson L H, Walsh K A, Neurath H, Titani K 1975 Proceedings of National Academy of Sciences USA 72: 16–19

Esnouf M P, Prowse C V 1977 Biochimica Biophysica Acta 490: 471–476

Esmon C T, Jackson C M 1974 The Journal of Biological Chemistry 249: 7791–7797

Esmon C T, Owen G T, Jackson C M 1974 The Journal of Biological Chemistry 249: 8045–8047

Esmon C T 1979 The Journal of Biological Chemistry 254: 964–973

Fujikawa K, Legaz M E, Kato H, Davie E W 1974 Biochemistry 13: 4508–4516

Han Y N, Kato H, Iwanaga A S, Komiya M 1978 The Journal of Biochemistry (Tokyo) 83: 223–235

Harpel P C, Rosenberg R D 1976 In: Spaet T (ed) Progress in hemostasis and thrombosis, 3. Grune and Stratton, New York, pp 145–189

Hathaway W E, Belhasen L P, Hathaway H S 1965 Blood 26: 521–532

Heimark R L, Kurachi K, Fujikawa K, Davie E W 1980 Nature 286: 456–460

Holmberg L, Ljung R 1978 Thrombosis Research 12: 667–675

Hougie C, Sargeant R B, Brown J E, Baugh R F 1974 Proceedings of the Society for experimental Biology and Medicine 147: 58–61

Jackson C M 1980 In: Suttie J W (ed) Vitamin K metabolism and Vitamin K-dependent proteins. University Park Press, Baltimore, pp 16–27

Jackson C M, Nemerson Y 1980 Annual Reviews of Biochemistry 49: 765–811

Jesty J, Esnouf M P 1973 Biochemical Journal 131: 791–799

Jesty J, Silverberg S A 1980 In: Mann K G, Taylor F B Jr (eds) Regulation of coagulation. Elsevier: North Holland, pp 205–215

Jesty J, Spencer A K, Nemerson Y 1974 The Journal of Biological Chemistry 249: 5614–5622

Katayama K, Ericsson L H, Enfield D L, Walsh K A, Neurath H, Davie E W, Titani K 1979 Proceedings of the National Academy of Sciences, USA 76: 4990–4994

Kingdon H S, Noyes C M, Lundblad R L 1977 In: Lundblad R L, Fenton J W, Mann K G (eds) Chemistry and biology of thrombin. Ann Arbor Science, Publishers Inc, Ann Arbor, pp 91–96

Kisiel W, Davie E W 1975 Biochemistry 14: 4928–4934

Kisiel W, Hanahan D J 1973 Biochimica Biophysica Acta 329: 221–232

Kurachi K, Fujikawa K, Davie E W 1980 Biochemistry 19: 1330–1338

Lanchantin G F, Friedman J A, Hart D W 1975 The Journal of Biological Chemistry 248: 5956–5966

Macfarlane R G 1964 Nature 202: 498–499

McKee P A, Mattock P, Hill R L 1970 Proceedings of the National Academy of Sciences, USA 66: 738–744

Magnusson S, Petersen T E, Sottrup-Jensen L, Claeys H 1975 In: Reich E, Rifkin D B, Shaw E (eds) Proteases and Biological Control. (Cold Spring Harbor Conferences on Cell Proliferation, Vol 2). Cold Spring Harbor, New York, pp 123–149

Miletich J P, Jackson C M, Majerus P W 1978 The Journal of Biological Chemistry 253: 6908–6916

Morita T, Jackson C M 1979 In: Suttie J W (ed) Vitamin K metabolism and Vitamin K-dependent proteins. University Park Press, Baltimore, pp 120–123

Neal G G, Prowse C V, Esnouf M P 1976 FEBS Letters 66: 257–260

Nelsestuen G L 1980 In: Mann K G, Taylor F B Jr (eds) Regulation of coagulation. Elsevier: North Holland. New York, pp 31–40

Nelsestuen G L, Broderius M 1977 Biochemistry 16: 4172–4177

Nemerson Y, Pitlick F A 1972 In: Spaet T (ed) Progress in hemostasis and thrombosis, 1. Grune and Stratton, New York, pp 1–37

Nemerson Y, Silverberg S A, Jesty J 1974 Thrombosis Diathesis Haemorrhagica 32: 57–64

Nemerson Y, Zur M, Bach R, Gentry R 1980 In: Mann K G, Taylor F B Jr (eds) Regulation of coagulation. Elsevier: North Holland. New York, pp 193–203

Nesheim M E, Myrmel K H, Hibbard L, Mann K G 1979 The Journal of Biological Chemistry 254: 508–517

Olson R E, Suttie J W 1977 Vitamins and Hormones 35: 59–108

Ong T C, Esnouf M P 1979 Thrombosis and Haemostasis 42: 325

Østerud B, Rapaport S I 1977 Proceedings of the National Academy of Sciences, USA 74: 5260–5264

Petersen T E, Thøgersen H C, Sottrup-Jensen L, Magnusson S, Jörnvall H 1980 FEBS Letters 114: 278–282

Prowse C V, Esnouf M P 1977 Biochemical Society Transactions 5: 255–256

Radcliffe R, Nemerson Y 1975 The Journal of Biological Chemistry 250: 388–395
Ratnoff O D, Colopy J E 1955 The Journal of Clinical Investigation 34: 602–613
Rosenberg R D, Jordan R, Oosta G M, Gardner W 1980 In: Mann K G, Taylor F B Jr (eds) Regulation of coagulation. Elsevier: North Holland. New York, pp 607–619
Schwartz M L, Pizzo S V, Hill R L, McKee P A 1973 Chemistry 248: 1395–1407
Schiffman S, Lee P 1974 British Journal of Haematology 27: 101–114
Silverberg M, Dunn J T, Garen L, Kaplan A P 1980 The Journal of Biological Chemistry 255: 7281–7286
Silverberg S A, Nemerson Y, Zur M 1977 The Journal of Biological Chemistry 252: 8481–8488
Stenflo J 1976 The Journal of Biological Chemistry 251: 355–363
Stenflo J, Dahlbäck B 1980 In: Suttie J W (ed) Vitamin K metabolism and Vitamin K-dependent proteins. University Park Press, Baltimore, pp 89–95
Stenflo J, Jönsson M 1979 FEBS Letters 101: 377–381
Studer A 1946 Contribution à l'étude de la Thrombokinase (1st Jubilee Volume Dedicated to Emile Christophe Bonett). The Roche Companies, Basel, pp 229–237
Suttie J W 1980 Federation Proceedings 39: 2730–2735
Switzer M E, McKee P A 1976 The Journal of Clinical Investigation 57: 925–937
Thøgersen H C, Petersen T E, Sottrup-Jensen L, Magnusson S, Morris H R 1978 The Biochemical Journal 175: 613–627
Titani K, Fujikawa K, Enfield D L, Ericsson L H, Walsh K A, Neurath H 1975 Proceedings of National Academy of Sciences, USA 72: 3082–3086
Tuddenham E G D, Trabold N C, Collins J A, Hoyer L W 1979 Journal of Laboratory and Clinical Investigation 93: 40–53
Vehar G A, Davie E W 1980 Biochemistry 19: 401–410
Walker F J 1980 The Journal of Biological Chemistry 255: 5521–5523
Wuepper K D 1972 In: Lepow I H, Ward P A (eds) Inflamation mechanisms and control. Academic Press, New York and London, pp 93–117
Zeldis S M, Nemerson Y, Pitlick F A, Lentz T L 1972 Science 175: 766–768

14. Congenital and acquired coagulation disorders

P B A Kernoff   E G D Tuddenham

INTRODUCTION

Anyone attempting to summarize progress in the fields of haemostasis or thrombosis over even a short period of time faces a truly daunting task. The rate and volume of publication in all sections of this field of enquiry have become prodigious. There are three journals in English alone devoted exclusively to haemostasis. Relevant articles appear in almost every issue of all the biochemical, general medical, haematological and pathological journals. CA Selects abstracts on blood coagulation (United Kingdom Chemical Information Service, The University, Nottingham, England) contain summaries of around 150 such articles fortnightly. Seminars in Thrombosis and Haemostasis, Progress in Haemostasis and Thrombosis, and Recent Advances in Blood Coagulation are some of the regular series of reviews published to cover this speciality. At least five major books on these topics have appeared in the past two years and two more multi-author works are expected to be published shortly. Out of this welter of information, what follows can only be described as a personal selection of advances that strike us as being of particular importance and general interest to haematologists. We also describe our own approach to certain key problems.

HAEMOPHILIA

Immunoradiometric measurement of the factor VIII procoagulant antigen (VIII:CAg) and its application to the antenatal diagnosis of haemophilia A

Interest in immunologic as opposed to functional assays for procoagulant factor VIII (VIII:C) was first generally aroused in 1968 when Hoyer and Breckrenridge demonstrated the presence of antigenically cross-reacting material (CRM) in the plasmas of a small proportion of haemophiliacs. They used, as have most later workers, human antibodies to factor VIII that are almost invariably directed specifically against factor VIII:C. CRM was detected by its ability to neutralize the anticoagulant effect of the human antibodies. Although undoubtedly specific, this type of inhibitor neutralization assay (INA) is severely limited by imprecision and insensitivity as well as being very laborious technically.

A great technical advance was achieved by Lazarchick & Hoyer (1978) in Connecticut and independently by Peake & Bloom (1978, 1979) in Cardiff. Both groups of workers succeeded in radiolabelling and purifying human antibody to VIII:C and used this to establish an immunoradiometric assay (IRMA). The technical details of the two methods differed markedly, but the end-product in each case was a sensitive, reproducible assay that could be used to measure the antigenic activity of VIII:C (VIII:CAg) in large numbers of samples without the excessive demands on technical dexterity that are a feature of INAs. The Lazarchick assay is a one-site fluid phase procedure utilizing ammonium sulphate for phase separation. It can be completed in 24 hours and is sensitive to 0.01 μ/ml. The Peake assay follows two-site solid phase methodology and is more sensitive (0.001 μ/ml) though taking five days to complete. Both types of immunoradiometric assay have now been set up in many laboratories.

Results so far are remarkably consistent. In summary, VIII:C correlates closely with VIII:CAg in normal plasmas and in von Willebrand's plasmas. VIII:CAg may be

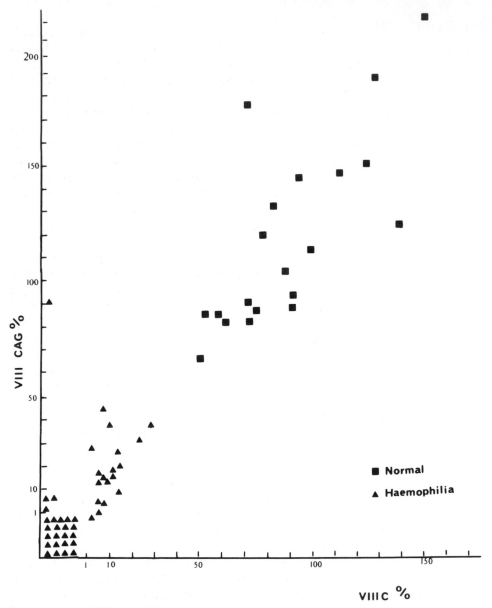

Fig. 14.1   Factor VIII:C and VIII:CAg levels measured simultaneously in normal plasmas and plasma samples from patients with haemophilia A (classic haemophilia).

found in the plasmas of even very severely affected patients with von Willebrand's disease, but is undetectable in most patients with severe haemophilia A. Lazarchick and Peake both identified two other main groups within haemophilia A — patients with detectable VIII:CAg that correlated with residual VIII:C and patients with much more VIII:CAg than VIII:C. This last group corresponds to those patients originally described as CRM+ or A+ by INA (Hoyer & Breckenridge, 1968; Denson et al, 1969). Peake also noted a fourth category of haemophiliacs with detectable VIII:C but no VIII:CAg. This appears to be an artefact of the two-site assay since only workers using that system have found this type of patient.

Figure 14.1 shows the results of VIII:C and VIII:CAg assays carried out in normals and haemophiliacs in our laboratory (Rotblat & Tuddenham, 1981). A very important feature of these assays is that they can detect VIII:CAg in serum and are not influenced by tissue or other thromboplastins. This opens the way to antenatal diagnosis, since normal fetal serum contains VIII:CAg, though at lower than adult levels. To date, only the group at Kings College Hospital, London, have consistently obtained fetal plasma suitable for VIII:C assay. Other groups have to work with clotted fetal samples contaminated by amniotic fluid. In this situation, VIII:CAg assay is essential and has proved as reliable in predicting factor VIII levels in newborn infants (Firshein et al, 1979) as have the VIII:C levels used by the Kings College group (Mibashan et al, 1980). The most recent figures presented by the Kings College group and by the workers at New Haven, Connecticut, indicate 100 per cent success in predicting normality in an aggregate of over 40 antenatal diagnoses. The Kings College group are also able to test factor IX levels by coagulation assay (IX:C). Initial results in a small group of carriers or potential carriers of Christmas disease appear promising. Holmberg and colleagues have claimed success in determining Christmas disease in an at risk fetus using an IRMA to measure factor IX antigen in a sample contaminated with amniotic fluid (Holmberg et al, 1980). Antenatal diagnosis of haemophilia has now definitely progressed to the point of being a reliable safe procedure in expert hands. Provision of the service will probably remain at regional centres since the total demand is not large and there is an absolute requirement for a highly competent team capable of ultrasonographic location of the placenta, fetoscopic sampling of fetal blood and laboratory assays for VIII:C and/or VIII:CAg.

Carrier detection in haemophilia A

This has now been the subject of a World Health Organisation memorandum (Akhmetali et al, 1977). This memorandum, which also refers to Christmas disease (haemophilia B), sets out guidelines for optimizing carrier detection by combining pedigree with laboratory data. A fundamental recommendation is that each laboratory undertaking this work should establish its own reference groups of normals and obligate carriers on whom VIII:C and VIII-related antigen (VIIIR:Ag) assays have been performed (IX:C and factor IX antigen assays in the case of Christmas disease). The reference groups need to be large enough (greater than 30) for valid statistical analysis. The reference data should be handled by a statistician in the first instance so that formulae or graphs can be constructed from which likelihood ratios can be derived for each future consultation. Clearly only large centres will have enough obligate carriers to make this exercise feasible, although smaller centres could pool resources and exchange samples (not data since all the assays have to be carried out in one laboratory for each reference set). The best that can be achieved even with this approach is a computed probability. Sometimes this will be very high for or against carriership, but in many cases odds against carriership may be uncomfortably short, e.g. 20:1. It is to these possible carriers as well as to the more certainly heterozygous women that antenatal diagnosis will be offered increasingly in the future. Certainty of carrier detection will have to await advances in genetic engineering such as isolation and cloning of the relevant genes for hybridization tests.

The treatment of patients who have antibodies to factor VIII

Circulating antibodies which neutralize factor VIII clotting activity (anti-VIII:C) are found in about 6 per cent of patients with severe classical haemophilia (Shapiro & Hultin, 1975) and may also arise in non-haemophilic patients, sometimes in association with various autoimmune disorders. These latter individuals are converted to a state of 'acquired haemophilia'. The presence of such antibodies can considerably complicate the management of bleeding episodes because patients are totally or relatively resistant to conventional treatment — i.e. the infusion of normal-sized doses of human factor VIII concentrate. Results of immunosuppressive therapy have generally been disappointing, except perhaps in a few patients with acquired haemophilia and low level antibodies (Green et al, 1980). Plasma exchange to reduce circulating inhibitor levels has become more practicable since the development of continuous flow cell separators (Slocombe et al, 1981) but the level of the logistic support required makes this latter approach too cumbersome for routine application. Interest in recent years has largely focused on the use of larger than normal doses of human factor VIII concentrate and on activated preparations of factor IX concentrate (Bloom, 1978). A very recent development is the introduction of a highly-purified preparation of porcine factor VIII which seems to have minimal thrombocytopenia-inducing effect. This review will be concerned with the therapeutic application of these various blood products. It should be emphasized at the outset that one of the major problems in this field has been, and is likely to continue to be, the difficulty in designing clinical trials to assess efficacy, evidence of which in most cases is largely based on clinical impression and anecdote. This problem is particularly relevant when attempts are made to estimate the relative cost-effectiveness of different treatment regimes, since some newer preparations are extremely expensive on a unitage basis and courses of therapy for individual bleeding episodes may cost many thousands of pounds.

Human factor VIII concentrate

When a patient with classical haemophilia and anti-VIII:C is not treated with factor VIII-containing preparations (or, more precisely, any preparation which contains VIII:CAg) levels of antibody usually fall progressively and, if sufficient time is allowed to elapse, the antibody may become undetectable. Factor VIII therapy given at this time is likely to be as effective in the short term as it would be in a patient without antibody. On about the fifth day after the start of therapy, antibody levels start to rise and the response to factor VIII infusion decreases both in terms of clinical effect and post-transfusion plasma factor VIII levels. Antibody levels usually peak between one and three weeks and fall to half-peak levels in one to two months (Biggs, 1978). Both peak levels of antibody and the rate of decline following the peak can vary considerably, however, both between patients and in individual patients on different occasions. Because of this variability, the classification of patients into 'high responders' or 'low responders' on the basis of their antibody response to treatment is, in our view, of limited value. Patients with acquired haemophilia do not generally show such a typical anamnestic response but instead their anti-VIII:C levels after treatment remain constant or may even fall.

In the past, it was a fairly widespread practice to limit transfusion of factor VIII to those patients who had very serious bleeding. Haemorrhages of more moderate severity, which included most haemarthroses, were often managed using conservative measures only. The rationale of this policy was that infrequent treatment would optimize the chances of the antibody level being low, and therefore the likelihood of the response being favourable, if and when transfusion with factor VIII was needed for a serious problem. Over the last few years, this policy has been largely abandoned in many centres both because factor VIII concentrate has become more available and because it has become evident that many bleeding episodes will respond to transfusion of larger than normal but still relatively modest doses of human factor VIII, whether or not a post-transfusion rise in the plasma factor VIII level can be detected. It has therefore seemed unreasonable to allow patients with antibodies to become incapacitated by recurrent untreated bleeding for fear of them becoming resistant to therapy at some unknown time in the future. Although it is clear that patients with high-level antibodies are less likely to show a favourable clinical response to factor VIII, particularly if the haemorrhage is severe, we find the anti-VIII:C level a very crude predictor of likely response. Our general first-line treatment for most bleeding episodes in patients with antibodies is therefore to use human factor VIII. The dose used depends on the severity of the bleed, the level of antibody and, most particularly, the patient's previous clinical responses. In patients who have joint or muscle bleeds of moderate severity, we find that a dose two to three times that which would be used in a patient without antibodies is often effective, particularly if it can be given shortly after the onset of bleeding. Patients who show a consistent response to this type of therapy may be maintained successfully on home treatment and several of our patients who have had periods of frequent recurrences of bleeding in particular joints have responded to limited-term prophylaxis.

The benefits of treatment of bleeding episodes with factor VIII may not be limited to the short term. Using extremely large doses of factor VIII on a regular basis, sometimes in combination with preparations of activated factor IX, Brackmann and his colleagues in Bonn have found that antibodies in some patients have disappeared, perhaps because of the induction of a state of immune tolerance. For largely economic reasons such 'superdose' therapy has rarely been practicable elsewhere. There is also some concern about possible long-term adverse effects. As treatment patterns have shifted towards the more active use of factor VIII in patients with antibodies, however, evidence has accumulated that much more modest doses of factor VIII, even when only given on a 'demand' basis to treat individual bleeding episodes, can also alter the immune response and cause a general decline in antibody levels over periods of months or years.

Activated factor IX concentrates
Concentrates of factor IX, also containing factors II, X and sometimes VII, were first

introduced for the treatment of Christmas disease. It has been recognized for many years that constituents of these concentrates may become 'activated' during the fractionation process, thereby rendering the concentrate potentially thrombogenic. Improvements in quality control over the years have resulted in factor IX concentrates which carry a very low risk of thrombosis or disseminated intravascular clotting (DIC) when used to treat patients with Christmas disease. In the early 1970s, several groups of workers reported that certain preparations of factor IX concentrate had the capacity to arrest bleeding when used to treat haemophiliacs with antibodies. It is possible that these preparations had become accidentally activated during fractionation. They caused shortening of clotting times of haemophilic plasmas containing antibodies and it was reasoned that this might be due to the content of activated factors or intermediates which could by-pass the need for factor VIII in the clotting cascade. A decrease in the availability of accidentally activated factor IX concentrates led to attempts to produce deliberately activated concentrates under controlled conditions. Such preparations are being used increasingly to treat haemophiliacs with antibodies. Two of these products are currently commercially available in the United Kingdom: FEIBA (factor VIII inhibitor bypassing activity, Immuno Limited) and Autoplex (Travenol Limited).

Many clinicians, including ourselves, are convinced that activated factor IX concentrates may sometimes be useful in the arrest or prevention of bleeding in patients with antibodies to factor VIII. It must be recognized, however, that claims of efficacy stem almost entirely from uncontrolled studies. Treatment failures, of which we have seen many, are rarely reported. Assuming that these preparations have a haemostatic effect, the active principle is at present unknown and therefore cannot be measured specifically. Methods of production are unpublished and vial contents are measured in arbitrary units which differ between different manufacturers. The clinician is therefore in the most unsatisfactory position of administering an unknown quantity of an unknown substance whose mode of action is speculative, whose efficacy is the subject of disagreement between experts, and which has the potential to cause serious side effects. The situation is made even more difficult because the costs of a course of treatment using these products in currently recommended doses (25–100 units/kg six hourly) may be high compared with human factor VIII (approximate current costs in the UK: FEIBA £0.20/unit, Autoplex £0.60/unit, factor VIII £0.10/unit). Dose-effect comparisons between different preparations are not available. For all these reasons, we do not regard activated factor IX concentrates as first-line treatments for haemophiliacs with antibodies. Where the clinical need is urgent and other measures have failed, however, we believe these products have a definite place in management.

Polyelectrolyte-fractionated porcine factor VIII concentrate
Antibodies to factor VIII occurring in patients with congenital or acquired haemophilia are rarely completely specific for human factor VIII, tending to cross-react to a variable degree with factor VIII of other species. In our experience, however, antibody activity is invariably less against non-human than against human factor VIII.

Factor VIII concentrates prepared from porcine plasmas have been available for clinical purposes since the mid-1950s. Over the last decade they have fallen into disuse, both because of the increased availability of human concentrates and because porcine preparations have had three major drawbacks — very poor solubility, a tendency to cause transfusion reactions, and a marked ability to provoke serious thrombocytopenia. It has long been recognized that if these problems could be overcome there would be a theoretical advantage in preferring porcine factor VIII concentrates for the treatment of patients with antibodies — namely that the factor VIII infused would be less susceptible to neutralization by antibody.

Of the problems associated with porcine concentrates, the thrombocytopenia-inducing effect has proved to be the most difficult to surmount. It is generally believed that this effect is due to 'platelet aggregating factor' (PAF) associated with the high molecular weight component of the porcine factor VIII complex (Evans & Austen, 1977). Factor VIII clotting activity can be fairly simply separated from PAF in small-scale laboratory experiments, but the same techniques have been unsuccessful when applied to bulk fractionation. The recent application of a novel fractionation technology involving polyelectrolytes (PEs) (Johnson et al, 1978), has resulted in the production of a highly purified porcine factor VIII concentrate (Hyate, Speywood Ltd) which contains only minimal quantities of PAF. This material is currently being subjected to clinical trial.

Clinical experience with PE-fractionated porcine factor VIII concentrate is necessarily limited at present. Such experience as we have had, however, is favourable. The solubility problem appears to have been overcome, and although occasional mild pyrogenic-type reactions have been noted with some batches, these have not so far been a significant clinical problem. We have seen no evidence of thrombocytopenia. Using single or multiple doses of 25–100 units/kg to treat bleeding episodes ranging from the most severe (e.g. an expanding neck haematoma) to the more moderate (joint and muscle haemorrhages), the clinical effect has been strikingly good, sometimes after therapy with human factor VIII has failed. As is the case with human concentrate, a therapeutic effect can be obtained without necessarily achieving high post-transfusion levels of factor VIII in the plasma. As might be expected, the dose-response relationship has been most favourable when the antibody level to PE porcine VIII has been low. Multiple courses of therapy have been given to some patients without evidence of loss of clinical efficacy. Immunogenic potential seems to be low, since most courses of therapy have not been followed by a 'classical' antibody response.

While the place of PE-fractionated porcine factor VIII in the treatment of patients with antibodies remains to be determined, present evidence suggests that the development of this preparation represents a real therapeutic advance. Cost-effectiveness will clearly depend on future pricing policies. At the present price (£0.15/unit) the product seems to have considerable advantages.

Hepatitis and liver disease in haemophiliacs and other patients treated with clotting factor concentrates

It is presumed that most instances of acute hepatitis in haemophiliacs are caused by transmission of infective agents in the various blood products used to treat bleeding episodes. The incidence of overt jaundice in haemophiliacs is low but the high proportion of asymptomatic or clinically mild cases has probably led to an underestimate of the true incidence of acute hepatitis. A majority of haemophiliacs have serological evidence of past infection with hepatitis B virus (McVerry et al, 1979).

Since it is well recognized that patients may suffer multiple attacks of acute hepatitis (Mosley et al, 1977), it may be concluded that several different infective agents are involved. One case report suggests, however, that multiple attacks of hepatitis may not always be attributable to infective agents (Myers et al, 1980).

In patients who are frequently transfused, there is little evidence that the risk of developing acute hepatitis is greater when using concentrates as opposed to cryoprecipitate, although occasional batches of concentrate are recognized to be 'hot'. Similarly, there is a lack of strong evidence that commercial concentrates, at least as regards those available in the United Kingdom, carry greater risks than the British products. The main factor determining the risk of hepatitis in an individual seems to be the extent of previous transfusion. Patients who have been infrequently or never previously transfused — e.g. patients with only mild disease, carriers of haemophilia, patients without congenital coagulation disorders — seem to be at high risk after concentrate transfusions. This is probably because they lack the immunity which heavily treated patients have acquired through repeated exposure to infective agents. Non-haemophiliacs with pre-existing chronic liver disease may be particularly likely to develop severe hepatitis — fatalities have been reported following the use of factor IX concentrates in such patients (Wyke et al, 1979).

Evidence has accumulated over the last few years that the majority of cases of post-transfusion hepatitis occurring in the non-haemophilic population are due neither to hepatitis A nor hepatitis B viruses, but to so-called 'non-A non-B' agents (Aach et al, 1980). It seems likely that this is also the case in haemophiliacs. Clinically, acute non-A non-B (NANB) hepatitis is generally milder than hepatitis B, but may be more likely to progress to chronic liver disease. There is evidence of at least two different types of NANB hepatitis, with differing incubation periods. Most instances occurring after administration of factor VIII concentrates, either to humans or chimpanzees, have a short incubation period of around 2 weeks (Hruby & Schauf, 1978). 'Long' incubation NANB hepatitis (7–10 weeks) has more often been associated with injection of factor IX concentrates. The antigenic characteristics of NANB agents have not yet been adequately elucidated, and serological tests are therefore not available for diagnosis. Recent reports have described an antigen/antibody system which is associated with 'long' incubation NANB hepatitis. This system is distinct from that causing the 'short' incubation variety (Thomas et al, 1981). That at least one of the NANB agents is a virus is supported by the finding of virus-like particles in a liver homogenate obtained from a chimpanzee infected with factor VIII concentrate (Bradley et al, 1979).

Most haemophiliacs receiving frequent treatment with blood products have persistent abnormalities of liver function tests (McVerry et al, 1979). While the causes of these abnormalities are not fully understood at present, it seems reasonable to assume that repeated transfusions are important in pathogenesis and that attacks of acute hepatitis, especially when caused by NANB agents, may be followed by chronic disease. In a group of 10 patients with NANB hepatitis who were followed prospectively, we found none with normal liver function after six months (Thomas et al, 1981). Histological studies of liver biopsy specimens at several Centres have shown a wide spectrum of abnormalities, including chronic active hepatitis, chronic persistent hepatitis, fatty infiltration, granulomata and cirrhosis (Spero et al, 1978; Preston et al, 1978). Histological appearances have rarely correlated with biochemical abnormalities or the clinical picture. As regards the latter, few patients under our care at the present time have clinical symptoms or signs suggestive of chronic liver disease. Therefore detection of hepatic disease in any individual depends on special investigations.

The long-term significance of persistent abnormalities of liver function tests or of histologically-proven chronic liver disease in haemophiliacs is unknown at present, as there is no precedent on which to base prognostic judgements. There is sufficient reason, however, to regularly assess liver function as part of the routine clinical management of patients with congenital coagulation disorders who receive blood product therapy. Our policy is to check liver function tests and hepatitis B serology at six-monthly intervals in all such patients. If abnormal liver function is detected, more frequent tests are carried out serially to assess chronicity over a six month period. If chronic liver disease is suspected, it is investigated in accordance with the normal practice in non-haemophiliacs — i.e. by full clinical evaluation, appropriate laboratory tests, radiography, ultrasound and scanning. Liver biopsy may be advised if it is considered that knowledge of the histological lesion is an essential pre-requisite for proper management of an individual patient. The most stringent precautions need to be taken to ensure firstly, that the patient is likely to benefit from the information derived from the biopsy and secondly, that the risks of the procedure are minimized by scrupulous attention to clinical assessment and observation, biopsy technique and coagulation control. As in other areas of haemophilia care, a multi-disciplinary approach to management is essential. We have found it advantageous to establish joint clinics with our hepatologist colleagues to review these problems, which are becoming of increasing concern to both physicians and patients.

Management of chronic liver disease in haemophiliacs is at present largely a matter of detailed assessment and surveillance although a minority of our patients have needed treatment with steroids. Various forms of anti-viral chemotherapy are currently under assessment in non-haemophiliacs and may in the future be indicated in haemophiliacs, particularly those with evidence of chronic carriage of hepatitis viruses. Prevention of NANB infection will depend to a large extent on the characterization of the responsible infective agents and the development of tests for these agents, goals which are likely to be achieved in the near future. Using such tests in a similar way to those currently available for hepatitis B, it should be possible to reduce the risk of infection by screening of blood donors and blood products. Development of vaccines is an additional possibility, although in the short-term the use of hyperimmune globulin to prevent infection in patients at high risk may be a more practicable proposition. Various approaches to sterilization of concentrates are also under evaluation, loss of clotting activity being the main problem which has to be overcome.

There is little doubt that in patients with severe haemophilia A or B, the benefits of therapy with coagulation factor concentrates far outweigh the potential hazards of acute and chronic liver disease. In patients with mild defects, however, it should be recognized that the risks of blood product therapy, particularly with concentrates, may be greater than was formerly appreciated and consideration should be given to the possibility of alternative forms of treatment — e.g. DDAVP, fibrinolytic inhibition and the use of cryoprecipitate made from small donor pools. Use of factor IX concentrates to correct the haemostatic abnormality in non-haemophiliacs with chronic liver disease is potentially dangerous and probably contraindicated when used merely to restore tests to normal prior to liver biopsy. Provided that the patient can tolerate the fluid load, fresh frozen plasma is safer and probably equally if not more effective. Similarly, fresh frozen plasma is preferable to concentrates when rapid reversal of the effects of oral anticoagulants is required.

Use of 1 deamino-8-D-arginine vasopressin (DDAVP) in the management of mild haemophilia A and von Willebrand's disease

Blood levels of factor VIII are responsive to many stimuli, including infusion of vasopressin. This substance produces a rapid increase in both VIII:C and ristocetin co-factor (VIII:RiCoF) in normal subjects. A similar effect was found after infusion of the vasopressin analogue DDAVP and as this agent has a lower incidence of unpleasant side-effects, it was tested in patients with moderately reduced factor VIII levels (mild haemophilia or von Willebrand's disease). The reason for seeking an alternative to factor VIII infusion to raise the blood level in this group of patients is that since they seldom receive treatment with blood products, infusion of concentrate carries a very high risk of transmitting hepatitis. Mannucci et al (1977) reported results in a total of 10 patients with moderate to mild haemophilia (factor VIII levels 2 to 18 u/dl) and two patients with von Willebrand's disease. They were given DDAVP intravenously prior to planned surgery and the increase in factor VIII monitored. They also received tranexamic acid pre- and post-operatively. By this means, surgery ranging from dental extraction to cholecystectomy was covered successfully and only one patient required cryoprecipitate for post-operative bleeding not responsive to DDAVP. This patient had the lowest factor VIII level prior to treatment (2 u/dl) and in view of the fact that his VIII level had only risen to 5 u/dl should probably have been treated with cryoprecipitate prior to surgery. Otherwise there were no untoward side effects and following this paper, many Centres have begun to use the drug for similar cases. Our practice for patients with baseline VIII:C of greater than about 15 u/dl is to infuse DDAVP 0.4 μg/kg two hours pre-operatively. If a satisfactory response — defined as the level that would have been aimed at with concentrate for the particular planned procedure — is obtained, then surgery is carried out without delay. Otherwise cryoprecipitate is used to obtain the desired plasma level of factor VIII. Tranexamic acid must always be used with DDAVP since DDAVP markedly enhances fibrinolysis by releasing plasminogen activator.

Factor IX antigen assays and their application to the detection of carriers of Christmas disease and factor IX variants

There have been many reports of immunologic assays for procoagulant factor IX antigen (IX:CAg) in the past 10 years. These assays have utilized four different methods: (i) INA using homologous antibodies (e.g. Elödi, 1975); (ii) electro-immunoassay (EIA) using precipitating rabbit antibodies (e.g. Orstavik et al, 1979); (iii) radioimmunoassay (RIA) using highly purified radiolabelled factor IX and rabbit antibodies (Thompson, 1977a); (iv) IRMA (Yang, 1978; Holmberg et al, 1980).

INA appears to be a more sensitive and precise method for the detection of IX:CAg than it is for VIII:CAg and is comparable to EIA using rabbit antisera down to 0.1 u/ml IX:CAg. It is clear that INA and EIA are detecting the same or closely related antigenic sites on the factor IX molecule. This contrasts sharply with the factor VIII antigens where INA corresponds to VIII:CAg and EIA to VIIIR:Ag. These two antigens of factor VIII are almost certainly located on different molecules and certainly the product of different genes (Graham, 1980). RIA for IX:CAg is more sensitive than EIA and INA but, of course, requires highly purified antigen. Thompson's RIA can detect 0.02 u/ml IX:CAg. The IRMA described by Yang can detect IX:CAg as low as 0.004 u/ml.

Several large surveys of patients with Christmas disease have now been undertaken using these methods (Kasper et al, 1977; Parekh et al, 1978; Thompson, 1977a). It is apparent that in the majority of kindreds at least some IX:CAg is detectable with the more sensitive methods. This means that truly CRM— kindreds are far less common than appears to be the case for haemophilia A. Thus Thompson (1977a), using RIA, found that IX:CAg was undetectable (<0.02 u/ml) in only two of 29 kindreds. Yang (1978) using IRMA, found readily measurable IX:CAg in each of three kindreds. However Kasper et al (1977) using EIA could not detect IX:CAg consistently in 45 out of 71 kindreds, and Parekh et al (1978) with a similar technique found 46 CRM— kindreds in a total of 98 Christmas disease families. Since EIA is only sensitive down to 0.01 u/ml it is highly likely that most of the families classified as CRM− or B− (groups IV and VI, Kasper et al, 1977), will prove to have detectable IX:CAg if studied with more sensitive methods. IX:CAg values are highly consistent in different affected males of the same kindred and have been used to try to improve the rate of carrier detection. Thompson (1977b) concluded that IX:CAg levels were of value in improving the prediction of heterozygotes. Likewise, Orstavik et al (1979) found that quantitation of IX:CAg was of value in the detection of carriers of both CRM+ and CRM− Christmas disease. A statistical study by Graham and associates (1979) also confirmed the value of IX:CAg assay in both types of kindred and found, somewhat surprisingly, that in CRM− kindreds the best separation of carriers from controls was obtained by measuring IX:CAg alone. Assay of IX:C did not improve discrimination.

The second major application of these assays has been to the characterization of variant factor IX molecules. The first good evidence that such variants exist was provided by the observation that some Christmas disease plasmas give prolonged prothrombin times with ox brain thromboplastin (Houghie & Twomey, 1967). It has been concluded that a variant factor IX molecule exists in these plasmas that interferes with the action of factor VIII on factor IX or factor X in the presence of heterologous tissue factor. This variant, called B^M, has proved to be the least common sub-group of Christmas disease, accounting for only five of 98 kindreds in one study (Parekh et al, 1978) and 15 of 71 kindreds in another (Kasper et al, 1977). On the basis of IX:C, IX:CAg and bovine thromboplastin times, Parekh and colleagues distinguished four main groups in 98 kindreds, i.e.: B− — no detectable IX:CAg (52); B^R— IX:CAg<0.65 u/ml (30); B+ — IX:Ag>0.65 u/ml (11); and B^M — as above (5). Kasper et al (1977) distinguished six groups by subdividing B^M according to degree of prolongation of bovine thromboplastin time (groups I and II). Her groups III and V correspond to B+ and B^R, and groups IV and VI to B−. There is a similar distribution of kindreds in the various subgroups in the two surveys.

One factor IX variant molecule has been highly purified for functional studies. Factor IX Chapel Hill (Chung et al, 1978), from a patient whose plasma contains 0.05 u/ml IX:C but 1.0 u/ml IX:CAg, has a similar molecular weight to normal factor

IX, the same N terminal residue (tyrosine), a similar amino acid analysis and 10 gamma carboxy glutamate residues. The major and presumably crucial abnormality is delayed activation by factor XIa in the presence of calcium ions. A specific defect has been localized in another genetic variant by Bertina & Veltkamp (1979). Their patient's factor IX is non-functional in coagulation and displays abnormal mobility on two-dimensional EIA in the presence of calcium. It is also not absorbed by aluminium hydroxide, therefore resembling the decarboxy factor IX induced by vitamin K deficiency or warfarin (PIVKA IX). It seems likely that the functional defect of this variant is due to failure of the protein to bind to phospholipid.

Clearly the study of factor IX molecular pathology has just begun and many further studies on the function of this molecule and its variants are likely in the future.

VON WILLEBRAND'S DISEASE

The condition first described by the eponymous Finn in 1928 continues to be the subject of intensive study and speculation. New and different classifications of the variant types have been propounded by almost every author who has published a survey of patients with the condition in recent years. The source of this variation undoubtedly lies in the complex genetics of the conditions grouped together under this heading. This is particularly well illustrated by the study of two large Carolina kindreds carried out by Miller et al (1979). By studying large numbers of related individuals in two isolated communities, they were able to show that a single gene for von Willebrand's disease could produce phenotypically almost every mathematically possible variation of the parameters they measured, including total normality. It is therefore not possible at present to recommend or expect to have adopted any single set of criteria for diagnosis or classification of this condition. Most workers would probably agree that diagnosis must rest on some combination of abnormalities from the following group: Bleeding time, VIII:C, VIIIR:Ag, VIII:RiCoF, VIIIR:Ag electrophoretic mobility and VIIIR:Ag multimer size. Our laboratory uses the classification of Miller et al (1979) for convenience and because it makes no assumptions about the genetic background of any individual case. Table 14.1 shows this classification, the numbers in each category found in the two Carolina kindreds, and the numbers of patients in each category attending our Centre in July 1979.

An important technical advance in studying the molecular size of VIIIR:Ag multimers was recently reported by Hoyer & Shainoff (1980). It has been realized since the early 1970s that molecules carrying VIII:RAg become highly dispersed on electrophoretic migration due to variation in size and that variant molecules of lower moecular weight lack functional VIII:RiCoF activity. Various studies have shown that VIIIR:Ag after partial purification exists as a series of multimers of increasing molecular weight from about 10^6 Daltons up 20×10^6 Daltons. The methodology described by Hoyer & Shainoff (1980) enables these multimers to be visualized and quantitated in very small aliquots of untreated plasma. Initial studies indicate that this will be a very useful tool in the study of varieties of von Willebrand's disease.

Another line of enquiry into the molecular defect in these patients' plasmas has been pursued by Gralnick et al (1977). They found a deficiency of carbohydrate content in the VIII:RAg of a patient with variant von Willebrand's disease. A more recent study by Zimmerman et al (1979) found normal carbohydrate in 15 such

Table 14.1 Phenotypic variants of von Willebrand's disease

Variant type	Bleeding time	VIII:C	VIIIR:Ag	VIIIR:WF	2 Carolina‡ kindreds	RFH*
1	+	+	+	+	8	21
2	+	+	N	+	–	1
3	+	+	+	N	–	–
4	+	N	+	+	–	7
5	N	+	+	+	7	12
6	+	+	N	N	–	–
7	+	N	+	N	–	–
8	+	N	N	+	2	3
9	N	+	+	N	1	–
10	N	N	+	+	7	5
11	N	+	N	+	1	–
12	N	N	N	+	13	4
13	N	+	N	N	4	2
14	N	N	+	N	5	–
15	+	N	N	N	6	–
16	N	N	N	N	11†	

N = normal
+ = abnormal
‡ = Data from Miller C H, Graham J B et al, 1979.
* = Mostly unrelated patients diagnosed as having von Willebrand's disease and registered at the Royal Free Hospital Haemophilia Centre, July 1979.
† = These were proven transmitters of a gene for von Willebrand's disease who were normal on laboratory testing.

patients but confirmed the reduction for the patient previously described by Gralnick and his colleagues. Thus carbohydrate deficiency of VIIIR:Ag is not a consistent abnormality in von Willebrand's disease.

FACTOR V DEFICIENCY

The correlation between plasma levels of factor V and bleeding tendency is poor. A patient with no detectable factor V in his plasma may be very mildly affected and only present with bleeding in later life following surgery. An explanation for this curious discrepancy has been provided by Miletich et al (1978a). Following up their observation that the binding site for factor Xa on platelets is actually platelet-bound factor V (Miletich et al, 1978b), these workers studied the binding of purified labelled factor Xa to platelets from patients with congenital factor V deficiency. In two of three patients with undetectable plasma factor V the binding of Xa to platelets was virtually absent. These two patients were severely affected clinically. The third patient with no plasma factor V, however, could bind Xa to his platelets (15 per cent of normal control) and was only mildly affected clinically. Two other patients with plasma factor V levels of 4 u/dl and 3 u/dl respectively, had greater ability to bind Xa to their platelets (34 per cent and 45 per cent of normal respectively) and had had correspondingly fewer bleeding episodes. The binding defect of patients' platelets could be corrected with the supernatant from thrombin treated normal platelets or by thrombin treated pure bovine factor V. Several possible explanations for the variable platelet binding in these patients can be advanced. The most likely one is that there can be residual factor V on these patients' platelets and that its quantity and degree of activation determine the efficiency of Xa binding, thrombin generation and hence clinical haemostasis. It now remains to prove this conjecture by directly measuring factor V on the surface of deficient patients' platelets.

ISOLATED DEFICIENCIES OF PLATELET PROCOAGULANT ACTIVITY

Occasionally patients are encountered with a moderate to severe bleeding tendency in whom standard tests of plasma coagulation and platelet function are normal. An in vitro defect becomes apparent only when platelet interaction with plasma coagulation is tested, as in prothrombin consumption or platelet factor 3 availability tests. One such patient was reported on by Weiss et al (1979). This woman's bleeding time, platelet count, platelet aggregability and adhesion, and plasma coagulation were all consistently normal. The platelet factor 3 test was prolonged and serum prothrombin time was short. The same patient was studied by Miletich et al (1979) and by using the methods alluded to above the platelet defect was localized to an inability to bind factor Xa, even in the presence of excess factor V. Presumably the defect is a deficiency of the platelet surface binding site for the factor V–Xa complex. That such a binding site exists has been proved by the work of Tracy et al (1979). Another study from Cardiff (Parry et al, 1980) describes ten patients belonging to three separate kindreds who have reduced prothrombin consumption in the presence of normal plasma coagulation and platelet aggregation. Platelet factor 3 availability was normal in these individuals so the disorder(s) seems to be distinct from that in Weiss's patient. Three of these individuals had a clinically significant bleeding tendency. One patient was studied in detail and the conclusion reached was that the defect involves delayed conversion of prothrombin to thrombin in clotting whole blood due to a plasma inhibitor. In one family the genetics were unequivocally autosomal dominant (male to male transmission). In vivo transfusion studies showed that both plasma and platelets needed to be given to correct the defect, in contrast to Weiss's patient who responded clinically to platelet infusion alone.

These reports underline the continuing importance of a test of 'global' haemostasis such as the prothrombin consumption index in the laboratory evaluation of patients with a history of bleeding.

FIBRINOLYSIS

Fibrinolysis, the process of dissolution of solid fibrin, is generally considered to be primarily dependent on the activation of the proenzyme plasminogen to the proteolytic enzyme plasmin. The possibility that non-plasmin proteases, particularly those derived from granulocytes, are of physiological and pathological importance is receiving increasing attention.

The fibrinolytic system has recently been extensively reviewed elsewhere (Davidson, 1977; Kernoff & McNicol, 1977) and this account is therefore confined to developments which have taken place over the last few years.

Antiplasmin

Plasmin has broad substrate specificity in vitro and a problem which has attracted interest for many years is why its in vivo activity, at least under most circumstances, should be restricted to fibrin digestion. The recent identification and characterization of the major circulating plasmin inhibitor, termed α_2-antiplasmin or fast-acting antiplasmin (Collen & Wiman, 1978), may help to resolve this problem. α_2-antiplasmin is a single-chain glycoprotein with a molecular weight of about 65 000 Daltons which differs immunochemically from all other known plasmin inhibitors. It reacts extremely rapidly with plasmin to form a stable stoichiometric 1:1 complex which is devoid of enzymatic activity. The level of α_2-antiplasmin in normal plasma is about 7 mg/dl ($1\,\mu$M), the range in normal subjects being 80 to 120 per cent of average normal. Levels are reduced in patients with severe liver disease and disseminated intravascular coagulation, and fall to very low levels during thrombolytic therapy with streptokinase. The principal biological function of α_2-antiplasmin seems to be the rapid neutralization of plasmin in the circulation. Only after complete activation of plasminogen (plasma concentration $1.5\,\mu$M) is excess plasmin neutralized by α_2-macroglobulin. Under most circumstances it seems unlikely that other plasma protease inhibitors play a role in plasmin inactivation. Formation of plasmin–antiplasmin complexes results in the emergence of neoantigenic sites which render the complexes antigenically distinct from the parent molecules. Quantitation of these neoantigens by means of haemagglutination-inhibition or latex agglutination tests allows assessment of in vivo fibrinolytic activation. Such tests are likely to become commercially available in the near future.

Physiological fibrinolysis

While plasmin formed in the circulation is rapidly neutralized by antiplasmin, it seems unlikely that this is the case on the surface of, or within the fibrin clot — unless, of course, plasmin is not the principal proteolytic enzyme responsible for physiological fibrinolysis. Over the years, several different hypotheses have been advanced to account for this apparent resistance of plasmin to inhibition (Kernoff & McNicol, 1977). Both plasminogen (especially in its partially degraded form) and endogenous plasminogen activator have a strong affinity for fibrin. It seems likely that the known ability of fibrin to markedly enhance activation of plasminogen to plasmin is due to the adsorption of plasminogen and activator on to the fibrin network. The interaction between plasminogen and fibrin is probably mediated through lysine-bonding sites on the plasminogen molecule. Availability of such sites on the plasmin molecule may not only be necessary for binding of plasmin to fibrin, and hence degradation of fibrin, but also for binding of plasmin to antiplasmin. It has been suggested that plasmin formed on the fibrin surface has its lysine-binding site(s) occupied in complex formation with fibrin, and can therefore react only very slowly with antiplasmin (Wiman & Collen, 1978). In contrast, plasmin which is released from digested fibrin, or plasmin which may be formed in the circulation, has available binding sites and is therefore rapidly neutralized by circulating antiplasmin. It is of relevance that antiplasmin can also be bound to fibrin, by means of cross-linking catalyzed by activated factor XIII (Sakata & Aoki, 1980). This might explain why cross-linked fibrin, whose formation is also catalyzed by activated factor XIII, has a reduced susceptibility to plasmin proteolysis as compared with non-cross-linked fibrin.

Congenital and inherited disorders of fibrinolysis

Growth of knowledge about the mechanism of blood coagulation has, to a large extent, depended on the recognition and characterization of patients with congenital deficiencies of clotting factors. It could be argued that the main justification for believing that coagulation is of any physiological importance is the association between the lack of certain clotting factors and the presence of severe clinical bleeding disorders. Surprisingly, there have been few reports of patients with congenital deficiencies of components of the fibrinolytic system and in most of these the correlation between the level of the deficient factor and the severity of clinical disease has not been particularly strong. One reason for this paucity of reports is probably that detailed assessment of fibrinolytic function has not generally formed part of the routine clinical work-up of patients with bleeding and thrombotic disorders. It is also true that many of the currently available tests are insensitive, non-specific and poorly reproducible. The recent introduction of new test systems utilizing immunological and biochemical techniques may lead to a more rapid rate of identification of fibrinolytic deficiency states.

The physiological importance of α_2-antiplasmin is suggested by a report of a 25-year-old Japanese man with virtually complete deficiency of the inhibitor in his plasma as assayed by both functional and immunological methods (Aoki et al, 1979). The patient had a life-long history of excessive bleeding, shortened euglobulin and whole blood clot lysis times, and normal plasma levels of other fibrinolytic inhibitors. Family members had approximately half normal levels of plasma α_2-antiplasmin, but were asymptomatic. There was a high incidence of consanguinity. The disorder therefore appeared to be inherited in autosomal recessive fashion. Antifibrinolytic drugs were helpful in management.

Associations between congenital abnormalities of fibrinolysis and thrombotic states are less clear cut. Jacobsen (1968) described an apparently inherited defect of plasma 'proteolytic capacity' but there was no increased tendency to thrombotic disease. One of us has studied a 48-year-old woman with virtually no functionally or immunologically-detectable plasma plasminogen (Kernoff & McNicol, unpublished data). This woman was identified in the course of a screening programme of patients with deep venous thrombosis, but had very mild disease and no previous history of thrombosis. She had a normal euglobulin lysis time. Although her two sons each had approximately half the average normal plasminogen level (measured functionally and immunologically), neither had any history of thrombosis and there was no family history suggestive of a thrombotic tendency. Aoki et al (1978) described a 31-year-old man with a 15 year history of recurrent thrombosis who had half-normal levels of plasma plasminogen when measured functionally, but normal levels when measured immunologically. A similar discrepancy between functional and immunological plasminogen levels was found in many other family members, including a five-year-old girl who had virtually no functionally-detectable plasminogen. None of these other family members, however, had any clinical history suggestive of a thrombotic tendency. Structurally abnormal plasminogen was demonstrated by biochemical analysis. It was suggested that the defect was transmitted autosomally as an incompletely recessive trait. Two further plasminogen variants, Chicago I and II, have been described by Wohl et al (1979). Low levels of plasminogen activity were associated with suboptimal plasmin generation rates. The patients from whom the plasma samples were obtained had histories of deep venous thrombosis but other family members did not, even though they had a similar in vitro abnormality. It seems that a deficiency or defect of plasminogen alone is unlikely to cause severe disease. Perhaps this is additional evidence that there are physiologically important non-plasmin mediated fibrinolytic pathways.

HEPARIN

Although heparin has been widely used as an antithrombotic agent since it was first introduced into clinical practice in the mid-1930s, it is only in recent years that its mode of action as an accelerator of the naturally-occurring coagulation inhibitor antithrombin III (AtIII) has been clarified (Rosenberg, 1977; Barrowcliffe et al, 1978). Growth of knowledge about the mode of action and structure of heparin has been accompanied by a series of clinical advances, most notably in the field of low-dose prophylaxis against venous thromboembolism (Thomas, 1978). It seems likely that future developments in the clinical use of heparin will be more firmly founded on a basis of scientific knowledge than has been possible in the past. Since the subject was last reviewed in this series, there have been advances in two particular areas of scientific knowledge which either are or seem likely to become of relevance to clinical practice in the short term — heparin fractions, and heparin-induced thrombocytopenia. Only these aspects of the subject will be considered here. For fuller accounts of advances which have taken place in the field over the last decade the reader is referred to the reviews cited above and Kelton & Hirsh (1980).

Heparin fractions and heparin analogues

Heparin available for clinical use is extracted from either porcine intestinal mucosa or bovine lung. Both forms of heparin are heterogeneous in several respects. With regard to molecular weight, commercial heparins contain molecules ranging from about 6000 to 25 000 Daltons. When fractionated, the effects of heparin on different components of the blood coagulation system differ according to the average molecular weight of the fraction used. Smaller molecular weight heparin (6000 to 7000) has a relatively greater capacity to potentiate the inhibition of activated factor X (anti-Xa effect) than it does to potentiate the inhibition of thrombin or overall clotting (as measured by APTT). Fractions with higher average molecular weights (15 000 to 20 000) have relatively less anti-Xa effect and more activity on overall clotting (Andersson et al, 1979). Heparin may also be separated on the basis of its affinity for At III into high and low affinity fractions which differ in their anticoagulant activities. Different fractions, as regards both molecular weight and At III affinity, have differing abilities to provoke and enhance platelet aggregation (Salzman et al, 1980).

These observations have not only yielded important new information on the mechanism of action of heparin at a molecular level but seem likely to be of clinical relevance. When heparin is used to prevent thromboembolism, it is generally considered that its anti Xa potentiating effect is of greater importance than its ability to enhance inhibition of thrombin or overall clotting, if only because factor Xa is potentially more thrombogenic than thrombin itself (Barrowcliffe et al, 1978). As regards potential to cause bleeding, it is likely that the effect on overall clotting is of greater importance than the effect on anti-Xa. To achieve maximum protection against thrombosis with minimum risk of bleeding, therefore, it would seem logical to prefer those heparin fractions which have the most effect on anti-Xa and the least on overall clotting — i.e. fractions of low molecular weight and high At III affinity. Clinical trials using such fractionated heparins are currently in progress.

Although it is doubtful whether heparin itself is normally present in human plasma, the presence of various related glycosaminoglycans on the cell surfaces of vascular endothelium and platelets suggests that these substances may be exerting some physiological antithrombotic function. Different glycosaminoglycans such as heparan and dermatan sulphate have anticoagulant activity and, to differing degrees, can potentiate At III activity. A semi-synthetic heparin analogue (SSHA) has also been described, which, in a limited clinical trial, has been found to be as effective as heparin in preventing deep venous thrombosis. Unlike heparin, SSHA has low in vitro activity. After sc injection, however, there is a marked increase in anti-Xa activity without a significant effect on overall clotting — a potential clinical advantage similar to that of fractionated heparin. The in vivo effect of SSHA may be due to the release of a substance that potentiates factor Xa inhibition (Thomas et al, 1980). There is evidence that heparin exerts some of its effect by this mechanism.

Heparin-induced thrombocytopenia

Thrombocytopenia associated with heparin therapy has been recognized for more than 30 years. The incidence has been reported to be as high as 30 per cent, although in most studies the incidence was considerably lower, in the range 0 to 10 per cent. The reasons for this discrepancy are not known. Route of administration is not an important factor. There is some evidence that bovine lung preparations are more likely to cause problems than mucosal heparins. Differences in molecular weights, contaminants or preservatives could be relevant but have not been studied in detail.

Thrombocytopenia is usually of only mild to moderate severity but may sometimes be of clinical importance. The onset may be noticed within hours of starting heparin therapy but is more usually delayed for several days. After stopping heparin, thrombocytopenia resolves within a few days. Thrombocytopenia is most often recognized because of the occurrence of a clinical complication — either thrombosis or bleeding. When such complications occur during heparin therapy they are usually attributed to inadequate or to excessive anticoagulation. It is well-documented, however, that both venous and arterial thrombotic events may occur in patients receiving heparin therapy in circumstances which suggest that heparin provoked the event. It is also well-recognized that patients whose heparin therapy is under theoretically good control may suffer apparently inappropriate and sometimes serious haemorrhage.

Suggested possible mechanisms for heparin-induced thrombocytopenia (HIT) include immunologically-mediated platelet aggregation and the development of DIC. The two possibilities are not mutually exclusive. The plasma of many patients with HIT contains a factor, characterized in some cases as a complement-dependent IgG antibody, which reacts with a heparin-platelet membrane complex to cause platelet aggregation and release (Ansell et al, 1980). Such a reaction could cause not only thrombocytopenia, but also thrombotic phenomena and DIC. Platelet release might also cause an acquired platelet functional defect which, together with thrombocytopenia, could contribute to inappropriate bleeding during heparin therapy. Pending the result of further investigation of these possibilities, it is a wise precaution to monitor the platelet count in any patient receiving heparin therapy.

FIBRONECTIN

The existence of a component of fibrinogen-rich plasma fractions which is cold insoluble but not thrombin clottable was first recognized over 30 years ago, and termed cold-insoluble globulin (CIg). It was suggested initially that CIg might be some form of fibrinogen, but more recent physical, biochemical and immunological data has shown that CIg is distinct from fibrinogen, factor VIII and other plasma proteins. It is now commonly referred to as plasma fibronectin (FN). In the last few years an immunologically identical protein, cellular FN, has been found widely distributed in association with cells and tissue of mesenchymal origin, basement membrane and loose connective tissue. Cellular FN, also known as surface fibroblast antigen (SFA), large, external, transformation-sensitive (LETS) protein, and cell surface protein (CSP), is one of the major externally secreted proteins synthesized by cultured fibroblasts and endothelial cells and forms an important component of the extracellular connective tissue matrix.

FN is a glycoprotein with a molecular weight of about 450 000 Daltons. Each molecule probably consists of two homologous sub-units of similar size (220 000 Daltons) linked by disulphide bridges. FN from different sources shows evidence of size heterogeneity, perhaps partly caused by limited plasmin proteolysis. Aggregates of high molecular weight may also exist. In the plasma of healthy adults, FN concentration is 300 to 400 μg/ml. Lower values are found in serum (probably because FN is incorporated into the fibrin clot) and in the plasmas of patients with DIC. FN has a high affinity for fibrin, fibrinogen and collagen and can be cross-linked by activated factor XIII both to other FN molecules and the COOH terminal region of the α chains of fibrin and fibrinogen. FN is an important and perhaps essential component of the heparin-precipitable fraction of normal plasma and the 'cryofibrinogen' which may be detected in certain pathological plasmas, especially those from patients with DIC. Cellular FN is strikingly diminished on the surface of cells which have been virally or chemically transformed.

The physiological and pathological functions of FN are not well understood at present. The affinity of FN for fibrin and collagen, its presence on cell surfaces, in the extra-cellular matrix and in plasma, and its synthesis by fibroblasts and endothelial cells suggests an important role in wound healing and tissue repair. FN is present in the α granules of platelets and partially released after stimulation with collagen or thrombin. Little or no FN is found on the unstimulated platelet surface. FN may be of importance in platelet–collagen and platelet–fibrin interaction. Lack of FN cross-linking to fibrin in patients with factor XIII deficiency may be the cause of the excessive bleeding and poor wound healing which are seen in that condition. Similarities between FN and serum α_2-opsonic glycoprotein (α_2 surface-binding glycoprotein) may imply a role in the clearance of soluble fibrinogen–fibrin complexes by the reticulo-endothelial system. The lack of FN on transformed cells may be relevant to tumour growth and metastasis. Study of these possibilities is currently under intensive investigation. The subject is more fully reviewed by Mosesson & Amrani (1980).

REFERENCES

Aach R D, Kahn R A 1980 Annals of Internal Medicine 92: 539–546

Akhmetali M A, Aledort L M, Alexaniants S, Bulanov A G, Elston R C, Ginter E K, Goussev A, Graham
    J B, Hermans J, Larrieu M J, Lothe F, McLaren A D, Mannucci P M, Prentice C R M, Veltkamp J J
    1977 Bulletin World Health Organisation 55: 675–702
Andersson L O, Barrowcliffe T W, Holmer E, Johnson E A, Söderström G 1979 Thrombosis Research
    15: 531–541
Ansell J, Slepchuk N, Kumar R, Lopez A, Southard L, Deykin D 1980 Thrombosis and Haemostasis
    43: 61–65
Aoki N, Moroi M, Sakata Y, Yoshida N, Matsuda M 1978 Journal of Clinical Investigation 61: 1186–1195
Aoki N, Saito H, Kamiya T, Koie K, Sakata Y, Kobakura M 1979 Journal of Clinical Investigation
    63: 877–884
Barrowcliffe T W, Johnson E A, Thomas D 1978 British Medical Bulletin 34: 143–150
Bertina R M, Veltkamp J J 1979 British Journal of Haematology 42: 623–635
Biggs R 1978 In: Biggs R (ed) The Treatment of haemophilia A and B and von Willebrand's disease.
    Blackwell, Oxford, chapter 9
Bloom A L 1978 British Journal of Haematology 40: 21–27
Bradley D W, Cook E H, Maynard J E, McCaustland K A, Ebert J W, Dolana G H, Petzel R A, Kantor
    R J, Heilbrunn A, Fields H A, Murphy B L 1979 Journal of Medical Virology 3: 253–269
Chung K S, Madar D A, Goldsmith J C, Kingdon H S, Roberts H R 1978 Journal of Clinical Investigation
    62: 1078–1085
Collen D, Wiman B 1978 Blood 51: 563–569
Davidson J F 1977 In: Poller L (ed) Recent advances in blood coagulation No 2. Churchill Livingstone,
    Edinburgh, chapter 4
Denson K W E, Biggs R, Haddon M E, Borrett R, Cobb K 1969 British Journal of Haematology
    17: 163–171
Elodi S 1975 Thrombosis Research 6: 39–51
Evans R J, Austen D E G 1977 British Journal of Haematology 36: 117–126
Firshein S I, Hoyer L W, Lazarchick J, Forget B G, Hobbins J C, Clyne L P, Pitlick F A, Muir W A,
    Merkatz I R, Mahoney M J 1979 New England Journal of Medicine 300: 937–941
Graham J B 1980 Lancet 1: 340–342
Graham J B, Flyer P, Elston R C, Kasper C K 1979 Thrombosis Research 15: 67–78
Gralnick H R, Sultan Y, Coller B S 1977 New England Journal of Medicine 296: 1024–1030
Green D, Schuette P T, Wallace W H 1980 Archives of Internal Medicine 140: 1232–1235
Holmberg L, Gustavii B, Cordesius E, Kristoffersson A, Ljung R, Löfberg L, Strömberg P, Nilsson I M
    1980 Blood 56: 397–401
Hougie C, Twomey J J 1967 Lancet i: 698–700
Hoyer L W, Breckrenridge R T 1968 Blood 32: 962–971
Hoyer L W, Shainoff J R 1980 Blood 55: 1056–1059
Hruby M A, Schauf V 1978 Journal of the American Medical Association 240: 1355–1357
Jacobsen C D 1968 Scandinavian Journal of Clinical and Laboratory Investigation 21: 227–237
Johnson A J, MacDonald V E, Semar M, Fields J E, Schuck J, Lewis C, Brind J 1978 Journal of
    Laboratory and Clinical Medicine 92: 194–210
Kasper C K, Østerud B, Minami J Y, Shonick W, Rapaport S I 1977 Blood 50: 351–366
Kelton J G, Hirsh J 1980 Seminars in Hematology 17: 259–291
Kernoff P B A, MicNicol G P 1977 British Medical Bulletin 33: 239–244
Lazarchick J, Hoyer L W 1978 Journal of Clinical Investigation 62: 1048–1052
Mannucci P M, Ruggeri Z M, Pareti F I, Capitano A 1977 The Lancet i: 869–872
McVerry B A, Ross M G R, Knowles W A, Voke J 1979 Journal of Clinical Pathology 32: 377–381
Mibashan R S, Peake I R, Rodeck C H, Thumpston J K, Furlong R A, Gorer R, Bains L, Bloom A L 1980
    Lancet 2: 994–997
Miletich J P, Majerus D W, Majerus P W 1978a Journal of Clinical Investigation 62: 824–831
Miletich J P, Jackson C M, Majerus P W 1978b Journal of Biological Chemistry 253: 6908–6916
Miletich J P, Kane W H, Hofmann S L, Stanford N, Majerus P W 1979 Blood 54: 1015–1022
Miller C H, Graham J B, Goldin L R, Elston R C 1979 Blood 54: 117–145
Mosesson M W, Amrani D L 1980 Blood 56: 145–158
Mosley J W, Redeker A G, Feinstone S M, Purcell R H 1977 New England Journal of Medicine 296:
    75–78
Myers T J, Tembrevilla-Zubiri C L, Klatsky A U, Rickles F R 1980 Blood 55: 748–751
Ørstavik K H, Veltkamp J J, Bertina R M, Hermans J 1979 British Journal of Haematology 42: 293–301
Parekh V R, Mannucci P M, Ruggeri Z M 1978 British Journal of Haematology 40: 643–655
Parry D H, Giddings J C, Bloom A L 1980 British Journal of Haematology 44: 323–334
Peake I R, Bloom A L 1978 Lancet 1: 473–475
Peake I R, Bloom A L, Giddings J C, Ludlam C A 1979 British Journal of Haematology 42: 269–281

Preston F E, Triger D R, Underwood J C E, Bardhan G, Mitchell V E, Stewart R M, Blackburn E K 1978 Lancet 2: 592–594
Rosenberg R D 1977 Seminars in Hematology 14: 427–440
Rotblat F, Tuddenham E G D 1981 Thrombosis Research 21: 431–445
Sakata Y, Aoki N 1980 Journal of Clinical Investigation 65: 290–297
Salzman E W, Rosenberg R D, Smith M H, Lindon J N, Favreau L 1980 Journal of Clinical Investigation 65: 64–73
Shapiro S S, Hultin M 1975 Seminars in Thrombosis and Hemostasis 1: 336–385
Slocombe G W, Newland A C, Colvin M P, Colvin B T 1981 British Journal of Haematology 47: 577–585
Spero J A, Lewis J H, van Thiel D H, Hasiba U, Rabin B S 1978 New England Journal of Medicine 298: 1373–1378
Thomas D P 1978 Seminars in Hematology 15: 1–17
Thomas D P, Barrowcliffe T W, Merton R E, Stocks J, Dawes J, Pepper D S 1980 Thrombosis Research 17: 831–840
Thomas H C, Bamber M, Murray A, Arborgh B A M, Trepo C, Scheuer P J, Kernoff P B A, Sherlock S 1981 Gastroenterology (in press)
Thompson A R 1977a Journal of Clinical Investigation 59: 900–910
Thompson A R 1977b Thrombosis Research 11: 193–203
Tracy P B, Peterson J M, Nesheim M E, McDuffie F C, Mann K G 1980 In: The regulation of coagulation (eds) Mann K G, Taylor F B. Elsevier/North-Holland: 237–243
Weiss H J, Vicic W J, Lages B A, Rogers J 1979 American Journal of Medicine 67: 206–213
Wiman B, Collen D 1978 Nature 272: 549–550
Wohl R C, Summaria L, Robbins K C 1979 Journal of Biological Chemistry 254: 9063–9069
Wyke R J, Tsiquaye K N, Thornton A, White Y, Portmann B, Das P K, Zuckerman A J, Williams R 1979 Lancet 1: 520–524
Yang H C 1978 British Journal of Haematology 39: 215–224
Zimmerman T S, Voss R, Edgington T S 1979 Journal of Clinical Investigation 64: 1298–1302

15. Modern trends in blood transfusion: the use of computerization

H H Gunson J Dunleavy

INTRODUCTION

Management of the modern blood transfusion service is complex. Large panels of donors must be maintained in order to allow for regular calling to blood collection sessions, which must be organized in such a manner that the supply of blood equates as nearly as possible with demand. Although the donation of whole blood is the basic commodity of the service, the trend in recent years has been to use blood components in clinical supportive therapy so that the patient can be treated with the appropriate product.

Figure 15.1 summarizes the major products obtained from blood donations, e.g. red cell preparations, platelet concentrates, cryoprecipitates, and fresh frozen plasma. Products such as the typing reagents are obtained from donations of blood or plasma from selected donors, whilst granulocytes are most effectively harvested using cell separators (Graw et al, 1971), or by filtration (Djerassi et al, 1972). The preparation of granulocytes for transfusion is finding increasing application in clinical practice and probably their use will be extended when their value can be unequivocally established (International Forum, 1980b). Panels of specially typed blood donors must be maintained to provide red cells or HLA-matched platelets for patients who have developed allo-antibodies. Transfusion centres also play a key role in the provision of plasma for the fractionation of coagulation factors, albumin and immunoglobulins (both from normal plasma and from donors with high levels of specific antibodies).

The trend towards blood component production has gathered momentum during the past decade, and has had a considerable impact upon transfusion centres, since it

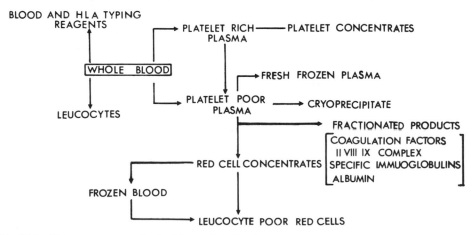

Fig. 15.1 Major components obtained from whole blood.

has been accompanied by an increased demand and an understandable requirement for the maximum available quality assurance. It will be appreciated that it has been necessary to devote more time to quality control and particularly to clerical procedures designed to ensure maximum safety of the product. It is not surprising, therefore, that consideration has been given to extending the automation which has been used for many years to include computerized data processing in an attempt to increase the safety of the blood products and to provide other information which can be helpful in blood transfusion service management. The principal aim in this chapter is to review the use of computers in the transfusion service, assessing their advantages and disadvantages.

One must not lose sight of the fact, however, that with increased activity and complexity an important aspect of the work in a transfusion centre is to prepare products which will have maximum clinical effectiveness. Space does not allow an exhaustive discussion of this problem, but to illustrate the factors involved, the preparation of red cell concentrates, platelet preparations and cryoprecipitates, and a discussion on quality control have been chosen for particular consideration.

CONCENTRATES

Whole blood and red cell concentrates

The preparation of many products entails the removal of plasma from the red cells within a short time after blood collection (Fig. 15.1). This results, inevitably, in the preparation of red cell concentrates for clinical use. Much depends on their administration in various clinical states if adequate supplies of other products are to be obtained. Experience has shown that in addition to administration of red cell concentrates to correct anaemia, when they are the product of choice, it is possible to use them effectively in the treatment of patients suffering mild or moderate blood loss. The properties of the red cell concentrates are important, however, if they are to be acceptable for such therapy. Valeri (1974a) demonstrated that providing the PCV did not exceed 70 per cent the red cell preparation flowed readily through the standard filter (170 μ) and through a microaggregate filter (40 μ) under pressure. The level of 70 per cent PCV should be regarded as an upper limit and many transfusion centres in the UK remove only 180 ml plasma from donations of 450 ml whole blood in order to achieve an average PCV of 60 to 65 per cent. Such red cell concentrates have been called 'plasma reduced blood' to distinguish them from 'concentrated red cells' with a PCV in excess of 70 per cent.

Dorner (1977) considered that 30 ± 5 per cent loss of blood volume could be treated by the use of suitable red cell concentrates and crystalloid solutions without the need for colloid plasma volume expanders. Hassig & Lundsgaard-Hansen (1978) recommended the use of red cell concentrates for the treatment of haemorrhage requiring a maximum of three to four units, supplemented with colloid plasma substitutes or crystalloid solutions to compensate the deficit in plasma volume. They estimated that patients with anaemia and those suffering from mild or moderate haemorrhage accounted for some 80 to 90 per cent of all transfusions. However, in a further study, Lundsgaard-Hansen (1978) found that 12.5 per cent of patients required additional infusion of albumin preparations. These findings agree with the earlier estimates of

Chaplin (1969) and Westphal (1972) that 70 to 80 per cent of transfusions can be given as red cell concentrates

The reluctance to use red cell concentrates in the treatment of blood loss can be partly overcome by the introduction of educational programmes (Hillman et al, 1979). However, it is important to achieve a realistic proportion of red cell concentrates since the accompanying infusion of plasma or albumin solutions has cost implications and the use of whole blood is a preferable alternative. In the experience of one of the authors (H.H.G.) a maximum of 60 per cent red cell concentrates gives an acceptable balance. If the volume of plasma recovered in such a policy is insufficient for the production of sufficient factor VIII concentrate, a limited programme of plasmapheresis can be undertaken. Removal of a larger volume of plasma from each donation of whole blood to achieve a PCV of 85 per cent, which has been suggested, will result in an even greater use of supplementary albumin (Lundsgaarden-Hansen, 1979). There may be use for a relatively small number of such red cell units if 40 to 100 ml of saline-adenine-glucose solution is added after the plasma removal (Hogman et al, 1978a) providing that the problem of haemolysis on storage can be resolved (Hogman et al, 1978b).

Preparation of platelet concentrates

It is important to recognize the variables involved in the preparation and storage of platelets (Table 15.1) so that an optimum yield of viable platelets can be obtained.

Table 15.1 Variables in platelet concentrate preparation and storage

Method of blood collection	Temperature
Type of anticoagulant	Duration
Centrifugation	pH
Resuspension	Type of plastic container

Blood collection

Atraumatic venepuncture and a smooth blood flow is a pre-requisite although Reiss & Katz (1976) established that a blood collection time of up to 12 minutes did not adversely affect platelet yields compared with less than eight minutes. Blood should be maintained at 20 to 24°C until the platelets are separated since exposure to cold results in loss of the normal disc shape (White & Krivit, 1967). Damage due to cold can be observed at temperatures of 17°C and appears to be complete at 13°C (Murphy, 1976). Such changes can occur within a few minutes (Zappia et al, 1976) and are associated with aggregation (Katlowe & Alexander, 1971). From his extensive investigations Murphy (1978) concluded that the maintenance of discoid shape implies platelet viability allowing morphological studies to assist in interpreting possible in vivo effects. It is advantageous to remove the platelet rich plasma from the red cells as soon as possible after blood collection, although Avoy et al (1978) showed that platelet yields were not significantly different when obtained from blood stored at 21° to 24°C for six hours compared with those when the blood was processed immediately after collection.

Choice of anticoagulant

EDTA induces a rapid transformation from disc to sphere and is an unsatisfactory anticoagulant (Murphy, 1978). Both acid-citrate-dextrose (ACD) and citrate-phosphate dextrose (CPD) are suitable for platelet preparation and yields are similar (Slichter & Harker, 1976a). These authors also found that the yield using acidified ACD was similar to that with ACD or CPD but its use reduced viability upon storage (Slichter & Harker, 1976b). The advantage of acidified ACD is that resuspension of the platelet preparation following centrifugation is readily achieved. Platelets concentrated from ACD or particularly CPD plasma can be uniformly resuspended if the centrifuged concentrate is allowed to remain undisturbed at room temperature for $1\frac{1}{2}$ hours before gentle mixing (Mourad, 1968).

Conditions of centrifugation

Slichter & Harker (1976a) found that 1000 g for nine minutes for the preparation of platelet rich plasma followed by 3000 g for 20 minutes to concentrate the platelets resulted in the highest yield. Other workers have used higher gravitational forces with reduced time, and Kahn et al (1976) after using eight different combinations of centrifuge speed and time concluded that satisfactory yields, i.e. greater than 7.5×10^{10} platelets from 230 ml plasma, could be obtained with a variety of conditions. On the other hand, Slichter & Harker (1976b) showed that higher speeds decreased viability, which was further reduced on storage.

Storage conditions

Platelet concentrates may be stored at 4°C or 22°C. Storage at 4°C results in a shortened survival in vivo to three days (Becker et al, 1973; Murphy & Gardner, 1979; Valeri, 1974a, b), although they are haemostatically active (Becker et al, 1973). In aspirin treated volunteers, platelets stored at 4°C were shown to be more effective in shortening the bleeding time compared with platelets stored at 22°C for the same period (Valeri, 1974b). However, in carefully controlled studies platelets stored at 22°C were superior to those stored at 4°C in shortening bleeding times in patients with thrombocytopaenia (Slichter & Harker, 1976b; Filip & Aster, 1978) and both viability and post-transfusion incremental counts are improved at this temperature (Murphy & Gardner, 1969; Slichter & Harker, 1976b). Storage at 22°C is generally preferred. Although there is a potential increase in risk of bacterial growth at this temperature the incidence of contamination is infrequent (Khan & Syring, 1975).

pH CHANGES DURING STORAGE

A change in platelet morphology occurs if the pH of the platelet concentrate is allowed to fall below 6.0 (Murphy et al, 1970). During storage of platelets at 22°C resynthesis of ATP will occur with the production of CO_2 and lactic acid; the latter will be produced more rapidly if there is inadequate oxygenation of the concentrate and maintenance of satisfactory oxygenation depends on several factors, i.e. external pO_2, the permeability and surface area of the container to oxygen and the concentration of the platelets (Murphy & Gardner, 1975). Slichter & Harker (1976b) recommend that 70 ml residual plasma is retained to ensure that the concentration of platelets is less than 1.7×10^{12} per 1. Agitation is beneficial to platelet viability when the concentrates are stored at 22°C (but unnecessary at 4°C) and possibly assists with oxygenation although the exact mechanism involved is uncertain (Murphy et al, 1970; Slichter & Harker, 1976b). The type of agitation may be important (Murphy, 1978).

Choice of plastic
The deleterious effect of a certain type of PVC on platelet viability was noted by Slichter & Harker (1976a). It is hoped that future development of different plastics for containers used to prepare and store platelet concentrates will extend the useful life of the preparations.

Cryopreservation
Cryopreservation of platelets can be achieved using the cryoprotective agent dimethyl-sulphoxide and after thawing such platelets are suitable for transfusion and will control bleeding (Murphy et al, 1974; Schiffer et al, 1976a, b, 1978). Schiffer et al (1978) showed that it was possible to platelet-pharese leukaemic patients with alloantibodies to obtain platelets during remission which could be stored frozen; subsequent relapses associated with thrombocytopenia could be treated with the autologous platelets. One hour post-transfusion recoveries range between 50 and 60 per cent (Schiffer et al, 1978; Valeri, 1974b). Freezing can be an effective method for storing HLA-typed platelets, particularly since it has been demonstrated that satisfactory post-transfusion increments can be achieved after storage in liquid nitrogen for a period of three years (Daly et al, 1979).

CRYOPRECIPITATES

Although many patients suffering from haemophilia A now receive lyophilized factor VIII concentrates, cryoprecipitates prepared from single units of donor plasma continue to be used. Opinion is divided in the advantages of the use of this material with respect to prevention of post-transfusion hepatitis (International forum, 1980b). Present evidence suggests that it is reasonable to treat mild haemophilia A with cryoprecipitate despite the disadvantages of that preparation with respect to its variable potency and the need for storage in the frozen state. To improve their usefulness, cryoprecipitates should be prepared to obtain maximum yield of factor VIII procoagulant activity (C). Also, information gained on the optimum conditions for the preparation of single unit cryoprecipitates can be used, with advantage, in the collection of fresh plasma for large pool fractionation since the initial step usually involves cryoprecipitation (Smith & Bidwell, 1979).

Important variables in the preparation of cryoprecipitate are: blood group, age of the starting plasma, rate and manner of thaw and choice of anticoagulant. Study of a particular variable is often difficult due to the problems in maintaining others constant. In comparative experiments it is important to assay pools of cryoprecipitates to counter the variable levels of factor VIIIC in individual plasmas.

Blood group
Preston & Barr (1964) showed that there was significantly higher factor VIIIC in group A plasma compared with group O, and it has been clearly demonstrated that this difference is also reflected in the cryoprecipitates prepared from plasmas from these groups (Gunson et al, 1978; Wensley & Snape, 1980) which is not surprising

since several workers have demonstrated a correlation between factor VIIIC in a given plasma and the cryoprecipitate prepared from it (Bennett et al, 1967; Graybeal et al, 1969).

Age of starting plasma

It has been known for many years that factor VIII is labile (Penick & Binkhous, 1956) but significant differences could not be found in factor VIIIC in cryoprecipitates derived from 4-hour and 18-hour old plasma (Gunson et al, 1978). However, Wensley & Snape (1980) demonstrated that an improved yield of factor VIIIC could be obtained when the plasma was less than two hours old. This is probably explained by a biphasic decay in factor VIIIC in plasma with an initial rapid partial loss of activity followed by slower decay (Stibbe et al, 1972; Vermeer et al, 1976).

Rate of thaw

Thawing of frozen plasma to harvest the cryoprecipitate is usually carried out at 4°C for a period of approximately 18 hours or at 8°C for 1½ to 2 hours. Advantages of rapid thaw have been shown by several workers (Brown et al, 1967; Gunson et al, 1978; Masure, 1969; Slichter et al, 1976; Vermeer et al, 1976) particularly if this is combined with shaking (Burka et al, 1975; Margolis, 1976) or with syphoning (Mason, 1978). The end-point of thawing is difficult to determine during rapid thaw. To overcome this problem and obtain the benefits from rapid thaw, Wensley & Snape (1980) successfully used a warm air cabinet with a high velocity air flow at 24°C until a temperature of 0°C was reached in a control pack. At that temperature a rapid reduction of the air temperature to 3°C was attained to prevent overthawing. Conducting the thawing in such a carefully controlled manner has resulted in a reduction by 65 per cent of the variability in yield compared with the previous method where the end point of the thaw was determined arbitrarily by timing (Wensley, personal communication).

Choice of anticoagulant

Several investigators have failed to demonstrate improved yields of factor VIIIC in cryoprecipitates prepared from CPD plasma with its higher pH compared with those from ACD plasma (Morrison, 1966; Graybeal et al, 1969; Shauberge et al, 1972; Slichter et al, 1976; Vermeer et al, 1976) despite the pH dependency of cryoprecipitation (Pool, 1967; Gilchrist & Ekert, 1968). In the study by Gunson et al (1978) experimental evidence suggested that CPD plasma may be advantageous, particularly when the starting plasma was less than 4 hours old. In a subsequent more carefully controlled experiment, Wensley & Snape (1980) were able to demonstrate significantly higher yields of factor VIIIC in cryoprecipitates prepared from CPD plasma throughout the range of 4 hours to 18 hours. They postulated that the initial destruction of factor VIIIC is less when blood comes into contact with CPD than with ACD, but thereafter the rate of decay is the same with both anticoagulants.

A consideration of the results from the above studies allows transfusion centres to take advantage of optimum conditions for the production of cryoprecipitates having maximum factor VIIIC activity, although the use of group A donations solely for this purpose is of limited value since this leads to imbalance of blood stocks. However, where it is practical to prepare cryoprecipitates from two-hour-old CPD plasma and controlled rapid thaw combined with syphoning, there are clear advantages to be gained in the yield of factor VIIIC.

In addition to its value in the treatment of haemophilia A cryoprecipitates are a useful source of fibrinogen (Bove, 1978).

Other products
Fresh frozen plasma is prepared by removing supernatant plasma from whole blood as soon as possible after collection (preferably within six hours). This product contains a multiplicity of coagulation factors and is finding increasing application in transfusion practice, particularly in association with massive blood transfusion. Demand is increasing and preparation of this material competes with the need to collect fresh plasma for the fractionation of other products. This can pose problems with respect to the maintenance of a programme based on the use of a 60 per cent proportion of red cell concentrates.

An important aspect of the work of a transfusion centre is to provide raw material for fractionation to produce coagulation factors, albumin and immunoglobulins. The need for factor VIII concentrates represents the driving force since after initial cryoprecipitation many other products can be obtained. It is important that every effort is made to obtain the maximum supply of plasma separated from within 6 to 18 hours and this may pose logistic problems. Whilst a detailed discussion of the factors affecting yield of factor VIIIC in the fractionation process cannot be considered the quality of the starting plasma is of paramount importance and requires considerable attention to detail.

QUALITY ASSURANCE AND CONTROL

Tests to determine the standards required for safety and clinical effectiveness of the product apply to reagents, equipment, and the product itself.

Reagents and equipment
A review of the quality control of reagents and equipment which meets the requirements for accreditation by the American Association of Blood Banks has been compiled by Guy et al (1977). Such requirements are not mandatory in the UK and a detailed description of the procedures to be undertaken will not be entered into here; however, as a general principle there should be a protocol in every laboratory which is followed meticulously to ensure that all reagents and equipment used to test a blood product are performing satisfactorily. Complete records must be kept, listing the results of the quality control tests performed. Participation in national or regional schemes for proficiency testing, whilst suffering the criticism that tests may be carried out in a special manner unlike routine work, can be valuable in detecting problems in the case of a persistent poor performer.

Blood products

Safety
There are several procedures which must be carefully checked to ensure that the product issued for clinical use is as safe as possible, consistent with present knowledge.

LABELLING

Each blood product must carry a label accurately describing the product, its reference number and the batch number of the container. It is particularly important that blood group labels are correctly applied; using manual methods much time is expended in ensuring that this criterion is met since several cross-checking procedures must be carried out to overcome human error when a mistake may occur infrequently.

TESTING FOR BACTERIAL CONTAMINATION

Bacterial contamination is a potential hazard in all blood products. It is neither practical or feasible to culture many products before administration, e.g. red cells, platelets. However, in addition to the monitoring of preparation areas and storage conditions, random culturing of a proportion of the blood products should be undertaken and closed systems of preparation used whenever possible. In this way information can be obtained with respect to performance, and perhaps the results will give an early warning of deterioration of standards. Representative units of a batch of certain products, such as those fractionated from pools of plasma, can be cultured and tested for pyrogenic activity prior to issue.

TESTING FOR HEPATITIS INFECTIVITY

The incidence of post-transfusion infection to the hepatitis B virus has decreased since routine screening for surface antigen (HBsAg) in blood donations and other products has been carried out routinely (Alter et al, 1972; Seef et al, 1975). However, despite use of the most sensitive tests for HBsAg, some patients still suffer post-transfusion B hepatitis. Such infections may arise from transmission of the virus in donor blood at a level too low for detection, but Hoofnagle et al (1978) obtained evidence that units of blood which were positive for anti-hepatitis B core (anti-HBc) in the absence of anti-HBs could be infective. Routine screening of blood donors for anti-HBc is not carried out at present, and this low risk of developing hepatitis (0.4 per cent in the above study) will not be detected.

Post-transfusion hepatitis of non-B character has been shown to be unrelated to other viruses which may induce hepatitis, e.g. hepatitis A, cytomegalovirus and Epstein-Barr virus (Prince et al, 1974; Alter et al, 1975; Geraty & Tabor, 1979). This illness has been called non-A non-B hepatitis and in addition to a sequelae of blood transfusion it has been reported following the infusion of factor VIII concentrates (Bradley et al, 1979; Craske et al, 1975) and factor IX complex (Wyke et al, 1979).

The true incidence of non-A non-B hepatitis is difficult to determine since, whilst the illness may be clinically severe, many infections may be asymptomatic and possibly remain undetected (Berman et al, 1979). At present the diagnosis is dependent on tests for exclusion of other viruses and the use of non-specific tests for liver function such as serum transaminase. Non-A non-B hepatitis, however, is clinically important since evidence is accumulating that chronic hepatitis may be a more common sequelae than after A or B hepatitis (Berman et al, 1979; Galbraith et al, 1979; Knodell et al, 1977). Circumstantial evidence that more than one agent is responsible for the production of non-A non-B hepatitis was obtained from examination of patients apparently suffering multiple attacks (Galbraith et al, 1979; Moseley et al, 1977), the variation in incubation period from two to nine weeks (Hoffnagle et al, 1977) and certain clinical differences between the disease induced by blood transfusion and the administration of plasma products. The disease can be transmitted to chimpanzees. In some experiments cross-challenging with viruses apparently causing different clinical syndromes have suggested that a single agent or a group containing a common antigen is involved (Tarbor & Gerety, 1979). However, one report clearly indicates experimental evidence for the existence of two viruses in the causation of non-A non-B hepatitis (Tsiquaye & Zuckerman, 1979) (see also p 307).

It is important that reliable diagnostic tests for the viral agents can be developed as soon as possible, since it has proved difficult up to the present time to obtain reproducible results in tests carried out in different laboratories (Zuckerman, 1980). It is also important, and the use of a diagnostic test will assist greatly, to assess the morbidity of post-transfusion non-A non-B hepatitis, particularly with respect to the repeated administration of blood products prepared from large pools of plasma, e.g. factor VIII concentrate.

SPECIFIC ACTIVITY

It is desirable, where possible, to obtain a measure of the specific activity of the product. With certain products this is feasible, e.g. measurement of factor VIIIC activity in batches of lyophilized concentrate, anti-D levels in Rh immunoglobulin. Not all products, however, lend themselves to individual assays. This is particularly true of cell components because of the inherent biological valuations encountered. It is possible to estimate the concentration of the cells in a unit of the product, e.g. PCV for red cells, total count of platelets. Whilst this is an important factor to asess in order that a prediction of the clinical response can be made, it will not give an accurate measure of the viability of the cells. In the absence of specific tests which can be readily applied, strict attention to the preparative method and observation of the clinical effect following transfusion often offer the only effective controls.

THE NEED FOR COMPUTERIZATION

Precision is essential in all aspects of the work of transfusion centres. With an overriding necessity to produce maximum clinical effectiveness and safety, scientific staff have found that their time has to be divided between carrying out and supervising technical procedures involved with product preparation and the no less important clerical procedures associated with labelling and documentation of the product. Many of the latter procedures are time-consuming and boring and may lead to inaccurate transcription of data; methods which will avoid transcription of data will eliminate this major source of error.

Also, management of Transfusion Centres requires access to statistical information in order to assess trends and decide future policy. Even within the day to day, up-to-date information of blood collection programmes, issues and inventory control are important. The increased demand for specially typed blood, HLA typed platelets, the need to correlate laboratory data with the donor record and the ability to trace donations which have led to undesirable clinical effects following transfusion have added to the requirement for detailed clerical procedures.

Computers can assist in the above. Programmes can be written which will ensure that all quality control procedures and safety checks have been carried out before the units of blood and blood products are labelled; this saves the time of scientific staff and ensures that they can apply their skills to technical procedures. The question of which procedures should be programmed cannot be answered in a uniform manner for each transfusion centre, and will depend upon the local problems which assume the greatest importance. Thus, it may be decided that maximum benefit would accrue from a computerized call-up of donors; alternatively the out-dating of blood may be given priority and computers used to define the many variables involved in inventory control. Computers can be of assistance also in the automatic transfer of data concerning the product to permanent records and this aspect has been facilitated by the recent introduction of automated grouping machines with added computer facilities.

It should be stressed, however, that careful thought must be given prior to the introduction of such systems; they must be designed in such a manner that the aims outlined above are realized and it is essential that flexibility is allowed to meet the individual needs of the transfusion centre. Even within a relatively small country such as the UK, geography and other factors result in differences within the regional transfusion centres and a national uniform system would be difficult to manage although this has been introduced in some countries (Messeter & Low, 1977). With advantage, however, a degree of standardization is desirable, with flexibility to allow for local demands.

Automated blood grouping

Following the work of Matte (1963), automated blood grouping using multi-channel cuvettes for the reaction mixtures was developed in a machine known as the 'Groupamatic'.[1] The machine comprises an electro-mechanical unit in which the agglutination reactions are carried out and an electronic unit for processing the results of agglutination tests and print-out of the group. Sample identification was achieved by means of a punched card fixed to the tube (Garetta et al, 1975). The need for integration of the automated grouping machines with additional data processing in transfusion centres led to the modification of the 'Groupamatic' in the form of attachment of a low-energy laser scanner to read barcodes (Allen et al, 1978).

In a parallel development, the continuous flow system used in the 'AutoAnalyzer'[2] was adapted successfully for ABO and Rh blood typing (Sturgeon et al, 1963; Sturgeon et al, 1965). The first machine was introduced into the UK in 1967 and has been widely used for large scale blood typing. This machine was only partly automated since the interpretation of the blood group depended upon visual inspection of a series of agglutination reactions on filter paper; also it suffered from the disadvantage that the sample tube was not positively identified. Rechsteiner & Benjamin (1976) incorporated an electronic readout system to the 'AutoAnalyzer' grouping machine and later Rechsteiner et al (1977) added a sample number reader, thus obtaining a fully automated system. Following trials of the upgraded machine modifications to the data processor were made and a laser scanner was incorporated; the machine is known as the 'Autogrouper 16C'. (Lockyer & Cotton, 1980.)

The reliability of both the 'Groupamatic' and 'Autogrouper 16C' have been assessed. Garetta et al (1974) and Nordhagen (1978) concluded that ABO and Rh typing could be accurately performed on the 'Groupamatic' and Salmon et al (1978)

[1] Roche Biolectronics.
[2] Technicon Instruments Ltd.

demonstrated that the machine was able to detect rare ABO phenotypes as well as the most accurate manual techniques. A proportion of groups, estimated to be 4 per cent (Gunson, personal observations) are not determined for various reasons. Similarly, Lockyer (1980) in testing 33 000 donor blood samples on the 'Autogrouper 16C' found incomplete results in 3.4 per cent.

Automated identification methods

Barcodes

A barcode comprises a series of vertical bars and spaces arranged in various combinations to represent different characters. There are several different barcode systems, each with different rules governing the representation of the characters. The CCBBA of the American Blood Commissions reviewed the different barcode systems and chose 'CODABAR'[1] as the most acceptable basic system for use in blood transfusion, basing their recommendations on the ease of printing the barcode, a suitable structure, ease and accuracy of reading (CCBBA, final report, volume 3). Using the CODABAR system modifications were made to meet more exactly the requirement of blood transfusion practice and the resultant code is known as the ABC

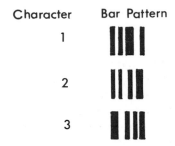

Fig. 15.2   Examples of bar pattern to represent characters using ABC symbol to modify CODABAR.

Table 15.2   The available numbers, letters and other characters available in the ABC modification of CODABAR

	CODABAR with abc symbol Characters								
Numbers	0	1	2	3	4	5	6	7	8	9
Letters	a	b	c	d						
Other Characters	−	+	:	.	/	$				

symbol. This symbol consists of four vertical black bars and three white spaces to represent a character. Each bar and each space may be narrow or wide. Different characters are represented by different combinations of thick and thin bars and spaces as exemplified in Figure 15.2. The numbers, letters and other characters which can be represented in CODABAR using the ABC symbol are shown in Table 15.2. Many countries have agreed to adopt the above system including the UK.

[1] Monarch Marking Systems Inc.

By combining the numbers, letters and other characters, a series of barcodes can be built up to represent donation numbers, blood groups and various blood products (American Blood Commission, 1979). In each instance an eye-readable number or description is included with the machine-readable code. Figures 15.3, 15.4 and 15.5a and b illustrate a set of donation numbers, examples of blood group and blood product labels respectively.

Fig. 15.3   Set of barcode labels to identify donations of blood and products.

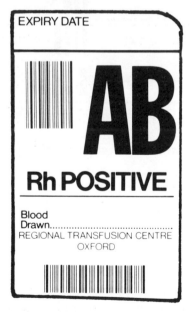

Fig. 15.4   Example of a blood group label with barcodes representing AB Rh positive and the transfusion centre of origin.

Devices which will interpret barcodes pass a beam of light across the code making use of the two levels of optical reflectance, viz. the black bars and white spaces. Both laser scanners, referred to above and barcode readers incorporating a light pen which can be hand held are used for reading the barcodes.

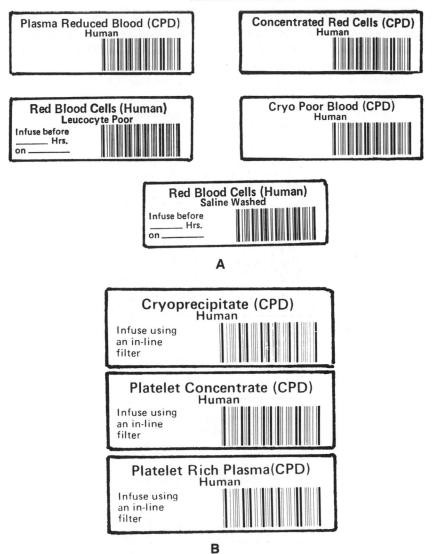

Fig. 15.5 Examples of blood product overstick labels: (A) Cellular components. (B) Products derived from plasma.

Optical character recognition
By printing eye-readable characters in a special font known as OCR the equipment reading a label can interpret characters which can also be recognized visually. This system has been developed for use in certain centres in Scandinavia.

Computer systems
There are several distinct aspects of blood transfusion practice which can be linked by data processing and for convenience of presentation they will be considered separately.

Blood collection schedules

Seasonal variations in the supply and demand of blood and blood products are well known to those working in Transfusion Centres. Pegels et al (1975) analyzed schedules of blood collection by programming the computer to predict stock levels, outdating and the ages of blood which will result from the schedule. Changes were made to the trial schedule to minimize variation in these parameters. Use of this iterative procedure proved successful in blood bank management and was beneficial economically.

Donor administration

Manual donor filing systems usually depend upon maintenance of individual donor cards. Management of card files, often in excess of 100 000 per Transfusion Centre, causes several problems. Thus:

(a) It is difficult and time-consuming to review all donor cards regularly or to produce essential statistical information for management of the blood collection.

(b) The donor card often contains a variety of information including administrative, laboratory and medical details. This may result in various departments requiring information simultaneously; thus cards are physically transferred from one department to another, or duplicate cards are prepared, with consequent difficulties in maintaining updating.

(c) Cards may be misfiled, which effectively causes their loss.

Adequate maintenance of donor card files requires considerable clerical effort. In one of the earliest developments in data processing, O'Hara & Josephson (1970) used a computer module which maintained donor records, enabled rapid searches to be made for donors, and carried out such functions as printing call-up cards and the preparation of statistical reports. The donor file carried all essential data concerning the donor, including blood groups, results of hepatitis tests and availability for donation.

Computers are efficient in inspecting large numbers of records quickly and accurately; donor records can thus be reviewed regularly to provide information on the whole file, and allow simultaneous access to the same donor's record from different locations. It is possible to ensure that records are not lost and maintain records of donors who do not attend regularly and with whom contact may otherwise be lost. Thus a more efficient use can be made of the donor panel which may help to alleviate recruitement problems and reduce costs.

The computer system can be used to hold information concerning detailed blood grouping for systems other than ABO and Rh and HLA types. Should a patient require specially selected blood a search can be made for suitable donations either already present in the bank available for issue, or those being processed in the laboratory, in the donor call-up for that day, or if time is available, during the succeeding few days. Alternatively, the main donor file can be searched and the donors called to the Centre.

Laboratory procedures for blood grouping

Accurately labelled units of blood and blood products which can be traced readily should there be undesirable clinical effects is clearly necessary. Mislabelling is usually caused by clerical errors which, as volume and complexity increases, can be minimized more readily using a computerized system compared with manual checks.

The introduction of modern blood grouping machines has provided impetus for computerization of laboratory aspects of blood banking and parallel developments are now proceeding in many blood transfusion centres. Allen et al (1978) introduced the 'Groupamatic' system with CODABAR reading facilities and print-out of the blood group and concluded that this saved time, reduced the tedium and proved to be free from errors. Brodheim (1978a, b) proposed an extension of these procedures to the labelling of blood packs and the elimination of those which were unsatisfactory for use. The system was based on the use of light pens to scan barcoded identification and group or special instruction labels.

To illustrate the use of a computer system in the laboratory processing of blood donations, a brief description will be given of that used in the Oxford Regional Transfusion Centre. It has been developed and modified from that described for the New York Blood Center above, and represented the first phase of a computerization programme to embrace donor administration and call-up, co-ordination of the preparation of blood products and control of issues. It can be described in three sections.

Procedure on blood collection sessions

The laboratory is dependent upon accurate information concerning donations being transmitted from sessions. During the collection of the donation, a barcoded label (Fig. 15.3) is attached to the main pack, satellite pack, the sample tube to be used for blood grouping, and the donor record card. Immediately adjacent to the label on the donor record card a barcoded label is affixed designating the appropriate blood group for the donor, if known. The eye-readable labels are used for identifying a clotted sample tube used for hepatitis testing, antibody and syphilis screening, and a card which is used for the selection of donations for the preparation of blood components.

At the end of each session a report is completed listing the range of donation numbers used at the session and detailing special information concerning individual packs, particularly those which should not be issued to the hospital, e.g. because of doubtful sterility.

Laboratory procedures

Grouping. Several procedures take place simultaneously:

(a) The details of the sessional report are keyed into the computer so that information can be stored concerning the range of donation numbers which will be expected after the grouping is complete and the numbers of any donations which must not be labelled with a blood group.

(b) For donors previously bled whose blood group is known, the barcode of the donation number and adjacent blood group on each donor record is scanned using a light pen so that the information can be held by the computer. (This procedure will be modified and streamlined when the donor records are computerized.)

(c) ABO group and Rh phenotype are determined using the 'Groupamatic' and the results are transmitted to the computer.

Donations from new donors and those whose group is unknown, are grouped on two separate occasions. Each result is transmitted to the computer.

(d) Tests for HBsAg, syphilis screening and irregular antibody screening, are carried out manually and the donation number of the positive results are entered via the keyboard into the computer file.

There must be no reason why a pack cannot be labelled at the end of this procedure. For a blood group label to be attached the essential criterion is that the ABO and Rh groups determined for that donation must agree with the known groups of a donor who has given blood previously or that the two groups performed on donations from new donors are in agreement. For those donations which do not fulfil these criteria a special instruction label is attached to the pack. Examples of three such labels are shown in Figure 15.6 and other labels which are available for this purpose are RED CELLS NOT FOR CLINICAL USE, and USE IN EMERGENCY ONLY. The latter label is attached to the pack on the infrequent occasions when blood has to be issued prior to completion of tests.

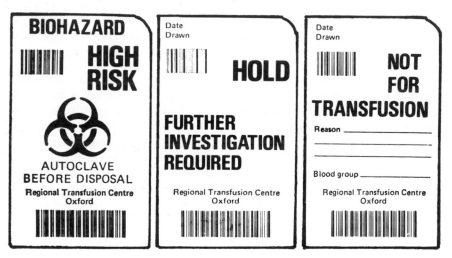

Fig. 15.6   Examples of special instruction labels.

Labelling. The following procedure is adopted for labelling of the pack using the information held by the computer:

(a) The operator scans the donation number on the main blood pack using a light pen.

(b) The computer assesses the information it holds concerning that donation. A check is made that there are two blood grouping results and that they agree; a search is made of other data to ensure that, despite correct grouping, there are no other reasons why the pack cannot be labelled with a blood group.

(c) If the computer search is satisfactory the ABO and Rh groups of the donation are shown on the visual display unit.

(d) The operator attaches the appropriate blood group label to the pack ensuring that the barcode of this label (Fig. 15.4) is adjacent to that of the donation number.

(e) The operator scans the barcodes of the donation number and blood group label in one sweep of the light pen. The computer programme allows a check that the correct label has been attached. Only if this has been done will the operator be able to label the next donation.

(f) If, for any reason relayed to the computer, a pack cannot be labelled with a blood group, scanning the donation number of the pack will produce the appropriate instruction for labelling. Again a check that the correct label has been applied is performed as in (e) above.

At the conclusion of the labelling procedure the computer prints out a summary detailing the numbers of each pack labelled with the various blood groups and special instruction labels.

This is an example of rigorousness of a computer system which, if well designed and properly applied, is superior to manual checking procedures since it is virtually impossible for the operator to bypass or miss safety checks. Also it confers safety with one operator; manual safety checks to be effective must be carried out by more than one person. Although this system was designed for use in the Oxford Region, the same principle can be used in other transfusion centres with modifications to suit local practices; the labels used have been standardized in the UK as a result of the efforts of a Working Party to advise the Regional Transfusion Directors on the introduction of barcodes.

Product preparation
Each product prepared from a donation of blood is labelled appropriately. The product labels available in the UK are listed in Table 15.3 and examples are shown in Figures 15.4 and 15.5. The name of the product is printed in red. The use of a light

Table 15.3 Blood labels available in the UK

Blood product overstick labels	
Platelet rich plasma (CPD)	Red blood cells (human)
Platelet concentrate (CPD) prepared at 22°C	saline washed.
Platelet concentrate (ACD) prepared at 4°C	Concentrated red cells (CPD)
	Plasma reduced blood (CPD)
Cryo-poor blood (CPD)	
	Cryoprecipitate (CPD)
Red blood cells (human) leucocyte poor.	
	Fresh frozen plasma (CPD)
Red blood cells (human) thawed and washed.	

pen system to record the products from each donation into a computer file removes the necessity for detailed clerical recording of product preparation with potential errors. Recall of the information concerning all the products made from a single donation can be achieved readily. Extension of this system to include fractionated products is feasible.

Issues of blood and products and stock control
An effective policy for issuing blood and blood products and stock control in hospitals is essential so that neither excessive shortages or outdating occurs. The first of these results in unscheduled deliveries with increased cost, and the second results in waste. Theoretical studies (Catassi & Peterson, 1967; Cohen & Pierskalla, 1975; Elston & Pickrel, 1965; Jennings, 1968; Yahnke, 1972) led to the preparation of working models demonstrating that, by assessing the method of ordering, the stock levels held for various types of blood and crossmatching policies it was possible to reduce shortage and outdating. An analysis of stock levels and shortage rates (the percentage of days on which a shortage occurs) was carried out by Brodheim et al (1976) and it was found that by maintaining stocks of blood at levels corresponding to the shortage rates it was possible to predict the number of unscheduled journeys required and therefore stock levels could be set and maintained for known periods by prescheduled journeys. On the other hand, Cohen & Pierskalla (1979) concluded that it was not necessary to utilize shortage rates to set inventory and emphasized that the importance and cost of outdating must be balanced with the cost of unscheduled journeys, since shortage rates and outdating are inter-related. Recycling of blood between hospitals (Abbott et al, 1978; Graf et al, 1972; Yahnke et al, 1973) has proved effective in reducing outdating and combining prescheduling of deliveries a reduction in outdating of over five-fold was achieved (Brodheim & Prastacos, 1979).

Clearly, the monitoring of stock control is a complex problem involving many variables. It will depend on the number, types and size of hospitals serviced and within this framework measures will not be successful if certain rules are ignored, i.e. unscheduled journeys only requested if the available stock is not sufficient for crossmatching needs, use of oldest blood first and recycling of units of blood on the prescribed date (Brodheim & Prastacos, 1979). To attempt to carry out the examination of such data without the aid of a computer would be difficult and time-consuming. This aspect of blood transfusion practice is, however, vitally important and one which requires further investigation. The cost of obtaining blood and its derived products cannot be ignored and waste must be reduced to a minimum.

The use of computers in hospitals
This is a large and complex subject and includes patient administration systems in addition to those in laboratories. Although many hospitals have introduced computer systems for various hospital and laboratory functions, few have provided facilities for the hospital blood banks.

However, it is hoped that eventually it may be possible to develop equipment that will use a barcoded patient identification wrist-band to enter the patient's identity into the computer. The barcoded donation number on the blood pack will be scanned at the same time. The computer will then check the information that it holds for both the patient and the donation to ensure that they are identical. Some hospitals have introduced barcodes other than CODABAR as part of their own computer systems, which will lead to problems. The need for rationalization and standardization is apparent.

A cautionary note
Conversion of a manual system to one which depends upon a computer is a difficult

task and it is important that the limitations of computers must be recognized. Several factors must be considered:

Ensuring safety. There may be a tendency to assume that automated systems are inherently safe. It is necessary to prove, however, that this is true. This can be exemplified by the experience with reading of barcode labels at the Oxford Regional Transfusion Centre. The number 3071019 was scanned using a light pen and the number was interpreted as 3071013. This number was attached to a primary blood pack and because of the substitution error the wrong group was shown on the visual display unit and the wrong label attached. Because the labelling procedure requires two scans (vide supra) the occurrence of this error on two consecutive scans would have led to the mislabelling of the pack. Errors in reading codes may be attributed to the barcode, the incorrect functioning of the light pen or laser scanner or an incorrect interpretation by the computer. In the instance cited above, investigation revealed that the label had not been printed to the exact specification of CODABAR.

This experience illustrates the need for quality control in these systems. Chances of error can be reduced by the inclusion of a check digit in the barcode but exact specifications must be prescribed for the printing and quality control of the labels by the manufacturer and the logic of the light pen.

Involvement of staff. The design and implementation of a computer system which operates satisfactorily requires a considerable degree of involvement of staff in the transfusion centre. The planning of the system should be looked at objectively; there is often a tendency to computerize an existing manual procedure which may not be as effective if new processes are introduced.

Development time scales. Development of computer systems, dependent on their complexity, may take months or years. The time between definition of a system and its implementation may cause frustration to staff when they compare the programme to the introduction of manual systems.

Availability of computer systems. Manual systems are always available; computer equipment may fail for technical reasons and it is vital that back-up procedures are available since the work of the transfusion centre must continue without interruption.

Inflexibility. Changes to a computer system require more effort and take longer than one might expect. Also, computer systems can be more rigid than manual procedures because input to the computer is defined by the programme and it is not always a simple matter to begin collating new data. On the other hand the rigidity may confer certain advantages; it is not possible to short circuit checking procedures which may be a tendency in manual systems when there is a very small proportion of detectable errors.

Despite the limitations outlined above the use of computers has proved beneficial to the management of transfusion services. Their primary use has been in checking procedures and the collation of data; simplification of these tasks has enabled all departments in the transfusion centre to concentrate on the procedures available to reach maximum efficiency with respect to donor call-up, blood collection programmes, preparation of blood products and inventory control. However, it must be stressed that in all aspects of the work quality control is an essential feature and the introduction of computers has extended its scope.

REFERENCES

Abbott R D, Friedman B A, Williams G W 1978 Transfusion 18: 709–715
Allen F H Jnr, Brodheim E, Hirsch R L, Steele D R, Ying W 1978 Transfusion 18: 716–721
Alter H J, Holland P V, Purcell R H 1972 Annals of Internal Medicine 77: 691–699
Alter H J, Purcell R H, Holland P V, Feinston S M, Morrow A G, Moritsugu Y 1975 Lancet 2: 838–841
American Blood Commission 1979 Arlington Virginia USA
Avoy D R, Ellisor S S, Nolan N J, Cox R S Jnr, Franco J A, Harbury C B, Schrier S L, Pool J G 1978 Transfusion 18: 160–168
Becker G A, Tuccelli M, Kunicki T, Chalos M K, Aster R H 1973 Transfusion 13: 61–68
Bennett E, Dormandy K M, Churchill W G L, Coward A R, Smith M, Cleghorn T E 1967 British Medical Journal ii: 88–91
Berman M, Alter H J, Ishak K G, Purcell R H, Jones E A 1979 Annals of Internal Medicine 91: 1–6
Bove J R 1978 Transfusion 18: 129–136
Bradley D W, Cook E H, Maynard J E 1978 Journal of Medical Virology 3: 253–269
Brodheim E 1978a Transfusion 18: 298–303
Brodheim E 1978b Revue Française de Transfusion et d'Immuno-hématologie 21: 681–692
Brodheim E, Hirsch R, Prastacos G 1976 Transfusion 16: 63–70
Brodheim E, Prastacos G P 1979 Transfusion 19: 455–462
Brown D L, Hardisty R M, Kosoy M H, Bracken C 1967 British Medical Journal ii: 79–85
Burka E R, Puffer T, Martinez J 1975 Transfusion 15: 323–328
Catassi C A, Peterson E L 1967 Transfusion 7: 60–69
Chaplin H 1969 New England Journal of Medicine 281: 364–367
Cohen M A, Pierskalla W P 1975 Transfusion 15: 58–67
Cohen M A, Pierskalla W P 1979 Transfusion 19: 444–454
Craske J, Dilling N, Stern D 1975 Lancet 2: 221–223
Daly P A, Schiffer C A, Aisner J, Wiernik P H 1979 Blood 54: 1023–1027
Djerassi I, Kim J S, Suvansri U, Mitrakul C, Ciesielka W 1972 Transfusion 12: 75–83
Dorner I M 1977 In: Myrhe B A (ed) A seminar on blood components and unum pluribus. American Association of Blood Banks. Washington Ch II, p 17–35
Elston R C, Pickrel J C 1963 Transfusion 3: 41–47
Filip D J, Aster R H 1978 Medicine 91: 618–624
Galbraith R M, Dienstag J L, Purcell R H, Gower P H, Zuckerman A J, Williams R 1979 Lancet 1: 951–953
Garetta M, Gener J, Muller A, Matte C, Moullec J 1975 Transfusion 15: 422–431
Garetta M, Muller A, Gener J, Matte C, Moullec J 1974 Vox Sanguinis 27: 141–155
Gerety R J, Tarbor E 1979 Infection 7: 208–209
Gilchrist G S, Ekert H 1968 Transfusion 8: 294–298
Graf S, Katz A, Morse E 1972 Transfusion 12: 185–189
Graw G G Jnr, Herzig G, Perry S, Henderson E S 1972 New England Journal of Medicine 287: 367–371
Graybeal F Q Jnr, Mooreside D E, Langdell R D 1969 Transfusion 9: 135–140
Gunson H H, Bidwell E, Lane R S, Wensley R T, Snape T J 1978 British Journal of Haematology 43: 287–295
Guy L R, Neitzer G M, Klein R E 1977 Transfusion 17: 183–194
Hässig A, Lundsgaard-Hansen P 1978 Vox Sanguinis 34: 257–260
Hillman R S, Helbig S, Howes S, Hayes J, Meyer D M, McArthur J R 1979 Transfusion 19: 153–157
Högman C F, Hedlund K, Zetterström H 1978(a) New England Journal of Medicine 299: 1377–1382
Högman C F, Hedlund K, Akerblom O, Venge P 1978(b) Transfusion 18: 233–241
Hoofnagle J H, Gerety R J, Tarbor E 1977 Annals of Internal Medicine 87: 14–20
Hoofnagle J H, Seef L B, Bales Z B, Zimmerman H J 1978 New England Journal of Medicine 298: 1379–1383
International Forum 1980a Vox Sanguinis 38: 40–56
International Forum 1980b Vox Sanguinis 38: 106–119
Jennings J B 1968 Transfusion 8: 335–342
Kahn R A, Cossette I, Friedman L I 1976 Transfusion 16: 162–165
Kahn R A, Syring R L 1975 Transfusion 15: 363–367
Kattlowe H E, Alexander B 1971 Blood 38: 39–48

Knodell R G, Conrad M E, Ishak K G 1977 Gastroenterology 72: 902–909
Lockyer W J 1980 Personal communication
Lockyer W J, Cotton B 1980 Personal communication
Lundsgaard-Hansen P 1979 Vox Sanguinis 37: 65–72
Lundsgaard-Hansen P, Bucher U, Tschirren B, Haase S, Kuske B, Lüdi H, Stankiewicz L A, Hässig A 1978 Vox Sanguinis 34: 261–275
Margolis J 1976 Proceedings of the XI Congress W.F.H., p 223–227
Mason E C 1978 Lancet 2: 15–17
Masure R 1969 Vox Sanguinis 61: 1–9
Matte C 1963 Revue Française de Transfusion 6: 381–402
Messeter L, Löw B 1977 Vox Sanguinis 33: 116–123
Morrison F S 1966 Blood 28: 479–482
Mosley J W, Redeker A G, Feinstone S M, Purcell R H 1977 New England Journal of Medicine 296: 75
Mourad N 1968 Transfusion 8: 48
Murphy S 1976 In: Spaet H (ed) Progress in haemostasis and thrombosis. Grune and Stratton, New York, Vol 3 p 289–310
Murphy S 1978 In: Schiffer C J (ed) Platelet physiology and transfusion. American Association of Blood Banks. Washington. Ch 2 p 7–15
Murphy S, Gardner F H 1969 New England Journal of Medicine 280: 1094–1098
Murphy S, Gardner F H 1975 Blood 46: 209–218
Murphy S, Sayar S N, Abdou N I, Gardner F H 1974 Transfusion 14: 139–144
Murphy S, Sayar S N, Gardner F H 1970 Blood 35: 549–557
Nordhagen R 1978 Revue Française de Transfusion et d'Immuno-hématologie 21: 363–368
O'Hara M, Josephson A M 1970 Transfusion 10: 215–220
Pegels C C, Seagle J P, Cumming P D, Kendall K E 1975 Transfusion 15: 381–386
Penick G D, Brinkhous K M 1956 American Journal of Medical Sciences 232: 434–442
Pool J G 1967 Transfusion 7: 165–167
Preston A E, Barr A 1964 British Journal of Haematology 10: 238–245
Prince A M, Brotman B, Grady G F 1974 Lancet 2: 241–246
Rechsteiner J, Benjamin C J 1976 Vox Sanguinis 30: 445–452
Rechsteiner J, Benjamin C J, Budding R W 1977 Vox Sanguinis 33: 108–115
Reiss R F, Katz A J 1976 Transfusion 16: 229–231
Salmon Ch, Gener J, Muller A, Garretta M 1978 Revue Française de Transfusion et d'Immuno'hématologie 21: 279–293
Shanberge J N, Gruhl M C, Ikemori R, Inoshita K, Chalos M K, Aster R H 1972 Transfusion 12: 251–258
Schiffer C A, Aisner J, Wiernik P H 1976a British Journal of Haematology 34: 377–385
Schiffer C A, Aisner J, Wiernik P H 1978 New England Journal of Medicine 299: 7–12
Schiffer C A, Bucholz D H, Aisner J, Wolff J H, Wiernick P H 1976 Transfusion 16: 321–329
Seef L B, Wright E C, Zimmerman H J 1975 American Journal of Medical Sciences 270: 355–362
Slichter S J, Counts R B, Henderson R, Harker L A 1976 Transfusion 16: 616–626
Slichter S J, Harker L A 1976a British Journal of Haematology 34: 395–402
Slichter S J, Harker L A 1976b British Journal of Haematology 34: 403–419
Smith J K, Bidwell E 1979 Clinics in Haematology 8: 183–206
Stibbe J, Hempker H C, Van Creveld S 1972 Thrombosis et Diathesis Haemorrhagica 27: 43–58
Sturgeon P, Cedergren B, McQuiston D 1963 Vox Sanguinis 8: 438–451
Sturgeon P, DuCros M, McQuiston D, Smythe W 1965 In: Technicon Symposia: automation in analytical chemistry. Mediad Inc. New York, p 515–520
Tarbor E, Gerety R J 1979 Transfusion 19: 669–674
Tsiquaye K N, Zuckerman A J 1979 Lancet 1: 1135–1136
Valeri C R 1974a In: Malinin T T, Zeppa R, Drucker W R (eds) Acute fluid replacement in the therapy of shock. A B Stratton New York, p 119–137
Valeri C R 1974b New England Journal of Medicine 290: 353–358
Vermeer C, Soute B A M, Ates G, Brummelhuis H G 1976 Vox Sanguinis 30: 1–22
Wensley R T, Snape T J 1980 Vox Sanguinis 38: 222–228
Westphal R G 1972 Annals of Internal Medicine 76: 987–990
White J G, Krivit W 1967 Blood 30: 625–635
Wyke R J, Tisquaye K N, Thornton A, White Y, Portmann B, Das P K, Zuckerman A J, Williams R 1979 Lancet 1: 520–524
Yahnke D P, Rimm A A, Makowski G G, Aster R H 1973 Transfusion 13: 156–169
Yahnke D P, Rimm A A, Mundt C J, Aster R H, Hurst T M 1972 Transfusion 12: 111–118
Zappia G C, Steiner M, Ando Y, Baldini M 1976 Transfusion 16: 122–129
Zuckerman A J 1980 Personal communication

Index

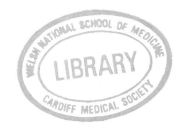